"*Attachment-Informed Grief Therapy* is a fascinating book! Kosminsky and Jordan have written a scientifically sound, clinically innovative, well-argued, and extremely informative volume. The authors show how insights from attachment theory and neuroscience are the keys that unlock the puzzle of healthy and disordered grief responses, and how, through understanding unmet attachment needs, attachment-related emotions and defenses, and the broaden-and-build repercussions of attachment security, grief therapists can help bereaved clients to manage their grief reactions and to find ways to move forward. I enjoyed reading this gracefully written and profound book and I strongly believe that it will become essential reading for clinicians, researchers, and students interested in the study and treatment of disordered grief."

Mario Mikulincer, *Professor of Psychology, Baruch Ivcher School of Psychology, Reichman University, Israel*

"In this remarkable revision of their ground-breaking volume, Phyllis Kosminsky and Jack Jordan penetrate still more profoundly into the developmental, interpersonal, and intersubjective neurobiological underpinnings of attachment that give rise and form to all grief. More than a compendium of clinical wisdom and contemporary theory and research, *Attachment-Informed Grief Therapy* provides resonant insights and concrete principles for helping clients read the deep text of their own needs in the wake of loss. Equally, it instructs the reader in how to become the secure base that allows survivors to integrate the rupture and realign the bond with a significant other who is present even in absence. I, for one, am a better therapist and companion to those who mourn for the gift of their vision."

Robert A. Neimeyer, *PhD, co-editor of* The Handbook of Grief Therapy *and director of* The Portland Institute for Loss and Transition

"The second edition of this important volume is a valuable resource for clinicians and researchers alike. Updating, expanding, and deepening their understanding of the interface between attachment styles and the processing of bereavement, Kosminsky and Jordan's integration of new findings from neuroscience adds an important dimension to their overview. The ample clinical material included is accompanied by rich and thoughtful consideration of the cases at hand. Accompanying these exemplary clinicians as they weave together theory, research and practice on bereavement will enrich the therapeutic encounter for therapists at all stages of their professional development."

Simon Shimshon Rubin, *PhD, director of the International Laboratory for the Study of Loss, Bereavement, and Human Resilience at the University of Haifa, Israel, and co-author of* Working with the Bereaved: Multiple Lenses on Loss and Mourning

T0372875

"Reading this book in one sitting, as I did, left me moved. It starts with a crystal-clear exposition of contemporary attachment theory and its neuroscience basis, defines and easy-to-understand attachment framework for helping bereaved people, and shows how sensitive therapy can help overcome physiological dysregulation and restore meaning. Convincing clinical illustrations are used throughout, contributing to an overall sense of two vastly experienced clinicians passing on deep theoretical and practical expertise to the next generations. Strongly recommended."

Jeremy Holmes, *MD, FRCPsych, University of Exeter, United Kingdom, and author of* Exploring in Security: Towards an Attachment-Informed Psychoanalytic Psychotherapy

"Grief, that harrowing experience after the death of a loved one, is again beautifully described in the second edition of *Attachment-Informed Grief Therapy*. What the authors have accomplished in this edition will continue to enrich how clinicians work with the grief-stricken and will provide them with an expanded knowledge of how attachment shapes the experience of grief in bereavement. And Kosminsky and Jordan do more. The rhythm of the writing combined with their clarity and deftness in explicating theory and neuroscience make *Attachment-Informed Grief Therapy* a book that is a pleasure to read."

Dorothy Holinger, *PhD, author of* The Anatomy of Grief

"In the second edition of this groundbreaking volume, Phyllis Kosminsky and John Jordan show us how to help our clients navigate the landscape of life, with all of its fault lines. Filled with deep empathy and wisdom, *Attachment-Informed Grief Therapy* is a book that will inform and inspire anyone who is in a position to offer support to people dealing with significant loss or with other difficult and painful losses."

Jakob van Wielink, *The School for Transition, The Netherlands, and co-author of* Loss, Grief, and Attachment in Life Transitions: A Clinician's Guide to Secure Base Counseling

"This volume provides a wonderful intergration of the concepts related to attachment, current theories of grief, and contemporary neuroscience. The book answered questions about attachment and therapy that I didn't even know that I had! It is an absolute must-read for any clinician who wishes to enhance their practice and provide sensitive and well-informed support to those who are grieving."

Darcy Harris, *PhD, professor, Thanatology Department, King's University College at Western University and co-editor of the Routledge Series in Death, Dying, and Bereavement*

"Finally! In an extraordinary blend of scholarship and clinical acumen, the rich store of information located in attachment theory/research has been retrieved and integrated with what the bereaved specifically require in the aftermath of significant loss. Synthesizing developmental psychology, traumatology, thanatology, neuroscience, and therapy research, Kosminsky and Jordan brilliantly elucidate the mourner's experience and needs, along the way operationalizing what clinicians must know to intervene successfully to promote healthy adaptation. Practical and cutting edge, this book makes a revolutionary contribution and will become required reading for those working with all kinds of loss."

Therese Rando, *PhD, BCETS, BCBT, founder and clinical director,*
The Institute for the Study and Treatment of Loss, Warwick Rhode Island,
and author of Coping with the Sudden Death of Your Loved:
A Self-Help Handbook for Traumatic Bereavement

"*Attachment-Informed Grief Therapy* is a must-read for grief counselors. This is a book that every therapist should have in his or her library and one they will consult regularly."

Kenneth J. Doka, *PhD, senior consultant to the Hospice Foundation of America and*
author of Grief is a Journey: Finding Your Path Through Loss

"This is an exceptional text! Written by two highly skilled clinicians, it presents the state of the art in attachment theory and bereavement in both a highly engaging and practical form. This book effectively bridges both research and practice and attachment and thanatology in a way that no other texts have previously done. Richly illustrated with clinical examples, this impressive book will enrich the understanding and skills of both beginning and experienced clinicians."

Christopher Hall, *MA, BEd, chief executive officer of the Australian Centre*
for Grief and Bereavement

Attachment-Informed Grief Therapy

Attachment-Informed Grief Therapy bridges the fields of attachment studies, thanatology, and interpersonal neuroscience, uniting theory, research, and practice to enrich our understanding of how we can help the bereaved. The new edition includes updated research and discussion of emotion regulation, relational trauma, epistemic trust, and much more.

In these pages, clinicians and students will gain a new understanding of the etiology of problematic grief and its treatment, and will become better equipped to formulate accurate and specific case conceptualization and treatment plans. The authors also illustrate the ways in which the therapeutic relationship is crucially important – though largely unrecognized – element in grief therapy and offer guidelines for an attachment informed view of the therapeutic relationship that can serve as the foundation of all grief therapy.

Written by two highly experienced grief counselors, this volume is filled with instructive case vignettes and useful techniques that offer a universal and practical frame of reference for understanding grief therapy for clinicians of every theoretical orientation.

Phyllis S. Kosminsky is a clinical social worker specializing in work with the bereaved, particularly those who have experienced a traumatic loss. Over the past 30 years, Dr. Kosminsky has provided bereavement counseling to individuals, conducted grief support groups, and provided trainings for mental health professionals in the treatment of normal and problematic grief. Her publications include journal articles, book chapters, and the book *Getting Back to Life When Grief Won't Heal.*

John R. Jordan is a retired psychologist in private practice in Rhode Island, where he specialized in work with survivors of suicide and other traumatic losses for almost 40 years. He was the clinical consultant for Grief Support Services of the Samaritans in Boston, Massachusetts, and the professional advisor to the Loss and Bereavement Council of the American Foundation for Suicide Prevention. He has published over 45 articles, chapters, and full books, including *Grief After Suicide: Coping with the Consequences and Caring for the Survivors* and *After Suicide Loss: Coping with Your Grief.*

Series in Death, Dying, and Bereavement

Series Editors: Robert A. Neimeyer, PhD
Portland Institute for Loss and Transition, Oregon, USA
Darcy L. Harris, PhD
Western University Canada, Ontario, Canada

Volumes published in the Series in Death, Dying and Bereavement are representative of the multidisciplinary nature of the intersecting fields of death studies, suicidology, end-of-life care, and grief counseling. The series meets the needs of clinicians, researchers, paraprofessionals, pastoral counselors, and educators by providing cutting edge research, theory, and best practices on the most important topics in these fields—for today and for tomorrow.

Superhero Grief
The Transformative Power of Loss
Edited by Jill A. Harrington and Robert A. Neimeyer

New Techniques of Grief Therapy
Bereavement and Beyond
Edited by Robert A. Neimeyer

Pediatric Palliative Care
A Model for Exemplary Practice
Betty Davies, Rose Steele, and Jennifer Baird

The Restorative Nature of Ongoing Connections with the Deceased
Exploring Presence Within Absence
Laurie A. Burke and Edward (Ted) Rynearson

Compassion-Based Approaches in Loss and Grief
Darcy L. Harris and Andy H. Y. Ho

Attachment Informed Grief Therapy
The Clinician's Guide to Foundations and Applications
Phyllis S. Kosminsky and John R. Jordan

For more information about this series, please visit https://www.routledge.com/Series-in-Death-Dying-and-Bereavement/book-series/SE0620

Attachment-Informed Grief Therapy

The Clinician's Guide to Foundations and Applications

Second Edition

Phyllis S. Kosminsky and John R. Jordan

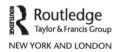
Routledge
Taylor & Francis Group

NEW YORK AND LONDON

Designed cover image: Kubkoo © Getty Images

Second edition published 2024
by Routledge
605 Third Avenue, New York, NY 10158

and by Routledge
4 Park Square, Milton Park, Abingdon, Oxon, OX14 4RN

Routledge is an imprint of the Taylor & Francis Group, an informa business

© 2024 Phyllis S. Kosminsky and John R. Jordan

First edition published by Routledge 2016

Library of Congress Cataloging-in-Publication Data
Names: Kosminsky, Phyllis, author. | Jordan, John R., author.
Title: Attachment-informed grief therapy : the clinician's guide to foundations and applications / Phyllis S. Kosminsky and John R. Jordan.
Description: Second edition. | New York, NY : Routledge, 2024. | Includes bibliographical references and index. | Identifiers: LCCN 2023027161 (print) | LCCN 2023027162 (ebook) | ISBN 9781032038469 (hardback) | ISBN 9781032038445 (paperback) | ISBN 9781003204183 (ebook)
Subjects: LCSH: Grief therapy. | Attachment behavior.
Classification: LCC RC455.4.L67 K67 2024 (print) | LCC RC455.4.L67 (ebook) | DDC 616.89/14--dc23/eng/20230921
LC record available at https://lccn.loc.gov/2023027161
LC ebook record available at https://lccn.loc.gov/2023027162

ISBN: 978-1-032-03846-9 (hbk)
ISBN: 978-1-032-03844-5 (pbk)
ISBN: 978-1-003-20418-3 (ebk)

DOI: 10.4324/9781003204183

Typeset in Times New Roman
by MPS Limited, Dehradun

In loving memory of Lucile Schoenfeld Glick (1928–1961) and Jay Milton Glick (1928–2011) and for JK, EK, YK, LE and SE. You guys are my favorite people in the world.

PSK

For Gladys C. Jordan (1918–2014) and Robert F. Jordan (1915–1974).

JRJ

CONTENTS

SERIES EDITOR FOREWORD

Attachment is instinctually programmed into us to ensure our safety and survival. From our earliest moments, our attachment experiences are the foundation of how we see the world, others, and ourselves, imprinting a template that will shape much of our lives. Attachment guides how we form relationships and the ways that we experience and express our deepest feelings. And, as the reader will find in this book, attachment influences the ways that we grieve the loss of a loved one and the ways in which we make meaning of loss and rebuild our lives.

The original volume of *Attachment Informed Grief Therapy* was a groundbreaking work of thanatology on both a theoretical and practical level. The book brought together, for the first time, advances in attachment theory and grief theory with the latest developments in neuroscience, while offering those who work with the bereaved a clear guide to applying theory to practice.

Since the publication of the original volume, researchers have gained a far greater understanding and appreciation of the impact of the infant-caregiver relationship on brain development, and employed new technologies to revolutionize our understanding of brain functions. In this second edition, Kosminsky and Jordan incorporate these new findings and illuminate connections between neuroscience, attachment, emotion regulation, and current theories and research in the field of bereavement. The sheer volume of new material in this book testifies to the speed and intensity with which these fields are expanding.

The book's new insights have direct implications for working with grieving clients who exhibit signs of an insecure attachment orientation, be it anxious, avoidant, or disorganized. The reader will find in this volume expanded sections that tell moving stories taken from the authors' own work with clients. Every therapist will have something to learn by "sitting in" on these sessions, each of which illustrates how to apply our deepening understanding of attachment to build a supportive bond with clients whose attachment systems have been dysregulated by grief.

As in the first volume, the authors come back time and again to the therapeutic relationship, the secure base upon which the client can begin the process of exploring new possibilities and rebuilding their lives after a debilitating loss. Expanding on their earlier work, Kosminsky and Jordan revisit the role of the therapist as a transitional attachment figure who helps guide the client through the confusing and often dark passages that must be navigated after the loss of a loved one. In this sense, the book brings needed attention to the human element of healing from grief, often overlooked in current approaches that focus on diagnostic categories, case formulations and manualized treatments. Often, what is lost in these approaches is the client and their story. By contrast, this volume shifts the focus from, in the authors' own words, *"What does the client have"* to *"What do they need?"* In this context, it is acknowledged that the past informs the present, and the therapeutic relationship serves as a liminal space where the present can open to the future. Within this space, the therapeutic relationship can help the client feel safe, cared for, and supported as they move from a world shattered by loss to a world of new hope and possibilities.

Another important addition to this volume is the exploration of the connection between attachment orientation and the potential for developing difficulties in grieving, including prolonged grief disorder (PGD), the newest grief-related diagnosis to be recognized in the American Psychological Association's Diagnostic and Statistical Manual (DSM-5). The authors provide attachment informed guidelines for offering support to individuals who meet the criteria for PGD, who have experienced traumatic loss, or whose grief may be complicated by other psychological factors.

Like its predecessor, this second volume is a seminal work and a necessary addition to the library of any clinician who wishes to enhance their understanding of the impact of grief and loss, and most especially, how best to support those who painfully grapple with the disequilibrium that occurs after the death of a loved one. It isn't often that I take the time to read a second edition word-by-word and cover-to-cover. However, with this book, I made the time because I found it so informative, insightful, comprehensive and – rare for a professional volume – moving and beautifully written. I am sure that you will find the same to be true.

Darcy Harris, PhD
Professor
Thanatology Department
King's University College at
Western University and Co-Editor
Routledge Series in Death,
Dying, and Bereavement

PREFACE TO THE SECOND EDITION

The first edition of *Attachment Informed Grief Therapy* grew out of a conference presentation that John Jordan and I made in 2012. In that presentation, we introduced our ideas about attachment theory as a framework for understanding peoples' response to loss and as a guide to interventions for working with the bereaved. At the end of the presentation, we were approached by our colleague Robert Neimeyer, who asked if we had considered writing a book on this topic.

In setting out to write the book we were motivated by the idea that integrating three distinct, but interrelated areas of research and theory had the potential to expand our understanding of grief and grief therapy. Our goal was to highlight the intersection of attachment theory, neuroscience, and contemporary grief models, and in so doing to demonstrate how, taken together, these bodies of knowledge shed light on questions that have been at the center of the field of death and dying since its inception. In particular, we sought to untangle the question of what complicates grief: how can we account for the extreme diversity of responses to loss, which ranges from sadness and longing to the kind of prolonged and intense suffering that many have argued merits the assignment of a clinical diagnosis? How can we identify grieving people who are likely to need professional help, and how are we to know what kind of help they need? These are questions that are at the front of mind for clinicians, many of whom responded with enthusiasm to the first edition of *Attachment Informed Grief Therapy* (Routledge, 2016). That response, and our awareness of the many extensions and updates to the core ideas presented in the book, provided the impetus for this second edition.

Over the course of the two years spent preparing this second edition, while we have done our best to keep up with publications addressed to attachment, neuroscience, grief, and the integration of one or more of these areas of theory, research, and practice, we are bound to have overlooked advances that will be evident to specialists in any one of these fields. We regret any oversights or oversimplifications. We hope that what we present from each of these three domains is enough to demonstrate the many points at which they intersect. Most of all, we hope that readers with an interest in bereavement will be excited, as we have been, to discover work in areas outside of their usual purview that have tremendous potential for enriching our understanding of grief and grief therapy.

The organizing principle of our book, which has not changed in the current volume, is that when we look at contemporary attachment theory, current models of grief, and findings about how the brain develops and how it functions, what we see is a convergence that serves to deepen our understanding of grief and its complications. Grief, we know, is a response to the loss of something precious to which we are emotionally attached. In general usage, grief refers particularly to the loss of a significant love relationship, usually through the death of that person, although it has long been understood that other types of interpersonal loss also produce a grief like response (Parkes, 2013).

Both of us enjoy sharing our ideas with colleagues and we continued to do so through the pandemic, although these presentations had to be made virtually rather than in person due to travel restrictions. While we prefer to meet face to face, we were nonetheless glad to be able to stay connected to professionals here in the U.S. and throughout the world. Interaction with our colleagues working in the field is what inspires us to deepen our knowledge and to find ways to bridge theory and practice. We hope that readers will find, within these pages, new insights about grief and grief therapy that will enrich their base of knowledge, strengthen their commitment to helping grieving people, and contribute to their confidence as healing professionals.

ACKNOWLEDGEMENTS

Phyllis S. Kosminsky

The field of death and dying attracts some wonderful people, and many of them have had a hand in bringing this book to completion. First on the list is Robert Neimeyer, who suggested we think about writing a book after hearing us give a presentation on attachment and loss at a meeting in 2011. That meeting was part of the annual conference of the Association of Death Education and Counseling, an organization that has been pivotal in my professional development. It was through my membership in ADEC that I met my co-author. Jack's skill as a clinician, particularly with suicide survivors, and his dedication to supporting the development of services for this population made for a very full plate when we began all of this a decade ago, and I am deeply appreciative of his willingness to be my partner in this project.

It is impossible to measure the contributions of colleagues with whom I have enjoyed years of conversation on many of the subjects discussed in this book. These include, but are no means limited to, all of my friends in ADEC and in the International Working Group on Bereavement and Loss, as well as my long-time colleagues at the Center for Hope/Family Centers. Thanks to Christopher Hall, whose invitation to deliver a paper in Australia was a great incentive for me to get my thoughts in order. Special thanks to Dr. Mary Vachon, who read and commented on several early drafts of the manuscript for the second edition. Her support and feedback helped me over the hurdle of beginning.

The editorial staff at Routledge has been consistently available and helpful with all of our questions and concerns. Special thanks to Anna Moore and Georgina Clutterbuck for their diligence and patience throughout the publication process.

It is traditional for writers to thank family members for their love and support, and I have received plenty of both from my husband Jay and my children, Lily and Eli. Since publication of the first edition, our family has gained two new members and I have gained access (along with additional love and support) to additional technical assistance and medical expertise. Thank you, Eli and Yuliya Kosminsky, and Drs. Lily and Sam Eisenberg for your expert – and kind - help with all things technical and medical. I seriously couldn't have done it without you. For the second edition of this book my husband Jay once again assumed his roles of first reader, first editor, and first re-writer, along with his most important role, which is loving me.

Without my clients I would not have my work, and I could not have written this book. Although I have taken pains not to identify them in the text, they know their stories and will no doubt recognize bits of them in these pages. To all of them: thank you for letting me share something of your journey with others. Most of all, though, thank you for allowing me to journey with you. Stories of loss are also stories of love. Every bereaved person is someone who has allowed themselves to be open to others, to risk being attached. They are some of the that most interesting, most courageous and most alive people I have had the privilege to know.

My father Jay Glick was, and continues to be, a source of strength, comfort, and inspiration for me. Thanks for everything, Dad.

John R. Jordan, Ph.D.

There are always too many people to thank for their impact and influence in bringing a project like this book to fruition. I can only mention a few of them here. First, my co-author, Phyllis Kosminsky, has been a wonderful collaborator on this book. When Phyllis and I discovered that we shared a mutual interest in attachment theory and interpersonal neuroscience, and that our thinking was remarkably in synch about the clinical implications of these important bodies of theory and research for grief therapy, we were off and running. The mutual learning and excitement that our conversations have generated has never faded, and we both hope that the reader will feel some of that energy as you read the book. Phyllis is an empathic soul, a gifted clinician, and an insightful thinker, and it has been my pleasure to share this journey with her.

Bob Neimeyer, the Editor of this Series, has been a long time mentor, colleague, role model, and friend of mine. His support of this book, and his general dedication to serving the needs of all people who are bereaved, have been and continue to be an inspiration to me. My many, many colleagues and friends in Association for Death Education and Counseling, and in the International Workgroup on Death, Dying, and Bereavement, have also been instrumental in the development of my thinking about these topics. It is because of the magnificent support and sharing that both of these organizations foster that I became a grief therapist early in my career, and I have never wanted to do anything else with my professional life. Likewise, in addition to my own experiences of loss, my true teachers about bereavement have been my clients. Their courage in facing the reality of their own loss, their openness in sharing their pain with me, and their willingness to allow me to serve as a transitional attachment figure at a very difficult time in their lives, have formed the real foundation for the content of this book.

Finally, I want to thank the people who have served as attachment figures in my own life. My children, Kate and John, are amazing, and are pursuing their own versions of service to others in their chosen paths in life. Their gift to me has been the privilege of being their father, and watching them blossom as they move into the world. My wife, Mary Ruby, has truly served as my secure base and safe haven for nearly fifty years – my gratitude for her patience with me, and my not infrequent bouts of frustration and complaining about the process of writing books, is boundless. And last but not least, the devotion to each other and to their children that my parents showed me growing up has been my template for family life even to this very day. My father's death in 1974 was too early in our relationship, but it was the pivotal loss in my own life that started me down the path of grief counseling. And my mother's ability to overcome the many adversities of her childhood and go on to become a loving wife and mother could not have served as a better model of "earned security" - my understanding of human resilience in the face of loss has its roots in her story. To both of them, I owe so much - including the insights that have allowed me to produce this book with Phyllis.

INTRODUCTION

As psychotherapists, we have devoted a good part of our professional lives to understanding the nature of grief and caring for people who are bereaved. At the same time, we have worked to come to terms with our own personal losses. Experiences and lessons from these two domains, the professional and the personal, have each in their own way contributed to the evolution of our thinking about the importance of attachment in life and the emotional and physical impact of loss. The questions that interest us – questions about love, loss, and healing – have occupied many other minds over the centuries, so on the one hand, there may be little that can be said about these subjects that is entirely new. On the other hand, developments in attachment theory, along with the burgeoning field of neuroscience that now underpins it, suggest to us new and compelling ways of thinking about these questions.

In what amounts to a kind of professional awakening for both of us, attachment theory has become integral to our work as grief therapists. We find ourselves incorporating insights from attachment theory and neuroscience into our work regularly, as it informs both our "macro" understanding of how our clients cope with their losses, and our "micro" understanding of what we are doing and why we are doing it in the moment-to-moment flow of grief therapy-

Insights from attachment theory have also helped us understand the meaning of our own losses. We each had a parent die early in our lives; PSK lost her mother at the age of 9, and JRJ lost his father at the age of 26; and we each lost our surviving parent in the two years prior to writing the

DOI: 10.4324/9781003204183-1

first edition of book. Attachment theory has significantly enhanced our understanding of our own reactions to loss, helping us to see the normality and universality of our own lifelong mourning processes. Our interest in attachment theory thus arises from a sense that this theoretical model has served us well in both in our professional and personal lives.

OTHER TRADITIONS THAT HAVE INFLUENCED OUR APPROACH

In addition to attachment theory, which forms the conceptual heart of this book, we have been influenced by several other intellectual streams. One of these streams is the development of interpersonal neuroscience. The remarkable surge in knowledge about the brain has seen the application of contemporary neuroscience to the understanding of all types of human relations, from romantic attachments to parenting to psychotherapy (Schore, 2012, 2019; Siegel, 2010, 2012, 2020). Another influence is traumatology, and the clinical advances that have helped us better understand the impact of traumatic events in people's lives, including early relational trauma at the hands of caregivers and traumatic bereavement in the course of adult lives (Allen, 2013; Herzog & Schmahl, 2018; Nelson & Gabard-Durnam, 2020). Lastly, we have been influenced by the changes that have emerged in the practice of general psychotherapy. Modern psychodynamic approaches, which have been powerfully influenced by attachment theory, offer a way to understand both the problems that clients bring to treatment and the role of the therapeutic alliance in promoting healing and bringing about change (Norcross & Lambert, 2018; Obegi & Berant, 2010; Schore, 2019). Developments in these fields of inquiry have gradually made their way–into the grief theory and research literature (Mikulincer & Shaver, 2008b; 2013; Smigelsky et al., 2019; O'Connor, 2019) and have been incorporated into recommendations on the practice of grief therapy (Sekowski & Prigerson, 2022; Shear & Gribbin Bloom, 2017).

ORGANIZATION OF THE BOOK

Attachment Informed Grief Therapy is divided into three broad sections. In Part I, we discuss the roots of attachment theory and describe its evolution from a theory of infant development to what Allan Schore has described as a "theory of regulation" (Schore, 2003a, 2003b). Chapter 1 introduces Bowlby's theoretical work and supportive research by the American psychologist Mary Ainsworth. In what was then a radical turn from psychoanalytic theory, John Bowlby put forward the idea of an inborn and biologically based attachment system that directs infants to seek proximity to their caregivers when distressed or hurt (Bowlby, 1982). Bowlby's thinking about attachment has become the basis for a remarkable and robust tradition of empirical research that continues to this day (Mikulincer & Shaver, 2017; Siegel, 2020).

The sustained appeal of Bowlby's core concepts is about more than intellectual curiosity and theory building: something about the idea that we as humans have a fundamental need for secure connection to others just feels right and helps us understand much of what we see in our own relationships, and those of our clients. We are drawn to the theory because it says something about our human nature that we intuitively believe to be true. That being said, Bowlby's ideas have not been without their critics. The exhaustively researched volume *Cornerstones of Attachment Theory* (Duschinsky, 2020) has made available a mother lode of new documentation that reveals the fine points of arguments and counterarguments about the utility and validity of attachment theory.

In Chapter 2 we trace the extension of attachment theory into the study of child, and then adult development and functioning in close relationships. Mary Main, a researcher in developmental psychology, advanced the field of attachment studies through the creation of the Adult Attachment Interview, a research method that has been widely used to identify the attachment orientation of adults (Main, Goldwyn, & Hesse, 1998; Main, Hesse, & Goldwyn, 2008). At about the same time, Peter Fonagy and his team introduced the concept of *mentalization*, the ability to think about our own and other people's behavior in terms of inner feelings, needs, and psychological defenses (Fonagy et al., 2002). The concept of mentalization has been extended to emphasize the importance of *epistemic trust* – the ability to take in and accept new information from others and from the world at large (Fonagy et al., 2014). Simply put, epistemic trust is what makes learning possible. In line with the view that grief is a process that involves relearning the world (Attig, 2011; Neimeyer, 2001, 2009), we propose that epistemic trust is a useful concept in our understanding of the value of grief therapy and in how we approach work with the bereaved.

In keeping with available research and our experience as clinicians, we have laid a strong emphasis on the importance of emotion regulatory capacity as a factor in how people cope with loss (Kosminsky & Jordan, 2016). We review research that has substantiated the role of emotion regulation in grief, and deficits in emotion regulation as a contributing factor to complicated grief.

Developments in research and theory in the social psychology tradition of attachment studies are also reviewed in Chapter 2 (Mikulincer and Shaver, 2017; Fraley & Roisman, 2019). With a focus on adult romantic relationships, social psychology research employs a different approach to instrumentation and measurement than developmental psychology, which is the focus of Chapter 3. While some writers have been critical of the lack of consistency in findings from these two branches of attachment research,

Duschinsky (2020) sees it as an unavoidable consequence of the divergent goals of questions being addressed and the methods employed.

Chapter 3 introduces the role of early attachment experience in the development of the child's capacity to maintain emotional equilibrium and to recover from emotional upset. Evidence concerning the lasting effects of early relational trauma has continued to mount, and the importance of emotion regulation as a factor in adaptation to loss has been supported by a substantial body of recent research. This research makes it clear that emotion regulation plays a large part in a variety of mental health problems, including adaptation to loss. Likewise, there is research related to the role of early relational trauma in complicated grief, as for example demonstrated by recent studies linking scores on the ACES (Adverse Childhood Experiences Scale) to complications in grief. These findings are two examples of research that has significant implications for our understanding of complicated grief and its treatment.

The work of theorists and researchers in the field of interpersonal neuroscience has strengthened the scientific foundation of attachment theory (Cozolino, 2017; Schore, 2019; Siegel, 2020). This chapter has been revised to include research made possible by technological advances that give us a clearer picture of the development, organization and functioning of the brain. Of particular clinical interest is the emergent focus of neuroscience research on "brain to brain" communication. Chapter 3, together with the preceding chapters on the evolution of attachment theory in developmental and social psychology, provides an empirical underpinning for the theoretical and clinical material presented in the rest of the book.

In Part II we set forth our thinking about the integration of attachment theory into the field of thanatology and the practice of grief therapy. In Chapter 4 we review two models of the mourning process that have particular resonance with attachment theory: the Dual Process Model of Bereavement (Stroebe & Schut, 2010, 2016) and the Two Track Model of Bereavement (Rubin et al., 2011, 2012). We discuss theory and research concerning the role of insecure attachment in problematic grief and the implications of variations in attachment orientation for the practice of grief therapy. Attention is given here to Stroebe and Schut's recent introduction of the concept of "grief overload", to refer to cases in which the weight and number of losses suffered intensifies grief and interferes with the process of healing as described by the model (Stroebe & Schut, 2016).

In Chapter 5, we explore the impact of the relationship with the deceased as a significant factor influencing the trajectory of bereavement. This includes both the kinship relationship (partner loss, child loss, etc.), and the nature of the ongoing internal relationship with the loved one after the death, i.e. their continuing bond with the deceased. We also suggest the need to expand our analysis of the relationship between attachment and loss. Bowlby's ideas were developed on the basis of observations of the reactions of children who have been separated from their attachment figure(s). This model applies to some losses, but not to others. In particular, it does not adequately explain the grief, helplessness, and guilt of parents who lose a child. These responses, we propose, are related to the loss of the parent's role as their child's caregiver.

Chapter 6 looks at the mediating effect of the nature of the death on how people respond to loss. Here we focus on the effects of traumatic bereavement – the death of a loved one in a sudden, unexpected, and often violent fashion – on how the mourner responds and how they cope. We discuss the nature of trauma in general, including some of the neuro-biology of the trauma response. We also discuss traumatic death from an attachment theory perspective by exploring the impact of dysregulation of affect and meaning making after traumatic deaths. These become major foci of clinical work in attachment informed grief therapy.

In Part III, we bring together all of the aforementioned information about attachment theory, neuroscience and bereavement in order to illustrate how this material can be of use to clinicians who provide grief therapy. Chapter 7 is a presentation of our own conceptualization of attachment informed grief therapy. This chapter includes a working definition of attachment informed grief therapy, and a clear explication of our assumptions about attachment, grief, and complicated grief. We then outline what we regard as the key components of attachment in-formed grief therapy and their importance in helping bereaved clients to heal, starting with the therapeutic relationship and including interven-tions to strengthen emotional self-regulation, restore or strengthen the capacity for meaning making, and facilitating the integration of new information and skills. These components are discussed in greater depth in Chapters 8–10.

In Chapter 8, we discuss the specific features that make for a strong therapeutic alliance in grief therapy, and also elaborate on what makes this relationship particularly important in work with the bereaved. In this chapter we also identify and describe five core capacities that we believe grief therapists need to have in order to foster an effective working alliance with bereaved clients. Chapter 9 concentrates on strengthening affect regulation in bereavement recovery and includes case examples and sug-gestions regarding specific techniques that can be used with clients to help them recognize and manage their grief related emotions. Chapter 10 continues the discussion of attachment informed techniques, illustrating the central role of meaning reconstruction in grief therapy and demon-strating the linkage between the ability to make meaning and the ability to mentalize. We conclude the book by commenting on the convergence of theory, research and practice in the fields of thanatology, attachment, and neuroscience, and identifying what we see as the rich potential for communication and collaboration going forward.

WHAT THIS BOOK IS, AND WHAT IT IS NOT

Attachment Informed Grief Therapy is not a book about a new model of therapy, or even a new protocol or set of techniques for grief therapy. Indeed, most of the ideas in the book have been drawn from what others are writing about in the more general psychotherapy literature. Likewise, most of the techniques are "agnostic" – that is, they do not belong to any particular school or approach to therapy or grief therapy. What we have tried to do here is to weave together ideas from several important clinical frontiers in psychotherapy, along with our combined experience as long-time grief counselors, to offer a way of understanding grief and grief therapy that will be useful to others who are doing the same work.

It is worth noting that we see differences between therapy that focuses on chronic attachment based problems in interpersonal relationships (Holmes, 2001, 2010, 2013; Wallin, 2007), and the practice of attachment informed grief therapy. These differences are inherent in the presenting problem of bereavement. Unlike dysfunctional attachment related patterns of thinking, feeling, and behaving that have their roots in early neglect, abuse, or trauma, the typical individual presenting for grief therapy has a real-time emotional injury, usually in the relatively recent past. It is difficulty in managing their response to this event that is usually the focus of treatment. This is not to say that addressing characterological issues is something outside the 3.1 scope of grief therapy. On the contrary, we spend a considerable amount of time working on these issues with clients, and we devote a good portion of this book to illustrating how bereavement is influenced by these difficulties. However, we also believe that clinicians must understand that the person in front of them is grappling with a real and unalterable challenge – the now permanent separation from someone who was important to the client. Ultimately, the goal of grief therapy is an adjustment to and acceptance of that change.

Another difference between grief therapy and conventional psychodynamic psychotherapy is the use of transference and countertransference. Specifically, while we propose that the relationship between therapist and client is paramount in both types of therapy, an explicit focus on the patient's transference is a significantly less frequent occurrence in grief therapy than in other types of psychotherapy, particularly psychodynamically-oriented treatment.

It is also worth noting here the distinction made by Worden many years ago between grief counseling and grief therapy. Worden regarded grief counseling as primarily referring to the supportive type of interventions suitable for mild to moderate bereavement related problems, and grief therapy to more intensive treatment for what has been called complicated grief (Worden, 1982, 2009, 2018) or more recently, prolonged grief disorder (DSMV-R). In the interest of simplicity, and because many of the examples provided in this book refer to complicated grief that has its roots in early attachment related dysfunction, we will use the term grief therapy throughout this book.

We also want to be clear about the extensive use of case material in our book. Of course, all of our case examples have been modified to protect the confidentiality of the individuals who are discussed. Some of the cases are, in fact, a composite of several people with whom we have worked, distilled into a single vignette that illustrates the ideas being discussed. Also, the gender of the client and the gender of the therapist have sometimes been changed. Readers should not assume that when the vignette refers to "she" it is referring to the first author, or "he" to the second. In some cases, the identity of the clinician in the vignette is indicated.

To conclude, what we present here as an attachment informed approach to orientation to grief therapy is not meant to replace or supersede other approaches to grief therapy. Instead, our focus is on the value of adding attachment theory to our understanding of the practice of grief therapy. Our goal is not to reinvent grief therapy, but rather to expand the reader's ways of understanding their bereaved clients, and the work they do with those clients. We believe that knowing something about how a person has learned to relate to others, and tuning into the hopes, expectations and needs that shape their attachments, can help us foster a healing experience for the bereaved person. It is our hope that what we share in this volume will provide the reader with a new lens through which to consider the nature of grief and the practice of grief therapy.

Part I

AN INTRODUCTION TO ATTACHMENT THEORY AND RESEARCH

The great source of terror in infancy is solitude.
William James, *The Principles of Psychology (1890)*

Attachment theory has drawn increasing interest over the past twenty years among researchers and clinicians in the field of bereavement (Currier et al., 2015; Mikulincer & Shaver, 2021; Shear & Shair, 2005; Smigelsky et al., 2019). Attachment style, and in particular the security or insecurity of early attachment bonds, has become a focus of research aimed at explaining the considerable variations that are observed in peoples' adaptation to the death of a significant other (Mancini et al., 2012; Meier, Carr & Neimeyer, 2013; Sekowski & Prigerson, 2021). In Chapters 1 and 2 we introduce the foundations of attachment theory, with particular attention to the role of early bonds in the development of attachment orientation or style, and associated aspects of social and emotional functioning across the lifespan. The impact of early relational experience on self-regulatory capacity will be further explored in Chapter 3, which focuses on contributions from neuroscience that are providing new insight into how the quality of caregiving in the first two years of life affects the development of the brain, particularly those parts of the brain that are most involved in emotional

DOI: 10.4324/9781003204183-2

processing (Schore & Schore, 2014; Siegel, 2021). Findings relating to the impact of early attachment experience on the capacity to respond flexibly in stressful situations rather than locking into rigid patterns of response will be highlighted, since these findings are directly relevant to emerging models of adaptation to bereavement.

1

FOUNDATIONAL CONCEPTS IN ATTACHMENT THEORY

Attachment is a risky business.

Our relationships with others are the source of our greatest comfort and joy and also the source of our deepest wounds. Our persistent efforts to form and maintain attachments despite the possibility of painful loss are a testimony to our need to belong and to feel known by another person. In short, we connect because we need to connect. We come into the world with an instinct to attach, and this instinct propels us to form connections that, if we are lucky, provide us with protection and nurturance in infancy, with solace in old age, and throughout our lives, with the gift of belonging.

Self-evident as these truths may seem, this perspective in fact owes much of its status as a cornerstone of psychological thought to John Bowlby, the British psychoanalyst and founder of attachment theory (Holmes, 2001). So many of Bowlby's ideas about attachment and loss have become embedded in our understanding of what factors are requisite for optimal development in childhood and optimal social and emotional functioning in adulthood that it is easy to lose sight of the fact that at the time of their introduction they were widely dismissed as radical, and worse, divisive to the field of psychology.

Bowlby challenged what was then the dominant psychoanalytic paradigm. In classic psychoanalytic theory, the infant's drive to attach to their mother or another primary caregiver was considered a secondary drive – a

DOI: 10.4324/9781003204183-3

behavioral response to the primary need for food, in infancy, and for sex, in adulthood (Bowlby, 1977). Bowlby turned this model on its head, proposing an overarching behavioral attachment system driving the need to connect with the mother, whether for food, protection, security, or other requisites of an infant's or child's survival.

Bowlby's theories arose from his early work as a psychiatrist in London's Child Guidance Center during World War II. During that period, he observed firsthand the impact on personality development of the deprivation of maternal care. His early work was further informed by research conducted by Harry Harlow and others documenting the central role of attachment in the personal and social development of other species (Harlow & Zimmerman, 1959; Lorenz, 1957). His personal experiences and knowledge of prior research on the subject of attachment led Bowlby to question the adequacy of what at the time was the predominant psycho-analytic model. He argued forcefully that attachment is "a fundamental form of behavior with its own internal motivation distinct from feeding and sex, and of no less importance for survival" (Bowlby, 2008, p. 27). Although it is most evident in early childhood, the need to maintain a connection to a familiar and safe individual "can be observed throughout the life cycle, especially in emergencies" (Bowlby, 2008, p. 27).

Bowlby did not discount the value of psychoanalytic theory regarding child development as conceptualized by Freud, and by his own clinical trainer, Melanie Klein (van der Horst, 2011). But he was critical of the "ivory tower" isolation of these thinkers and faulted them for failing to consider the actual circumstances of children's lives. In fact, it was the observation and analysis of these circumstances that initially inspired Bowlby to advance an understanding of child development based not only on drive theory but also on observation of the effects of lived experience - particularly adverse ex-perience – on emotional well-being, social functioning, and physical health (Wallin, 2007). Among these environmental factors, Bowlby believed, was the damaging effect on children of being separated from their primary caregivers, a common practice in England during World War II.

Working as a psychiatrist in London's Child Guidance Center during this period, Bowlby spent three years studying delinquent boys, and was able to gather evidence concerning the impact of early separation and loss on development and behavior. His report on "Forty-four Juvenile Thieves and their Characters and Home-Life" (Bowlby, 1944) documented the cata-strophic effects of protracted early separation on development. Subsequent accounts of Bowlby's report have drawn attention to his observations regarding social and economic factors associated with higher rates of delinquency in disadvantaged youth, factors that he identified as being at the root of attachment related behavioral problems. These aspects of his analysis received little notice at the time (Duschinsky, 2020). Similar concerns in-formed Bowlby's reportage when he was commissioned by the World Health

Organization to study the impact of homelessness on children in the aftermath of World War II (Bowlby, 1951). Bretherton (1992) notes that contemporary summaries of Bowlby's ideas neglected the role of social networks and other environmental factors on the development of healthy mother-child relationship (Bretherton, 1992).

Bowlby's major conclusion, grounded in available empirical evidence, was that to grow up mentally healthy, "the infant and young child should experience a warm, intimate and continuous relationship with his mother (or permanent mother substitute) in which both find satisfaction and enjoyment" (Bowlby, 1951, p. 13). Bowlby's theory amounted to a new conceptualization of what drives the infant to attach to their mother and what happens when the connection is lost. Bowlby's observations about the effects of separation led him to identify a sequence of responses that he interpreted as *the bereft children's attempts to cope with a reality beyond their understanding or control*. These patterns of response became the centerpiece of Bowlby's writing about attachment and loss. In the decades following this work, Bowlby identified a similar sequence of responses as characteristic of normal mourning in adults (Bowlby, 1977).

FUNDAMENTALS OF AN ATTACHMENT PERSPECTIVE

The Attachment Behavioral System

Bowlby proposed that human beings have an instinct for attachment that can be observed from infancy. This instinct can be observed in the way a child attaches to their primary caregiver, usually the mother, and how the child responds when the caregiver is needed and not immediately available. From these observations, Bowlby posited the existence of an *attachment behavioral system*, the goal of which is to provide protection and a sense of comfort and security for the child. is, the nearness of the caregiver provides the child with physical protection, and with a psychological sense of safety that allows them to engage in play, exploration, and interaction with others, comfortable in the knowledge that the caregiver is nearby and available.

The attachment behavioral system is activated when the child feels uncomfortable or afraid and the caregiver is not immediately available or responsive. The resulting separation distress is expressed in behaviors that are designed to restore proximity and allow the child to return to a comfortable internal state (Bowlby, 1982). If proximity is not restored, the child will become increasingly agitated. In the event that the caregiver returns and comforts the child, the system is deactivated, or "resets", and the child resumes their activities. If the caregiver does not return, the child's protests will intensify. Eventually, however, the failure of repeated attempts to achieve reunion will result in the abandonment of this strategy. The child will become increasingly distressed and frustrated and will ultimately disengage entirely. Bowlby labeled these three stages of attachment system activation protest, despair, and detachment (Bowlby, 1960). These behaviors, and the anxiety that sets them in motion, are "part of the inherited behavior repertoire of man":

> When they are activated and the mother figure is available, attachment behavior results. When they are activated and the mother figure is temporarily unavailable, separation anxiety and protest behavior follow... (Finally) grief and mourning will occur in infancy whenever the responses mediating attachment behavior are activated and the mother figure continues to be unavailable.
>
> (Bowlby, 1960, p. 10)

The panic of a young child who needs and cannot find their caregiver is a corollary of their dependency. Their sustained and high decibel attempts to restore proximity are an expression of the imperative to remain close to the person on whom their survival depends. The subjectively felt, and objectively realistic need for a caregiver, and the protest that ensues when the caregiver is not available, are inborn features of our species. Once triggered, the child's need to reconnect with the caregiver takes precedence over any other activity. Play, exploration, social interaction, all part of other behavioral systems that parallel the attachment behavioral system, are suppressed, while the child frantically tries to reestablish contact.

Bowlby predicted that the child's characteristic response to separation from the caregiver would be related to what the child has learned to expect regarding the caregiver's availability or unavailability. Children who have learned to expect that they will be able to reconnect with the caregiver when needed – who have a "secure base" – will be more inclined to engage with the world outside. The securely attached child is able to give full attention to play and exploration, comfortable in the expectation that the caregiver will return if needed. The child's behavior alternates between intervals of independent activity and periodic reunion with the caregiver. The flexibility of their behavior is a hallmark of attachment security.

The same base of security will be reflected in the range of emotion expressed by the child. For the securely attached child *what you see is what I feel*. A child who is not confident of the caregiver's availability or responsiveness will be intent on behaving in a way that will engage the caregiver, and this vigilance with regard to the caregiver will limit the attention available for independent activity. The child's emotional expression will be similarly limited and will be based on the child understanding of the caregiver's preferences. For the insecurely attached child, *what you see is what I think you want me to feel*.

Bowlby's hypotheses regarding the role of attachment security in infant's response to separation from their caregiver served as the foundation for research by his colleague Mary Ainsworth. These propositions regarding variations in attachment security and concurrent variations in behavioral flexibility and emotional expression would later reappear in Bowlby's writings about adult attachment and adult grief.

Individual Differences in Attachment System Functioning

Beyond describing the basic elements and functioning of the attachment behavioral system, Bowlby was interested in identifying and accounting for differences in how this system operates in individuals. As a clinician, Bowlby wanted to understand how the quality of early attachment relationships factored into people's ability to manage their emotions, to form healthy relationships with others, and to cope with the variety of stressors with which life presents us. If early relational security frees us to engage with the world and to weather life's storms, how does the lack of security restrict engagement, constrict development, and compromise functioning in childhood and beyond?

Bowlby theorized that the attachment behavioral system is on standby as long as the child does not feel threatened or unsafe, at which time internal alarms sound and the child protests the caregiver's lack of availability. For Bowlby, the nature of the caregiver's response at these times is a crucial moment in the development of attachment beliefs and behaviors. *In focusing his attention on differences in the quality of caregivers' responses and relating these to observable differences in a child's behavior, Bowlby laid the groundwork for a theory of attachment that explained not only the general characteristics of the attachment behavioral system, but also the role of early relational experience in accounting for differences in attachment orientation in adults.*

Primary and Secondary Attachment Strategies

Like little investigators, young children collect data about the likely outcome of their contact seeking behavior, learn to anticipate how different bids for attention will be met, and adjust their behavior accordingly. The *primary strategy* for signaling a need for the caregiver's attention is *protest* in the form of piercing wails that seem perfectly pitched to induce a response from any adult within range. If it turns out that protest is a successful strategy for reestablishing proximity with the caregiver, the child will continue to employ this as their primary strategy in the future. However, if this strategy is not successful – if the caregiver does not return, or if she shows signs of being impatient, angry or rejecting in response to the child's distress – the child will adapt one of two *secondary strategies* in an effort to reduce discomfort (Bowlby, 1982).

The first of these Bowlby identified as *hyperactivating* (akin to what has just been described as protest, in Bowlby's vernacular) or *deactivating* (Main & Hesse, 1990; Mikulincer et al., 2003). Children who employ a hyperactivating strategy will escalate their attempts to restore proximity: they will cry louder and harder, will thrash, pound, and in general, increase the intensity of their distress signals in an effort to attract the attachment figure's attention and care (Bowlby, 1982). When the caregiver returns, the child may attempt to maintain proximity by clinging, crying, and otherwise signaling distress and protest at any signal of imminent separation. In contrast to these hyperactive efforts to get, and keep, the caregiver's attention, deactivating strategies may be less apparent to an observer in that they involve the suppression of behavior and, in Bowlby's view, the suppression of affect. That is, deactivating strategies involve a *shutting down of the awareness of discomfort* when repeated attempts to seek comfort have not produced the needed response from: that is, secondary strategies are learned behaviors that reflect the child's experience with the caregiver the caregiver, as well as a shutting down of signaling behavior designed to produce a reunion with the caregiver.

The child's development of a secondary strategy represents their perception of the best-case approach to restoring and/or maintaining proximity. A child who judges that their caregiver is responsive when available, but whose availability in an emergency cannot be counted on, is likely to employ a hyperactivating strategy, in effect pulling out all the behavioral stops to keep the caregiver close by (Cassidy & Kobak, 1988). The same principle applies to deactivating strategies, which are viewed as an expression of what the child has come to understand is the caregiver's dislike of outward signs of distress. In these cases, the child has learned to expect better outcomes if signs of need and vulnerability are hidden or suppressed, proximity seeking efforts are weakened or blocked, and the attachment system is deactivated despite a sense of security not being achieved... "(Mikulincer & Shaver, 2007). Deactivating strategies serve to down regulate or turn off the attachment system; their "primary goal is to avoid frustration and distress caused by caregiver unavailability" (Mikulincer & Shaver, 2007).

Throughout his explanation of the attachment system Bowlby emphasized that a child's attachment behavior, even when it is contrary to that which is generally observed, is purposeful and in some sense strategic; it represents the child's accommodation to their caregiving environment. Bowlby's disinclination to categorizing as pathological behavioral accommodations to psychologically distressing circumstances is also evident in is writing on defenses and dissociation.

Suppression, Defensive Exclusion, and Dissociation

I am introducing the generic term 'to segregate' and 'segregated process'; they denote any process that creates barriers to communication and interaction between one psychic system and another.

(Bowlby, c. 1962, unpublished work, in Duschinsky, 2020, p. 75)

In another departure from contemporary psychoanalytic thought, Bowlby challenged the classic explanation of psychological defenses. As represented in the psychoanalytic literature, defenses involve selective inattention to the environment; taken to the extreme this inattention manifests as dissociation. In a short unpublished book from 1962 entitled "Defences that follow loss: Causation and Function", Bowlby advanced the idea that defensive strategies are subject to differing degrees of conscious control, and can be useful in some circumstances, buffering the individual from affect that would otherwise overwhelm them (Reisz et al., 2018; Duschinsky, 2020). Bowlby's alternative view of defenses built on the idea of "segregated systems" the purpose of which is to "create barriers to communication and interaction between one psychic system and another" (Bowlby, 1962, in Duschinsky, 2020, p. 78). A segregated system is one that does not accept information from another source, and potentially, from *any* other source. This can occur because what might otherwise be useful information is experienced as unacceptable or incompatible with currently held beliefs or values.

Under the umbrella concept of segregation, Bowlby coined the term *defensive exclusion*, and outlined several situations in which this strategy could be beneficial to the individual, one of which is in the aftermath of significant loss. In Bowlby's view, a potential benefit of selective exclusion is to avoid emotional overload. While intermittent avoidance of thoughts and feelings related to a loss is a feature of normal grief (Stroebe & Schut, 1999) there is a danger in using this strategy over time.

> What is perhaps less clearly recognized is that the underlying mechanism of selective exclusion itself becomes deranged. Instead of being sensitive, efficient and reversible, it becomes stuck in a condition that is at once restrictive, erratic and rigid.
>
> (Bowlby, 1962, in Duschinsky, 2020, p. 78)

While operating to protect the individual against overwhelming affect, defensive exclusion also interferes with integration of a loss by compartmentalizing, rather than integrating information, affect and behavior. A widow whose husband of 48 years died three months ago described her approach to managing her grief:

Anne

I avoid thinking about the time before he got sick when things were good because it just makes me sad. If pleasant memories come into my mind I immediately think about how he looked at the end, with the feeding tubes and the breathing tubes. Then I can feel relief that he's gone.

Defensive exclusion features throughout Bowlby's published and unpublished writing and is an important part of his ideas about infant attachment (Reisz et al., 2018). In the context of early attachment behavior, defensive exclusion is the "terminal strategy" that a child adopts to avoid the painful feelings associated with a caregiver's unavailability or unresponsiveness. Defensive exclusion involves the suppression of emotion *below the level of consciousness*. That is, the child, having concluded that protesting their fear and aloneness will not bring the desired response, not only stops expressing their dismay, but also stops *feeling* it. Suppressing painful emotion becomes the primary way of surviving in an environment that does not provide needed support and protection. Problems arise when this approach to managing feelings continues into adulthood. Without the information provided by emotions, it is difficult for a person to know what they want, to identify what is meaningful to them or to know whether a relationship is healthy or unhealthy. In a therapist's office, these are the clients whose response to any question about how they feel is "I don't know", and who seem unable even to identify what they *might* be feeling, or what someone else might feel under the same circumstances (Kooiman et al., 2004). For some people this may be an artifact of early defensive exclusion, a theme to which we will return when we discuss the role of emotion tolerance in coping with loss.

Internal working models

Bowlby used the term internal working model to designate a cognitive framework comprising mental representations for understanding the world, self, and others. Through the ongoing collection and consolidation of information on the availability and responsiveness of their caregiver, a child develops an internal working model of that relationship. This will become the first, but not the only, relationship model that a child will develop. Bowlby posited that children formulate not just one, but multiple working models, depending on their experience with different people, and he proposed that these working models play an ongoing part in how a person interacts with others later in life. For example, a child who has a problematic relationship with their mother, but a positive and secure relationship with their father, may grow up to be someone who is more at ease with men than with women. The working models developed early in life have a lasting, though by no means absolute, influence on the value people place on relationships, their feelings about what kinds of relationships they can expect to have or deserve to have, and their understanding of how to go about getting their need for connection other people met.

During the same period that Bowlby was doing his foundational work on attachment, Colin Murray Parkes, another British psychiatrist, was making observations about the course of normal and problematic grief in adulthood (Parkes, 1972). Parkes argued that although bereavement was not generally regarded as an "illness", it was associated with a range of physical and emotional symptoms. Among the bereaved psychiatric patients he treated Parkes had found substantial evidence of serious and prolonged grief related symptomatology (Parkes, 1972, 2013). Parkes became convinced that the course of a person's bereavement was impacted by two sets of factors: those related to the nature of the bereaved's relationship with the deceased, and those related to the nature of the death (Parkes, 2013). Realizing the relevance of Bowlby's work on attachment to his own studies of bereavement, Parkes joined Bowlby's research unit at the Tavistock clinic in 1962. This collaboration led to the publication of a joint paper delineating four phases of grief during adult life (Bowlby & Parkes, 1970).

In later studies (Parkes, 1998; Vanderwerker et al., 2004) Parkes used retrospective data collected through subject interviews to investigate the role of early attachment security on bereavement. Parkes reasoned that a trusting and secure relationship with parents would be associated with trusting and secure relationships in adulthood and would further be reflected in the nature of the individual's grief following the loss of these relationships. In short, Parkes, along with Bowlby, was among the first to suggest, and to substantiate, the lifelong impact of early attachment security and in particular, the connection between attachment and loss. The role of attachment security as a major influence on the response to loss continues to be a foundational construct in the research and writing of Parkes (Parkes, 2013; Parkes & Prigerson, 2010).

Mary Ainsworth and the Development of an Attachment Classification For Infants' Patterns of Response

John Bowlby is often referred to as the "father of attachment theory", a characterization that some recent commentators argue does not do justice to the contribution of the American psychologist Mary Ainsworth. Ainsworth was the first to provide attachment theory with a scaffolding of empirical support, in the course of which endeavor she introduced a research protocol that is still used today (Duschinsky, 2020). Ainsworth's collaboration with Bowlby involved a combination of naturalistic, in-home observation of young children and caregivers, and observation in a laboratory setting. Her methods are still used in research settings where the goal is to observe and codify parent-child interactions and their effect on child development, and in research/clinical environments where the goals extend to modifying caregiver behavior to provide greater relational security to the infant (Steele & Steele, 2008).

Although she is best known for her work with Bowlby and her laboratory studies, Ainsworth began her research in Uganda, in what was the first ever naturalistic, longitudinal study of infants in interaction with their mothers (Ainsworth, 1967). Among her observations were differences in what she identified as the behavior exhibited by infants when their mother was not available (Duschinsky, 2020). After returning to the United States, Ainsworth settled in Baltimore and enlisted 26 pregnant women who agreed, after the birth of their children, to be observed in their homes in four hour sessions over the course of the first year (Ainsworth et al., 1978). From the age of six months, infants showed a clear preference for their mother over other adults, sought their mother when they were distressed, and in the majority of cases, required the security of her presence in order to engage in exploration and play. The connection between the mother's presence and an engaged, playful child did not hold in all cases, however. Some children appeared to cling to their mothers, while others appeared largely disinterested in her presence. Some children only wanted to play, while others could not tear themselves away from their mothers and showed no interest in exploring their environment.

Ainsworth began to formulate her own theory about the role of attachment in development. She posited that it was not only attachment *per se*, but the *quality* of the attachment relationship, mediated primarily by communication between the caregiver and the child, that accounted for the differences she observed in children's social and exploratory behavior. In order to test these assumptions, and with the children in the home-based study now 12 months old, she created a laboratory environment, the "Strange Situation", where she and colleagues could study the behavior of a mother and child together in a pleasant, toy filled room. The researchers (who were not physically present in the room) would (a) observe the two together, (b) observe the behavioral response of the child when the mother, through prearrangement, left the room and put the child in the care of a stranger, and (c) observe the mother and child together again after the mother returned. Each of the 26 mother/child pairs was observed. The majority of the children in the Strange Situation played when the mother was present, cried when she left, were comforted and calmed when she returned, and soon after her return went back to exploration and play. However, there were exceptions, just as there had been exceptions in the home observations. Some children collapsed when their mothers left the room, were inconsolable when they returned, and remained indifferent to their environment. Others seemed to be largely unaffected either by their mothers' presence or her absence.

Ainsworth's classification of attachment patterns designated three categories of attachment. She classified as *secure* those children who were able to tolerate separation, and to seek consolation and comfort from the mother. Their flexibility in moving between exploration and attachment was supported by a secure bond with their mother, the context of which was a sense that she would be there when needed, so that temporary separations did not cause unmanageable and sustained distress.

Children categorized by Ainsworth as *insecure* in their attachment demonstrated two distinct rigid patterns of behavior. She described these as *anxious/ambivalent* or *avoidant* with regard to attachment. Anxiously attached children clung to their mothers and showed little or no interest in exploring their surroundings. When the mothers of these children were in the room, Ainsworth observed, they discouraged exploratory behavior, and the children complied. They remained despondent for the duration of the brief separation, and upon reunion, clung harder and cried more, as though they wanted to do everything possible to avoid another separation. Avoidantly attached children, on the other hand, paid little attention to their mothers when they were present and appeared disinterested in them when they returned after a brief separation. Both of these patterns of behavior were interpreted by Ainsworth as adaptations to the mother's verbal and nonverbal cues. In the case of avoidantly attached children, what appeared as indifference was actually the suppression of behavior that was ineffective or counterproductive in engaging a mother who communicated, with words, gestures and body language, discomfort and disapproval of the infant's outward signs of distress. Subsequent studies, in which the physiological arousal of these infants was measured, supported Ainsworth's assumption, showing that the apparent calm of avoidant children does not accurately reflect their internal state (Sroufe & Waters, 1977; Cassidy & Shaver, 2008). Neither the anxious nor the avoidantly attached children appeared to be relieved by their mother's return. "It was as if, even in their presence, these infants were seeking a mother who wasn't there." (Wallin, 2007, p. 20).

Strange Behavior in the Strange Situation: Mary Main

Based on her review of hundreds of hours of tapes from the Strange Situation (Main & Hesse, 1990), Main found confirmation of many of Ainsworth's observations. She also identified a group of young children whose behavior did not seem to fit any of Ainsworth's categories. Consistent with Ainsworth, Main noted that on the whole, insecurely attached children exhibited consistent patterns of behavior, reflecting either an avoidant or anxious attachment to the caregiver. For example, children who cried and clung to their mothers did this consistently; children who avoided their mothers also did this consistently and did not cry or cling. The very rigidity of these behavior patterns, in Main's view, was a marker of attachment insecurity, and contrasted with the more variable and flexible behavior of securely attached children (Main, 1996). But what Main saw when she looked at the tapes was another category of children whose behavior was impossible to describe in simple terms; the behavior of these children was not rigid, but it was *odd*. This small subgroup, which she classified as *Disorganized*, did not employ any one, fixed strategy for getting their attachment needs met. Sometimes they cried, sometimes they avoided the mother. And sometimes they engaged in a range of strange behaviors that had not previously been reported. A sample of 200 unclassifiable Strange Situation videotapes revealed an array of

> anomalous or conflicted behaviors in the parent's presence, as evidenced, for example, in rocking on hands and knees with face averted after an aborted approach; freezing all movement, arms in air, with a trancelike expression; moving away from the parent to lean head on wall when frightened; and rising to greet the parent, then falling prone.
>
> (Main, 1996, p. 239)

These behaviors, Main proposed, were a response to the erratic and extreme behavior of the child's caregivers, which ranged from angry and punitive to overly intrusive and clingy. Having no access to coherent memories of maternal interactions to guide their behavior, these children behaved in seemingly random and often jarringly contradictory ways. Unable to settle on a preferred strategy and deprived of the external help they needed to regain emotional equilibrium, they remained agitated and upset, and had little energy or interest left over to devote to exploration or play. Main's interest in this group of children, and their comparably unsettled and overwhelmed caregivers, led her to a new way of thinking about, and studying, early attachment experience and the intergenerational transmission of attachment orientation.

Mary Main: A Move to the Level of Representation

Until the 1980s, most attachment research had to do with attachment security in young children, and with the relationship between attachment security or insecurity and features of the parent-child bond observed in the Strange Situation. In 1985, Main, Kaplan and Cassidy published a study that included an assessment of adult attachment, and that introduced a used a newly developed research instrument, the Adult Attachment Interview (AAI). Although the AAI poses questions about the respondent's childhood, assessment is based *not on what the respondent says but on how they say it*, in other words, on qualities of discourse that have been shown to reflect a respondent's *internal representation* of attachment (Main et al., 1985).

Using the AAI in conjunction with Strange Situation observations, Main and her colleagues were able to make a connection between the behavior of infants categorized as disorganized and the early relational experiences of their mothers. Main found that a majority of the mothers of disorganized infants had experienced early relational abuse themselves as children, had a limited capacity to regulate their own emotions, and as a result were easily overwhelmed by their infants' distress and demands for attention. She concluded that these mothers were not only frightening *to* their infants, but frightened *of* them; of their crying, their neediness, their vulnerability (Main & Hesse, 1990).

These observations signaled a change in Main's analysis, from an explanation of the transmission of attachment style simply based on maternal *behavior* to one emphasizing an *internal orientation to attachment on the part of the caregiver that derived from their own early childhood experience.* Notably, Main proposed that it was not the experience itself but the *adult's internal representation of that experience* that was reflected in their parenting behavior. Over the past 25 years the AAI has been used in hundreds of studies documenting this intergenerational transmission of attachment style (Bakermans-Kranenburg & van IJzendoorn, 2009; Duschinsky, 2020). The AAI will be discussed further in Chapter 2.

Together, Ainsworth and Main provided the foundation for our understanding not only of variations in attachment style, but for individual differences in the capacity to tolerate painful emotions, the ability to cope in the face of stress, and the potential for recovery from significant loss. Subsequent research has identified the role of attachment in everything from general psychological health (Dozier et al., 2008), to romantic attachment (Hazan & Shaver, 1987), to the degree to which a person believes that life has meaning (Mikulincer & Shaver, 2012). Much of this research has served to strengthen Bowlby's claims about the critical importance of good early care for infants and children, and of a social environment that supports parents' ability to provide children with the best, most secure base at their most tender stage of development.

ADULT BEREAVEMENT THROUGH THE LENS OF ATTACHMENT

We move now from an overview of the factors that impact attachment orientation and behavior in children and adults, as conceptualized by Bowlby, Ainsworth, Main, and others, to consider what Bowlby had to say about the nature of bereavement in adults. Although Bowlby was initially interested in understanding the impact of attachment and loss of attachment in infancy and childhood, he believed that the instinct for attachment persisted throughout life, and with it, the distress occasioned by separation. This aspect of attachment so interested Bowlby that he devoted the third volume of his trilogy *Attachment and Loss* to bereavement and grief (Bowlby, 1980).

In this volume Bowlby articulated two ideas that are particularly relevant to an attachment perspective on grief therapy, and to which we will return in the chapters that follow. First, he argued that the seemingly irrational or immature behavior exhibited by many people in reaction to the loss of an attachment figure was in effect rooted in the same behavioral system that drives infants to maintain proximity to caregivers. In infancy this drive provides a survival advantage to those who can attract and hold onto the attention of caregivers. In other words, we come into the world with a strong felt sense of the importance of keeping track of our primary attachment figures, and a biologically encoded propensity to panic when they become unavailable. Seen in this light, the protest and searching behavior of many bereaved people takes on a deeper and clearer meaning.

In addition to describing the normative aspects of adult response to loss through death, Bowlby proposed a framework to account for atypical, disordered forms of mourning, describing a continuum from "chronic mourning" to "prolonged absence of mourning" (Bowlby, 1980). According to Bowlby, chronic mourning is characterized by an inability to move from a state in which awareness of the death, with its attendant fear, pain and yearning, interfere with the mourner's ability to engage in his normal, everyday tasks. This description of chronic mourning, and the characteristic suppression of functioning associated with it, may remind the reader of Bowlby's description of an infant who is preoccupied with reestablishing a tolerable level of proximity to a caregiver. While such a reaction is normal in the early stages of grief, it becomes problematic when it interferes with reengagement with life to the point where the bereaved individual becomes increasingly isolated and hopeless about the prospect of recovery (see the discussion of continuing bonds with the deceased in Chapter 5 for more on this). Here too, the parallel to an infant's response to separation is apparent. The chronically bereaved person, determined to regain connection with the deceased and unwilling to accept that this is impossible, puts all their energy into denial, protest, and despair, leaving little available for the tasks of reconciliation and rebuilding that are intrinsic to adaptive grieving. With reference to the discussion of hyperactivating and deactivating strategies previously, the chronic mourner can be seen as engaging in activating strategies, motivated by a seeming conviction that if they protest long and loudly enough, the deceased will return (Mikulincer et al., 2013).

Another version of what can be seen as an activating strategy is described by novelist Joan Didion in her account of the sudden collapse and death of her husband. Didion's "year of magical thinking" (Didion, 2007) involved exhaustive efforts to uncover the details of her husband's final hours, his condition on arriving at the hospital, the observations of everyone who worked on him, and the precise cause of his death. Retrospectively acknowledging the futility of these efforts, Didion sees them as her way of refusing to accept her husband's death, and instead focusing on the possibility of bringing him back:

> Whatever else had been in my mind when I so determinedly authorized an autopsy, there was also a level of derangement on which I reasoned that an autopsy could show that what had gone wrong was something simple ... It could have required only a minor adjustment – a change in medication, say, or the resetting of a pacemaker. In this case, the reasoning went, they might still be able to fix it.
>
> (Didion, 2005, p. 137)

In contrast, a person using a deactivating strategy will do whatever they can to avoid being reminded of the loved one, will deny strong feelings about the loss, and will suppress these thoughts when they arise. They may deny the importance of the relationship and reject any suggestion that the loss is affecting them in any significant way. Any suggestion that they may want to take some time from their normal schedule of activities will be rejected, as will any overtures of sympathy or offers of help. The level of disengagement from feelings about the loss may be so complete that the person does not in fact experience them on a conscious level, although they continue to affect their state of mind, and could be triggered without warning by reminders of the deceased (Bowlby, 1980). Bowlby believed that sustained suppression of emotions relating to grief had the potential to manifest itself as negative emotional or physical symptoms. As discussed in Chapter 4, this supposition is supported by research and clinical reports (Meier et al., 2013) although other researchers have challenged the assertion that every grieving person must experience and work through bereavement related distress (Bonanno & Boerner, 2008).

SUMMARY

Bowlby's theories about attachment grew out of his observations of children who were separated from their caregivers for medical reasons, for purposes of behavioral reform, or as a result of war or other extreme circumstances. What he observed led him to conclude that such separations deprived children of an essential source of security and comfort, the need for which was as basic as the need for food and shelter. A fundamental tenet of attachment theory is that children have an instinctive need to maintain connection with their primary caregiver, most often (but not always or exclusively) their mothers. Loss of that connection triggers behavioral responses that vary in intensity and form, but which have the common goal of reconnection. The same instinct to maintain connection is present in adults, and the same response to loss of connection that causes such distress in young children is manifested in bereaved adults.

Bowlby was the first to recognize the importance of early experiences of separation and loss on development and to suggest that these early experiences continue to have an impact on a person well into adulthood. *Further, the loss of a significant person in adulthood will evoke many of the same feelings, reactions, and even behaviors that accompanied separation from a security-enhancing attachment figure in childhood.* Bowlby's ideas about the attachment behavioral system, the normative nature of a child's response to separation, and the parallels between separation distress in infancy and adult bereavement have provided a conceptual framework for research and theory related to the role of early attachment experience in adult bereavement.

The work of Bowlby, Ainsworth, and Main regarding the importance of attachment in early childhood development and in the mental health and relational capacity of adults has inspired generations of researchers, many of whom have looked at questions that bear directly on our understanding of the nature of grief and its complications. How does maternal caregiving impact attachment security? Is attachment style in childhood predictive of attachment style in adulthood? Can attachment orientation change over time? Does insecure attachment create problems in cognitive, emotional, or social functioning that might complicate adaptation to grief? These are some of the questions we will explore in the next chapters.

2

BUILDING ON THE FOUNDATION:
THE SECOND WAVE OF
ATTACHMENT THEORY
AND RESEARCH

The experiences of childhood are the primordial soup of our identity. Ill equipped as we are in the first years of our lives to make sense of what is going on around us, or to distinguish what is real from what is imagined, we stumble through, dependent on the direction and attention of others. Given the depth of our dependence, the unrivaled intimacy of our first human relationships, and our own very limited ability to understand the behavior of our caregivers, it is not surprising that so many of our childhood memories are as incomprehensible as they are indelible.

Wallin (2007), commenting on the enduring effects of early experience, advises therapists to recognize that "much of the thinking, feeling, remembering, and behaving that we observe in our patients (and ourselves) has arisen and persists in order to preserve outdated – but all too enduring – internal working models of attachment" (p. 36). Many therapy clients, including those who seek help following a significant loss, find that the confusion they experienced as children has persisted into adulthood. Perhaps they have tried to retrace their steps in an effort to understand why they fear intimacy, why they have trouble with criticism, and if they are bereaved, why the prospect of living without a partner or

DOI: 10.4324/9781003204183-4

sibling is so terrifying. In Bowlby's view, although the lessons of child-hood can be reworked and modified, their impact is never entirely erased, and we retain, throughout life, vestiges of our early experiences, for better or for worse. Such were Bowlby's assumptions, and his assumptions have served as an inspiration and a challenge to generations of researchers and clinicians up to the present time.

Following Bowlby and Ainworth's lead, early attachment theorists and researchers concerned themselves with the role of attachment in the development of infant-caregiver relationships and the response of young children to separation from their caregivers. Beginning in the 1980's, the field expanded to include research by social psychologists interested in how the theory could be applied to adult relationships, particularly what were referred to as "romantic relationships." Duschinsky (2020) has described attachment theory as "one of the last of the grand theories of human development that still retains an active research tradition" (p. vii). The accuracy of this assessment is suggested by the research presented in this chapter, in Chapter 3, a summary of attachment related findings from neuroscience, and in Chapter 4, a review of attachment theory and research that have had a significant impact on discourse related to the nature of grief and its complications.

We begin this chapter with a further look at the work of Mary Main, and from there, focus on the contributions of Peter Fonagy and colleagues. Main and Fonagy have directed their efforts to enhancing our under-standing of the intergenerational transmission of attachment orientation, and the adverse effects of early relational trauma. Their methods, which are the methods generally employed in attachment research by develop-mental psychologists, make use of the Adult Attachment Interview (AAI) and other interview-based methods.

As discussed in Chapter 1, Main's account of the development and operation of internal working models related to attachment is referred to as a "move to the level of representation" to signify a shift from an em-phasis on observable differences in attachment related behavior to an emphasis on the assessment of internal models of attachment. The idea of "moves" as a way of describing the evolution of attachment theory is also reflected in descriptions of Fonagy's work as a "move to the level of concern" an allusion to Fonagy's research on the central role of menta-lizing, "the ability to hold another's mind in mind," in the development of relational security in young children and requisite to the capacity for empathy and mutual understanding in adults (Benbassett, 2020).

Next we review the work of social psychologists, including Hazan and Shaver (1987), Bartholomew and Horowitz (1991) and Mikulincer & Shaver (2017, 2019). Social psychologists have been primarily interested in adult attachment, particularly intimate partner relationships, and have utilized self-report measures such as the Experiences in Close Relationships inventory as the methodology of choice. This branch of attachment research has produced a substantial body of evidence concerning the impact of attachment orientation on a range of cognitive, emotional, and social processes as well as factors related to attachment in romantic relationships. Studies of how people's attachment orientation varies from one relationship to another are also primarily the domain of social psychologists (Thompson et al., 2021).

In the third part of this chapter, we turn our attention to current concepts and research concerning the effect of early attachment experience on the development of core capacities for emotion regulation, capacities that are requisite to healthy adaptation to loss. Beyond its function as the mechanism by which babies elicit essential care, the attachment system is involved in the development of the young child's ability to regulate their inner experience and outward display of emotion, manage stress, and experience a sense of self agency (Fonagy et al., 2014; Zeegers, et al., 2017). Secure relationships with caregivers support the development of these core self-regulatory capacities. Conversely, adverse early attachment experiences compromise the development of these capacities.

Given the differential impact of secure vs. insecure attachment experience, it might be expected that the incidence of problems in emotional social health and functioning would be higher among people who were not advantaged by a secure caregiving relationship early in life. Here again, research supports these assumptions (Duschinsky, 2020; Fraley & Roisman, 2019). The implications of this connection between early attachment experience, emotion regulation, and adaptation to loss, will be revisited throughout the remainder of this book.

DEVELOPMENTAL PSYCHOLOGY: MARY MAIN AND THE ADULT ATTACHMENT INTERVIEW

Main began her investigation of attachment as a graduate student of Ainsworth, during which time she spent many hours observing infants and mothers and viewing tapes of their behavior in the Strange Situation lab. But she is best known for the development of the Adult Attachment Interview (AAI), the creation of which generated a second wave of attachment research focused on identifying the roots of disorganized attachment. Main believed that parents' secure or insecure states of mind with respect to attachment are transmitted to children through the manner in which they care for their children, and with the creation of the AAI, introduced a methodology for testing this hypothesis that was unlike anything previously used in attachment research.

As discussed in Chapter 1, Main believed that taking a straightforward history of a mother's childhood would not allow the interviewer to assess her *internal representation* of that experience. And it was that internal representation that Main considered crucial in shaping the mother's, and ultimately the infant's, state of mind with regard to attachment. As her work progressed Main came to recognize that the lives of people with similar kinds of childhood stories can follow very different trajectories. In particular, some people who experience early abuse or neglect grow up to be calm and capable adults who raise healthy, well-adjusted children, while others cannot seem to break free of destructive bonds to the past. Main interpreted these variations as evidence that what influenced adult attachment behavior was not simply a person's early experience, their history, but their *internal narrative* of that history. She set herself the task of devising a method of gathering information that would allow her to get beneath people's practiced narratives about their past, to assess not only what the person had actually experienced, but what meaning they had made of that experience, and their resulting state of mind with regard to attachment.

Accessing Internal Working Models of Attachment

The question of how to assess an individual's state of mind regarding attachment is a bit like the question of how to measure the distance to the stars. Direct measurement is impossible, and the investigator must instead rely on ingenuity and invention to make an indirect assessment. Main designed the Adult Attachment Interview to capture indirectly, by reflection and inference, respondent's internal models regarding early attachment experience and present relationships (Main, 1996). Although the AAI is used to gather information about the respondent's childhood, Main made a point of emphasizing that what is being evaluated is *not* the security or insecurity of childhood relationships but rather the individual's "*current overall state of mind with respect to attachment*" (Allen, 2013, p. 14).

To understand the significance of Main's conceptual and instrumental innovations, consider a typical initial meeting with a client. Along with a discussion of "what brings you in" the clinician generally solicits information concerning the client's family history, current relationships, and significant life events. Asked about the nature of their family of origin, it is not uncommon for a client to respond with something like "it was just a normal family". Asked to elaborate about relationships with parents, typical responses include "We got along fine" or "I know my father loved me" or "I know my mother did the best she could." Over time, of course, deeper feelings may emerge. But even then, to Main's way of thinking, what we are hearing is a narrative that does not tell us much about how the individual's early experience has influenced their thoughts, feelings and behaviors related to attachment.

The AAI is a semi-structured interview in which respondents are asked to characterize their relationships with primary caregivers, to recount any experiences of early loss or trauma, and most importantly, to reflect on how they see their early experiences as having affected their development and current thoughts feelings and behavior related to attachment. The content and organization of the AAI are designed to slip past the respondent's conscious filters, to "surprise the unconscious" so that what emerges is something more than a well-rehearsed narrative. By posing questions in a calm but persistent manner, the interviewer takes the respondent back to "highly emotional events from early childhood that he or she will not ordinarily have discussed or reflected on, and to which, in some cases, he or she may not even have conscious access" (Steele & Steele, 2008).

A clinical example from the practice of the first author may help readers to relate to this concept. The client, a man in his forties whose father had recently died, described a chaotic childhood in which his parents traveled frequently, and he and his brothers were left at home alone. Being the youngest, he regularly found himself the target of his brothers' verbal and physical aggression. When asked how he felt about this at the time, and if he ever said anything to his parents about his older brothers' attacks, his first reply was nonresponsive to the clinician's question.

James

My parents loved us. But my mother always came first and we understood that. My father did whatever she wanted to do. The kids in the neighborhood would always come to our house ... we shot off fireworks and had fights. I sat in the corner a lot ...

A follow up question about whether he ever told his parents about the abuse elicited this response:

I think I did say something. But they made like it was no big deal. We stuck together and outside of the family no one was allowed to hurt us. We stood up for each other but sometimes what happened at home was worse than what happened at the outside.

These responses, according to the coding scheme developed by Main, would be considered evidence of an "Insecure-Dismissive" pattern of response "suggestive of a speaker with firm or even rigid defenses aimed at keeping actual childhood attachment experiences of rejection or neglect out of conscious awareness, or at least, out of the AAI conversation ... we presume, to prevent the speaker from becoming upset ..." (Steele & Steele, 2008, p. 10). In interviews coded as dismissing, the speaker's "attachment concerns are pushed aside ... sometimes with limited anger, but without indices of sadness, hurt, or vulnerability" (Steele & Steele, 2008, p. 10).

The AAI was developed as a research instrument, and its use in research requires in depth training (Hesse, 2008). However, the questions contained in the interview have proven extremely valuable as a guide to gathering information about early attachment experiences, as well as experiences of loss and trauma, which makes it particularly relevant to work with the bereaved (Thomson, 2010). While a basic familiarity with the manner in which the interview is to be conducted is recommended, formal training is not required to use the AAI in this manner (Steele & Steele, 2008; Levy & Kelly, 2009; Talia et al., 2019).

In the first section of the AAI interview, the respondent is asked to list five adjectives they would use to describe the relationship they had with their mother in childhood. This list of adjectives is read back one at a time to the respondent, who is asked to provide the interviewer with memories that illustrate each adjective chosen. This procedure is then repeated for the relationship with the father, and for any other significant attachment figures (for example, a grandparent or stepparent). The protocol next calls for questions about which parent the respondent felt closer to and why, what the subject would do when emotionally upset, or physically hurt or ill, and how the parent (mother first, then father) responded at such times (Hesse, 2008). The next section includes questions about experiences of rejection, separation, and discipline. Once these events are recorded, the respondent is asked to reflect on the effects of these experiences on his or her adult personality, whether they believe any of them had a negative impact on their adult development, and why they believe their parents may have behaved as they did. Further questions explore whether a person has lost a family member or someone else who was close to them, and if so, how the death occurred, their reactions to it at the time, their feelings about it then and in the present, and other details. Similarly detailed follow up questions are posed regarding any experiences of abuse or trauma mentioned in the interview.

In a research setting, the AAI interview is recorded and transcribed, and a trained coder classifies respondents into one of three categories of attachment that parallel (but are not precisely equivalent to) Ainsworth's infant typology: "secure-autonomous" (corresponding to "secure"); "insecure-dismissing" (corresponding to avoidant) and "insecure preoccupied" (corresponding to anxious/ambivalent) (Main, 1996). A second classification captures the extent to which respondents are "unresolved" with respect to trauma or loss. This second classification has particular significance for clinical work with the bereaved, in that it appears to overlap to a considerable extent with descriptions in the bereavement literature of complicated grief (Sekowski & Prigerson, 2022).

Interpreting the AAI

The AAI coding system is based on a set of assumptions about *how* information is communicated, rather than the information itself (Hesse, 2008; Main et al., 2008). The coder focuses not so much on what the person says as on the way they say it, and how their thoughts are ordered. The primary element the coders look for is the degree to which the narrative contained in the subject's answers is coherent, internally consistent, and responsive to the questions posed. Coherence in the narrative is closely related to the concept of *behavioral flexibility* in the Strange Situation (Main, 1996, 2000). As previously noted, Main proposed that the rigid patterns of behavior exhibited by some infants were evidence of insecure attachment. She contrasted this with the more flexible responses observed in securely attached infants. Main made a similar assumption about the connection between attachment security and *attentional flexibility* in adults, and this assumption is reflected in the AAI coding system. Adults classified as secure-autonomous are those who are able to shift their attention fluidly from describing attachment related experiences, to responding to requests to evaluate the influences of these experiences. In contrast, *attentional inflexibility*, as evidenced in a subject's dismissal of the importance of past attachment experiences, or their preoccupation with these experiences, is evidence of an insecure state of mind with respect to attachment (Hesse, 2008).

As noted above, in addition to classifying an individual as secure, insecure-dismissing, or insecure-preoccupied, the AAI interview and coding scheme are designed to elicit evidence regarding experiences of loss and trauma, and to determine the extent to which of these experiences continue to impact the subject's thinking and behavior. A classification of "unresolved with respect to loss" is assigned when a respondent's narrative of early loss and/or trauma is disjointed, tangential, and otherwise lacking in coherence and consistency (Hesse, 2008). This classification is associated with a range of psychological difficulties, including problems in recognizing and regulating emotion (Girme et al., 2021); depression (Fischer-Kern et al., 2022; personality disorders (Liotti, 2014; Fonagy et al., 2013) and complicated grief (Granqvist, Sroufe, et al., 2017; Sekowski & Prigerson, 2022). In sum, the AAI "examines whether adults have developed a psychologically mature account of early attachment experiences and their ongoing impact on personality" (Roisman, 2009, p. 122) – something that that has been described as a "reflective" stance on experience (Talia et al., 2022).

By administering the AAI to mothers of infants observed in the Strange Situation, Main and her colleagues were able to establish a strong correlation between the attachment security of a mother and that of her child (Main et al., 1985). In a later study, Main 1996). Main found that three out of four of the parent/infant pairs had the same attachment orientation. Among the most surprising results from research during this period was the finding that infant behavior in the Strange Situation could be *predicted* based on a mother's responses to the AAI *before the child was born* (Fonagy et al., 1995).

As fascinating as these early results were, they were only the beginning, and they raised new questions, one of which was sufficiently compelling that it led Main and her colleagues to set out on a new round of investigation that would lead to substantial modification of the measurement and classification of attachment orientation. In compiling their laboratory and interview data, Main and her colleagues were surprised to find that the long-term effects of early adverse experience on attachment security were far from uniform. Their findings showed that while many adults who report early abuse or neglect present as having an insecure, and even disorganized attachment style, some who describe comparably painful childhoods grow into adults with a secure attachment orientation. Main's proposed explanation for these variations involved the assumption that *it is not only experience that shapes the individual, but what they are able to make of that experience.* Main conjectured that respondents who were able to respond in a coherent, emotionally controlled way to questions about past adverse experience possessed two underlying capacities: the capacity to think about they were saying as they said it, and the capacity to exert conscious control over their responses to potentially emotionally evocative questions just as those put to them in an AAI interview.

In her elaboration of the precipitating factors of disorganized attachment, Main introduced the terms *metacognition* and *metacognitive monitoring* to describe the processes by which we examine our own minds and the minds of others. She proposed that a speaker with the ability to regulate their speech even when describing a traumatic experience has in effect achieved some mastery over it. In responding to questions posed in the Adult Attachment Interview, this individual is able to reflect on a traumatic experience in a coherent manner, without diverging from the question at hand or becoming emotionally dysregulated. Analyzing the transcripts of mothers whose infants demonstrated the kind of unusual behavioral patterns associated with disorganized attachment, it became increasingly clear that what the parents of disorganized infants had in common were "various indications of what was ultimately termed 'lapses in the monitoring of reasoning or discourse'" (Hesse, 2008, p. 570). In short, these narratives tend to veer off course, with breaks in logic or coherence suggestive of "temporary alterations in consciousness or working memory" (Hesse, 2008, p. 570). Lapses in the monitoring of *reason* are manifested in statements that violate our usual assumptions about causality or time and space, as when a speaker makes a statement indicating that a "person is believed simultaneously to be dead and not dead in the physical sense" (Hesse and Main, 2000, p. 112):

> It was almost better when she died, because then she could get on with being dead and I could go on with raising my family.
>
> (Hesse & Main, 2000, p. 112)

> "This statement" the authors note "implies that death is an activity that can be 'gotten on with'."
>
> (Hesse & Main, 2000 p. 112)

Lapses in the monitoring of *discourse* are cited when the narrative is hard to follow, disjointed, excessively detailed or metaphorical, suggesting that the speaker has entered into "peculiar, compartmentalized or even partially dissociated/segregated states of mind":

> We went to the hospital, let's see. I think it was the grey Buick, and I sat in the back to the right of my mother. I was wearing jeans and polo shirt, well not jeans, but you know, khakis, and we turned first down West Street, and then there was a kind of a lot of traffic, so we took ...
>
> (Hesse and Main, 2000, p. 113)

Hesse and Main suggest that this kind of unresponsive or fragmented narrative may be evidence of unresolved trauma, and they propose that in these cases, the interviewer's questions "may have sparked or induced a momentary but dramatic alteration in the speaker's mental state" (Hesse & Main, 2000, p. 113).

In explaining the significance of this observation with respect to the attachment experience of the infant, Hesse and Main suggest that it is reasonable to assume that parents who respond in this fashion in the interview setting are apt to experience "state shifts" when caring for their own children:

> (These parents) may at times become peculiarly frightened in response to aspects of the environment that are unconsciously associated with a traumatic event. Having entered such a state, the parent might exhibit anomalous forms of threatening, frightened, or overtly dissociated behavior, and the apparent inexplicability of such behaviors may, like overtly agonistic threats or direct maltreatment, be alarming to the infant.
>
> (Hesse & Main, 2000, p. 113)

Research employing the AAI has provided a great deal of evidence for Main's hypotheses concerning the association between unresolved trauma and breakdowns in meta-cognitive monitoring in mothers, and disorganized attachment in infants (Granqvist et al., 2017; Ivengar et al., 2019; Paetzold & Rholes 2017; Zeegers et al., 2017). A recurring factor identified in this research is fear on the part of the caregiver, as posited by Hesse and Main (2000). Jacobvitz & Reisz (2018), in their review of this research, conclude that the frightening behavior observed in the interactions of disorganized mothers with their infants arises from their altered mental states, including dissociation and depersonalization.

There is now little question of the link between the attachment security or insecurity of caregivers and that of their children, and of the particular risk to children of caregiver's unresolved trauma and loss. Does this mean that we are faced with an endless and inviolable cycle of disorganization and trauma carried from one generation to the next? Thanks to Main, and others who built upon her work, we know that the answer is "no." But why not?

Earned Security: Accounting for the Differential Impact of Early Neglect and Trauma

The answer, Main proposed, lies in the evidence provided by the mother's responses to the AAI, and in particular, the ability to speak coherently and logically about early life, including incidents of loss and trauma. Main noted that some mothers who reported significant early neglect and trauma were able to describe these experiences without lapsing into disorganized or illogical discourse; they were able to stay present, avoiding the lapse into an altered state described above. In effect, these women had been able, by the time they reached adulthood, to develop a more secure attachment orientation – what Main termed "earned security" (Main, 1996). As an example, Main reasoned that if a person can understand that their mistreatment in childhood was not their fault, if they can understand that the harsh words punitive actions of a parent did not reflect who they were as a child or who they are as an adult, this may serve to moderate what might otherwise be the damaging impact of early neglect or abuse. Moreover, if someone is able to understand some of what drove a parent to behave as they did, the overall sense of unfairness, resentment and anger can also be moderated, and therefore may not be carried over into other relationships later in life. A person who has learned to reflect on and consider the thoughts and the motives of others is a person who is less likely to react impulsively at the smallest hint of another person's apparent disregard or anger. As one researcher put it, adults who have developed a "psychologically mature account" of their early attachment experiences and how they continue to impact their personality are better equipped than those who have not done so to manage a variety of stresses, including the stress of parenthood, and to remain present and in control when responding to what can be the challenging behavior of young children (Roisman, 2009, p. 122).

As an example, consider Lorraine, a bereaved client who has struggled to understand what drove her now deceased father to abuse her and her sister verbally and physically. Why, she has asked again and again, is there so much misery and dysfunction in her family? Over time Lorraine has come to see the circumstances that contributed to her father's violent behavior and can reflect in a coherent manner on the events that precipitated her father's descent into alcoholism and violence. Lorraine had a younger brother who died at the age of four.

Lorraine

After my brother died, my father was never the same. He started drinking more than ever, coming home drunk. They had another baby – my sister. My father was terrible to her, hit her, yelled at her, and she's had problems with drugs and alcohol her whole life. I always blamed him. But as I think about it now – my brother was four years old. And my dad and he were really close. I can't imagine how it must have devastated him to lose his only son. Maybe if my sister had been a boy, things could have been different in my family.

For this client, understanding gained through metacognition had the effect of moderating arousal, allowing her to reflect on her father's behavior without becoming dysregulated.

In work that supported and amplified Main's ideas about how understanding mediates the effect of early adverse experience, Peter Fonagy and his colleagues took on the task of operationalizing and measuring metacognitve functioning. In studies with mothers and infants, this work established the crucial role that a mother's capacity to *understand what is in the mind of her child* plays in providing a secure base (Fonagy et al., 2002), and by extension, the crucial role that empathy plays in all intimate relationships.

PETER FONAGY: FROM A THEORY OF MIND TO A THEORY OF OTHER MINDS

Mentalization Theory: Origins

Fonagy's work is grounded in the concept of *mentalizing,* the capacity to reflect on and interpret one's own behavior and that of others based on an understanding of internal mental states. Elaborating upon a concept that originated in psychoanalytic theory, Fonagy and colleagues described mentalizing as a prewired human capacity (Fonagy et al., 1991), the development of which is subject to environmental factors. Mentalization overlaps with, but is distinct from mindfulness, attunement and other more familiar terms related to the ability to "hold another mind in mind." (Siegel, 2010; Siegel & Bryson, 2020).

Mentalization theory evolved from the observation in developmental psychology that a growing child learns to recognize that *they have a mind that is separate from the minds of other people,* including their caregiver(s). Moreover, the child begins to understand that *other people's behavior, as well as their own behavior, can be understood in terms of their internal mental states.* In plain English, the growing child comes to recognize that "My mother and I are separate beings. I have a mind that is different than my mother's mind. Her thoughts are not the same as my thoughts." Later comes the discovery – or what may initially be better described as a felt sense – that my mother *understands what is in my mind* and can respond to my needs even when I haven't directly expressed them. The child, in this case *feels felt* (Siegel, 2010; Siegel & Bryson, 2020) an elegant phrase that points to the feeling that slowly develops in children who have experienced a secure, empathically attuned attachment with their caregiver(s). This revelation will gradually lead to the discovery that it is also possible for the child to understand what is in someone else's mind. The development of mentalizing capacity, in other words, is a dyadic process: the attuned, responsive care of a mentalizing caregiver promotes security and primes the child to develop their own mentalizing capacity.

This developmental process rests on the parent's ability to attune to the child's emotions and to communicate that attunement to the child: I see you, I hear you, I understand what you are experiencing. It also depends on the parent's *affective mirroring*.

> Over time, through contingently matched affect mirroring that is gradually internalized, the child first develops an awareness of his/her subjective internal state, which sets the stage for increasing self-awareness, increasing control of internal states, and, ultimately, self-regulation. Empirical research across developmental stages, outcomes, and settings supports the importance of parental mentalizing for child socioemotional development.
>
> (Sharp & Fonagy, 2008)

Fonagy and colleagues proposed that a mother's ability to mentalize is crucial to the development of attachment security in her child. They reasoned that a mother who is able to hold in mind the thoughts and feelings of her child is more likely to be able to understand her child's intentions and behaviors. This understanding enables her to respond in a measured way to the child's behavior. The child whose mother responds with warmth and understanding rather than with anger is more likely to be securely attached, and this relational security provides a fertile ground for the development of the child's own capacities for mentalization and self-regulation, and for the further secure attachments with peers and romantic partners (Fonagy et al., 1991).

To advance this work and operationalize the concept of mentalizing, Fonagy introduced the term *reflective functioning* to describe the psychological processes underlying mentalizing capacity. Drawing from questions included in the AAI protocol, Fonagy and his colleagues constructed and validated a sub-scale, the Reflective Functioning Scale, which yields an assessment (RF) from-1 (totally lacking in mentalization or grossly distorting the mental representations of others) to 9 (exceptional RF, in which interviews show unusually complex, elaborate, or original reasoning about mental states) (Bakermans-Kranenburg & van IJzendoorn, 2009).

The work of Fonagy and his team established mentalization/reflective functioning as the *core capacity* that enables caregivers to provide a secure base for their children, even if their own early attachment experiences were insecure or traumatic (Fonagy et al., 2013). In a study examining the role of the parents' reflective functioning in relation to their children's attachment orientation, Fonagy found that among parents whose self-narratives led to a classification of "insecure" on the AAI, those with high Reflective Functioning scores were more likely to have securely attached children than those with low Reflective Functioning (Fonagy et al., 1995). In accounting for this finding, the investigators suggest that mothers who are high in reflective functioning can make sense of their own attachment experience and also to hold their child's internal affective experience in mind. The combination of coherence of their own childhood narrative and *the capacity to understand their child's behavior with respect to his or her feelings* supports the mother's ability to respond empathically, thereby providing her child with a sense of validation, security and safety.

Based on their meta-analysis of research on parenting factors related the quality of parent-child relationships, Zeegers et al. (2017) report that parental mentalization, "the degree to which parents show frequent, coherent, or appropriate appreciation of their infants' internal states ... exerts both direct and indirect influences on attachment security ...

> Parents' ability to "tune in" to their babies' thoughts and feelings predicted the most optimal relationships ... when interacting with their babies. These findings highlight the role of parents' attunement to their young children's mental states in shaping the parent – child relationship ... and highlight the relation between parental mentalization and both attachment security and sensitivity.
>
> (p. 1246)

Let us pause here and point to a theme that will recur in our discussion of attachment as a factor in how people respond to and cope with significant loss. Theory and research concerning mentalizing emphasize the role of mentalizing capacity in emotion regulation: when mentalizing capacity is compromised, the ability to regulate one's emotions is also compromised (Allen et al., 2011; Euler et al., 2019). Taken together, mentalizing deficits and associated problems in emotion regulation represent a transdiagnostic factor in most personality disorders (Beauchaine & Cicchetti, 2019) and in other problems in mental health that appear to be related to a breakdown in the individual's ability to self-regulate (Allen, 2013; Malik et al., 2014). This breakdown is most evident in situations in which the individual's ability to monitor and modulate their emotions is overtaxed by stressful or traumatic conditions or events. The death of a significant person in one's life is obviously one such stress inducing situation. The complications that arise in adaptation to loss in general, and certain types of loss in particular, are prime examples of what happens when a person's regulatory capacity is overwhelmed. Grief, loss, and trauma present complex and painful challenges to the individual's capacity for emotion regulation. Once we understand the role that mentalizing capacity plays in emotion regulation, its relevance to our understanding of how people cope with loss, and the difficulties that arise for a significant number of our clients, becomes clear, as does the need to address deficits in mentalizing as part of treatment in these cases.

A related topic is the identification of mentalizing capacity as *an essential clinical skill* (Allen, 2021). Our own approach to grief therapy and the skills involved in providing it is in accord with this view, as detailed in Chapter 7.

Expanding the Concept of Mentalization

In a series of papers, Fonagy and his colleagues revised the concept of mentalization while retaining much of its original function as a signifier and component of secure attachment. These revisions relate, first, to what the researchers identify as the factors that provide the scaffolding for healthy emotional development (Fonagy et al., 2013).

Figure 2.1 represents the authors' initial model of the role of early parent-child attachment in the development of mentalizing capacity. Parents with high levels of attachment security provide a secure base to their children, encouraging exploration and the development of cognitive and socio-emotional capacities (Luyten et al., 2020).

In a recent review of the mentalizing approach to psychopathology and psychotherapy theory, Luyten et al. (2020) explain how the model has been revised to reflect research on human development. In contrast to their initial formulation, which emphasizes the role of the parent's mentalizing capacity in promoting this capacity in the child in the context of a secure attachment

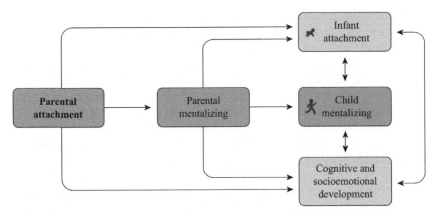

Luyten P, et al. 2020.
Annu. Rev. Clin. Psychol. 16:297-325

Figure 2.1. Parent-Child Attachment and Development of Mentalizing Capacity.
Source: Luyten et al., 2020, Annual reviews Inc. Reprinted with permission.

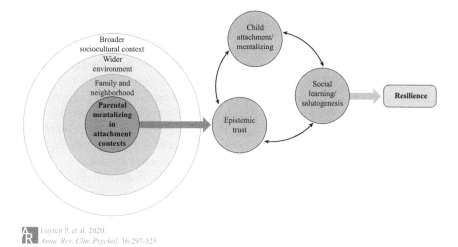

Luyten P. et al. 2020.
Annu. Rev. Clin. Psychol. 16:297-325

Figure 2.2. Development of Mentalizing Capacity.
Source: Revised; Luyten et al., 2020, Annual reviews Inc. Reprinted with permission.

bond, the revised model, shown in Figure 2.2, takes account of a broad range of factors, including the family and neighborhood, the wider environment, and the general sociocultural context (p. 300). Interestingly, this later formulation has much in common with Bowlby's position (radical at the time, and since then largely unrecognized) regarding the role of factors not directly under the caregiver's control, which either support, or undermine, the possibility of providing the kind of responsive, consistent care that supports a child's development. (Thompson et al., 2020; Hunter & Flores, 2021).

In this revised view of the development of mentalizing capacity, social and environmental factors, in conjunction with attuned caregiving, provide a secure setting in which the child is able to learn from, understand, and trust others. The child who enters the world thus prepared is primed for the development of *epistemic trust,* the "capacity to trust others as a source of information" (Luyten et al, 2020, p. 319). Attachment security supports the development of mentalizing capacity and epistemic trust, strengths which help the child, and later the adult, to "recalibrate thoughts and feelings when faced with challenging adverse circumstances either him/herself and/or in interaction with others through co-regulation, thus fostering resilience" (Luyten et al., 2020, p. 319).

Studies with nonclinical populations have demonstrated the importance of mentalizing as a health promoting resource (Fonagy et al, 2017; Luyten et al., 2020). In the first large scale study of mentalization and emotion regulation with a nonclinical sample, Schwarzer et al. (2021) collected data on 500 adults. Data from self-report measures of emotion regulation and measures of mentalizing capacity indicate that the ability to perceive and understand one's own mental states (self-focused mentalizing) "explains a significant amount of variance in maladaptive emotion regulation in the current sample, indicating a buffering effect of mentalizing capacity on using maladaptive forms of emotion regulation" (Schwarzer et al., 2021, p. 35). These "maladaptive" regulatory strategies are manifested in symptoms ranging from substance abuse and eating disorders to emotional states of irritability and aggression. Schwarzer et.al. conclude that these findings support the hypothesized association between mentalizing capacity and emotion regulation, and at the same time draw attention to the importance of mentalizing as a capacity that enables the individual to manage stress-related affective arousal.

Talia et al. (2022), in the first investigation of the in-session discourse of psychotherapy patients classified as unresolved with respect to loss or trauma by trained AAI coders, found that epistemic trust was lacking in *both* the patient and the therapist. The researchers identified two subgroups of U/d patients. Patients in the first group were found to be nonresponsive to the therapist's questions and often diverted attention from the subject being discussed. They appeared to be disinterested in whether or not the therapist found their account credible, and similarly disinterested in what the therapist had to say. The second group of U/d patients offered responses that were credible but failed to provide the listener with any details about the consequences of their experiences. These patients frequently interrupted their narratives mid-way or made contradictory statements without explanation or qualification. (Talia et al., p. 11). In discussing their findings, the researchers observe that these communication patterns suggest deficits in the speakers' capacity to mentalize (think about other people's mental states) and a lack of empathy or concern for other people's wellbeing.

Let us pause again to consider the relevance of "epistemic trust" to our understanding of grief and grief therapy. Bereavement has been described as a process through which the griever relearns the world. Neimeyer (2009) and Attig (2011) are prominent representatives of the view that grief involves reconstruction of identity and meaning, work that can only be possible if the griever is open to taking in new information and considering new possibilities for living. We will have more to say about mentalizing and epistemic trust in relation to bereavement in Chapter 4. In Part III, we will discuss the restoration of mentalizing capacity as a therapeutic goal in work with the bereaved and the closely related process of meaning reconstruction after loss.

SOCIAL PSYCHOLOGY: INVESTIGATIONS OF ADULT ATTACHMENT

Hazan and Shaver: Adult Romantic Relationships

In Bowlby's writing, the term "attachment relationship" refers to the child's relationship with a primary caregiver, the person most depended on for nurturance and protection (Bowlby, 1977, 2005). In the 1980s, Hazan and Shaver advanced the idea that this term can also be used to characterize emotionally intimate ("romantic") relationships between adults (Hazan & Shaver, 1987).

In support of this view, Hazan and Shaver identified what they saw as the many similarities between infant/caregiver relationships and the relationship between adult romantic partners: the feeling of security felt by each member of the dyad when the partner is nearby and responsive; the discomfort experienced when the other is inaccessible; and what the authors describe as the mutual fascination and preoccupation of romantic partners with one another, a state of absorption that is comparable to the sustained, intense gaze shared by a mother and her infant (Hazan & Shaver, 1987). According to Hazan and Shaver, if romantic relationships qualify as attachment relationships, we would expect to see the same kinds of variation in adult response to separation that Ainsworth observed in infant-caregiver relationships. That is, an attachment model of romantic relationships would predict that some adults are secure in relation to their partners, others are insecure, and when separated, these insecure adults will behave in either an anxious or avoidant manner similar to the infants observed by Ainsworth in the Strange Situation.

To investigate their suppositions about adult romantic relationships, Hazan and Shaver asked subjects to choose from among three statements the one that best represented their feelings and behavior in close relationships. These statements were formulated to reflect a secure orientation to attachment ("I find it relatively easy to get close to others ... I don't often worry about being abandoned or about someone getting too close to me"), an avoidant orientation ("I am somewhat uncomfortable being close to others ...") or an anxious/ambivalent orientation ("I find that others reluctant to get as close to me as I would like ... I often worry that my partner doesn't really love me or won't stay with me ...") (adapted from Hazan & Shaver, 1987). The distribution of attachment in their adult sample was comparable to that found among infants and children in the Strange Situation. That is, 60% of adults chose the statement representing secure attachment, about 20% identified with the avoidant statement, and the same percentage identified with the statement that emphasized anxiety as a corollary of intimacy with others.

Their initial studies using this methodology supported what the researchers proposed was the association of variations in attachment in adult relationships with factors identified in attachment theory, including beliefs about love and relationships and recollections of early experiences with parents (Hazan & Shaver, 1987). For example, follow-up interviews with people who chose the "secure" response were more likely to describe their relationship with parents as warm, and to characterize their parents' relationship with each other as harmonious. Anxious and ambivalent adults were more likely to report conflicted relationships with and between their parents. People self-identified as avoidant in their romantic relationships typically described their mothers as cool and rejecting. They were fearful of too much intimacy and skeptical about the longevity of romantic love (Hazan & Shaver, 1987).

Hazan and Shaver's research was followed by hundreds of studies of adult attachment, some of which supported their model and others that challenged or modified it. Shaver himself remarked upon a number of limitations in the original model (Fraley & Shaver, 2020). Chief among these was the "implicit assumption that all romantic relationships were attachment relationships" and what he and Fraley identified as a failure "to provide a means of separating attachment from non-attachment relationships (Fraley & Shaver, 2020, p. 140).

Subsequent studies by others in the field also called into question the three-category model proposed by Hazan and Shaver. Based on their studies of adult attachment Bartholomew and Horowitz (1991) proposed that individual differences in adult attachment reflected *two underlying dimensions*: attachment related *anxiety* and attachment related *avoidance* (Bartholomew & Horowitz, 1991). In a further refinement of adult attachment classification Bartholomew and Horowitz advanced the idea that the working models of adults consist of two parts, one dealing with *thoughts about other*s, and the other dealing with *thoughts about the self.* These two dimensions (anxiety/avoidance and thoughts about the other/thoughts about the self) yield the four categories of attachment proposed by Bartholomew and Horowitz and shown in Figure 2.3.

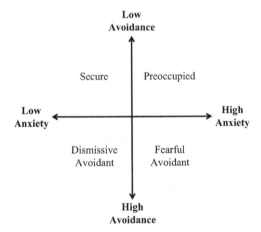

Figure 2.3. Attachment Styles.
Source: Adapted from Bartholomew & Horowitz, 1991.

Note that in Bartholomew's and Horowitz's model, the avoidant category in Hazan and Shaver's three category model is divided into two categories, "fearful" and "dismissive" avoidance. Whereas people in the fearful-avoidant category avoid close relationships with others because they are afraid of being hurt, people in the "dismissive-avoidant" category do so because they prefer not to rely on others for comfort or help. Bartholomew and Horowitz's model also includes a category of people who are high in dependence and low in avoidance ("preoccupied"): these individuals worry about the availability of others in close relationships.

Bartholomew and Horowitz: The Experiences in Close Relationships Scale (ECR)

Based on this model, Bartholomew and Horowitz developed the Relationship Questionnaire Clinical Version (RQ-CV), which consisted of four sets of statements similar to those used by Hazan and Shaver. An updated version of this scale, the Experiences in Close Relationships Scale (ECRl; subsequently revised as the ECR-R) is among the most widely used self-report measures of attachment (Lopez, 2019). The ECR-R provides subscale scores on each of the two orthogonal categories of anxiety and avoidance.

In an update to his 2009 review, Lopez (2019) highlights the "robust pace of research … including noteworthy conceptual work connecting the construct of adult attachment security to indicators of optimal functioning and therapeutic change" (p. 267). He concludes that attachment research has yielded a substantive body of evidence in support of Bowlby's core assumptions about the roots of attachment security and its importance in every stage of life.

FACTORS THAT CORRELATE WITH THE DEVELOPMENT OF SECURE ATTACHMENT

We return now to questions regarding the origin, transmission, and maintenance of attachment orientation. Over the past 20 years, the availability of large data sets and the development of increasingly sophisticated methods of data analysis have enabled researchers to offer new insight into the mechanisms of attachment, their operation, and the stability of relational models established in the earliest years of life.

Lopez (2009) has suggested the utility of organizing study findings into three domains of inquiry: Developmental and Family Histories; Cognitive-Affective Patterns and Coping Processes, and Types of Interpersonal Problems and Relationship Difficulties. These domains "parallel likely arenas of therapeutic exploration, and as such may hold particular promise as guideposts for the differential assessment of clients' adult attachment organization" (Lopez, 2009, p. 99).

Developmental and Family History Correlates

A fundamental assumption of attachment theory is that responsive, attentive, and loving caregiving promotes attachment security in children. This assumption has been supported by decades of research (Mikulincer & Shaver, 2007; Fonagy et al., 2014) and by several longitudinal studies (Grossmann et al., 2005; Fraley et al., 2013). The question of whether attachment security or insecurity in childhood persists into adulthood is more complex. The experiences of childhood constitute a significant, but not exclusive, influence on identity and functioning in adulthood (Bornstein, 2014; Fraley & Roisman, 2019; Mikulincer & Shaver, 2019).

That said, the advantages of a good beginning are undeniable. As Bornstein (2104) tells us, "the start does not fix the course or outcome of development, but it clearly exerts an impact on both" (p. 145). Children who have the kind of secure base that Bowlby describes develop internal resources that help them learn, interact, and productively manage their feelings in the short term, and in many cases, for the rest of their lives. Children who are secure in their attachment relationships tend to feel more secure in their adult relationships (Shaver et al., 2005), are less likely to report higher levels of depressive symptoms (Hankin et al., 2005) and tend to cope more effectively in response to stressful events (Borelli et al., 2019; Groh et al., 2017).

Early attachment experience has traditionally been the research domain of developmental psychologists, who have employed interview-based measures such as the AAI to assess parents' state of mind with respect to attachment. Recently, however, social psychologists, whose main interest had been adult romantic relationships, have used self-report measures (such as the ECR-R) to look at how parents' attachment styles influence parenting behaviors, emotions, and cognitions.

A review of research on the relationship between parents' attachment styles and self-reported and observed parenting behaviors (Jones et al., 2015) includes findings that are highly relevant to our understanding of the development of core capacities for social and emotional functioning. These capacities play a major part in how people form, and later cope with the loss of close relationships. For example, Jones et al.'s research suggests that mothers with a secure attachment style are better able to cope with the demands of parenting than are insecure mothers, are more likely to seek parenting support when needed, and in general, report less stress than parents with an anxious or avoidant attachment style (Jones et al., 2015). These findings complement AAI based research on the impact of attachment security or insecurity on maternal attunement and responsiveness (Hesse, 1996).

Mikulincer and Shaver (2019), commenting on personality and social psychological studies of the continuity of attachment patterns from infancy to adulthood, report that these investigations have consistently found attachment security to be a "fundamental building block of psychological resilience and mental health."

> The early attachment experiences of insecure people often involve unstable and inadequate distress regulation, which interferes with the development of inner resources needed for coping successfully with stressors. This impairment is particularly likely during prolonged, highly demanding stressful experiences that require active support-seeking and actual confrontation with a problem. In such cases, attachment insecurity can become extreme, damaging not only a person's own physical and mental health but also that of key relationship partners.
>
> (Mikulincer & Shaver, 2019, p. 6)

Cognitive–Affective Correlates

A recurring theme in analyses of differences in how people adapt to loss is the importance of flexibility and adaptation. Lopez writes:

> The more favorably organized internal working models of people with a secure attachment style or state of mind are also presumed to optimize their capacity for open, flexible cognitive processing and memory retrieval of attachment information, thereby facilitating more competent affect regulation.
>
> (Lopez, 2009, p. 101)

The conclusion reached by Lopez on the basis of his 2009 review has been supported by another decade of research that highlights the role of attachment security in the development of adaptive cognitive and affect related capacities that are particularly needed in times of stress, bereavement being a prime example.

Based on studies using the AAI, Fonagy, Main and others have reported correlations between attachment security and cognitive functioning, including meta-cognition, meta-processing and mentalization (Fonagy et al., 2014; Kampling et al., 2022) and affective regulatory capacity (Fonagy ct al., 2014; Main, 1996). Individuals classified as having a secure-autonomous state of mind with respect to attachment can access, retrieve, and appropriately describe both positive and painful attachment related memories without becoming overly emotional or lapsing into tangential or excessively detailed narratives. Their ability to engage in this way is grounded in an integrated, resilient self-structure that enables the individual to move fluidly between self-reflection and self-soothing as necessary. This capacity for flexible attention, as we will see in Chapter 4, is associated with adaptive coping in response to loss.

Support for the role of attachment security in cognitive functioning and affect regulation has also come from social psychological studies of adult attachment. One early study (Mikulincer & Florian, 1998) concluded that secure attachment functions as an inner resource that helps to cushion the blow of stressful events, including interpersonal losses. Other investigators have reported that securely attached individuals are more likely to seek support from others than avoidantly attached individuals (Davis et al., 2003). This finding is directly relevant to adaptation to bereavement, since there is an established link between the availability and utilization of social support and a positive trajectory of healing from loss (Kaniasty, 2012; Li et al., 2022).

Attachment security has been linked to the development of an array of capacities related to stress management, constructive coping, and optimal adjustment, with the opposite results being observed in individuals with avoidant or anxious attachment styles (Verhage et al., 2016). Davis, Shaver, and Vernon (2003), in a study of physical, emotional and behavioral reactions to relationship break up, found that in general, stressed secure adults demonstrate adaptive forms of coping and, when necessary, enlist the emotional support of others. In a complementary finding, Mikulincer and Shaver found that when faced with attachment related distress, preoccupied adults are more likely to ruminate on their emotions, thereby exacerbating their distress, while avoidant adults tend to engage in distancing coping behaviors such as denying the distressing impact of a negative event, minimizing their need for help from others, and inhibiting emotional displays (Mikulincer & Shaver, 2007).

Social Competencies and Relationship Problems

Attachment theory and research offer insights regarding many of the interpersonal problems that bring people into treatment, including treatment following the loss of a loved one. As suggested by the preceding discussion of cognitive and emotional capacities, people with a secure attachment orientation are more likely to possess the relational skills that support mutually satisfying and emotionally balanced adult relationships. In contrast, people with a predominantly preoccupied, anxious attachment orientation are likely to be hyper-vigilant about a partner's availability. Such a person's excessive demands for reassurance and support may damage their relationships. The fear of separation driving such behavior in an anxiously attached person would also be expected to manifest in a prolonged and intense grief response following the loss of a partner.

Findings from both interview and self-report studies confirm these suppositions. For example, in research using self-report measures, Shaver and colleagues (Shaver et al., 2005) found that people with high levels of attachment anxiety demonstrated a need for excessive reassurance in their relationships, and that this created problems in their relationships. As expected, problems arose in relationships of avoidantly attached people because of their perceived aloofness and indifference to partners (Gross &

John, 2003). Consistent with previous research and based on their own meta-analytic review of 132 eligible studies, Candel and Turliuc (2019) concluded that there is a negative relationship between attachment insecurity and relationship satisfaction. The proliferation of popular books and articles detailing the potential pitfalls of insecure attachment in adult relationships and suggesting corrective behavioral measures attests to the expansion of interest in attachment theory beyond academic and research circles (Heller, 2019; Levine & Heller, 2019).

Based on his review of findings from developmental and social psychology studies across these domains, Lopez has proposed four "Profiles of Adult Attachment Organization: Secure, Preoccupied, Dismissing and Fearful, shown below in Table 2.1 (Lopez, 2009). These categories roughly correspond to the categories of Secure, Anxious, Avoidant and Disorganized, which for simplicity's sake, will be consistently used in the remainder of this book.

Table 2.1 Summary of Adult Attachment Organization Correlates across Three Clinically Relevant Domains

Developmental/family history	Cognitive–affective processes	Social competencies/ relationship problems
Secure attachment organization		
• Favorable early parental bonds; positive, differentiated parental representations • Stable, satisfying relationship histories • Less childhood adversity • Mature, integrated personality orientation	• Enhanced capacity for self reflection; flexible cognitive processing of attachment information • Greater access to both positive and negative affect, memories; more adaptive coping • More resilient, coherent, positive self-structure	• Higher-quality self-disclosure • More collaborative problemsolving orientation • More stable, satisfying intimate relationships • Need-contingent support seeking, caregiving
Preoccupied attachment organization		
• Less warm, more enmeshed parental relationships • Parental representations as both punitive and benevolent • Dependent personality orientation	• Reflective capacities impaired by negative associations • Reactive, emotion-focused coping; low self-esteem • Less open to assimilating new information about others	• Excessive reassurance seeking; controlling • Seeks but devalues social feedback • Poor caregiving skills
Dismissing attachment organization		
• Early parental bonds as less warm and caring	• Poor recall, integration of attachment memories	• Low self-disclosure; viewed as aloof, detached

(Continued)

Table 2.1 (Continued)

Developmental/family history	Cognitive–affective processes	Social competencies/ relationship problems
• Less differentiated, more punitive parental representations • Counterdependent personality orientation	• Distancing, denial, and distraction as coping strategies • Suppresses attachment related affect; defensive self-esteem	• Unlikely to seek social support when stressed • Neither seeks nor values social feedback
Fearful attachment organization • More disrupted, traumatic early bonds • Well-differentiated, malevolent parental representations • More likely exposure to physical/sexual abuse • Socially avoidant personality orientation	• Chronic vulnerability to stress • Tendency to dissemble, dissociate when faced with attachment-related threats • Self-critical depression; low self-esteem	• Passive, unassertive, exploitable • Poor social and supportseeking skills • Less satisfying and stable intimate relationships

Source: Lopez (2009) Clinical Correlates of Adult Attachment Organization. Annual Reviews, Inc.

A MOVE TOWARD COHERENCE IN THE STUDY OF ATTACHMENT

As part of the continuing effort to bring coherence and clarity to the field of attachment research, the editors of *Attachment: The Fundamental Questions* (Thompson et al., 2020) invited a diverse group of experts to weigh-in on a series of questions that are of general interest within the field. Of the questions addressed, the following are particularly relevant to grief and loss.

- What kinds of relationships qualify as "attachment relationships?"
- How do internal working models develop and how do they influence adult attachment functioning?
- How does security buffer people from illness and support coping with stress?
- How does emotion regulatory capacity function as a mediating factor in grief response?

The book opens with several chapters that illustrate how specialized terms related to attachment are used inconsistently by developmental and social psychologists. A recurring theme is the lack of consistency and clarity in Bowlby's own use of terminology. Commenting on his discussion of Internal Working Models, for example, Thompson finds it "surprising that Bowlby did not devote greater attention" to delineating core concepts (p. 398). Differences in language usage and in the understanding of foundational concepts in attachment theory can be confusing, and the essays collected in this volume provide a helpful orientation to the field, identifying points of divergence and convergence in theory and research.

Defining Attachment Relationships and Attachment Security: What Kinds of Relationships Quality as "Attachment Relationships"?

Contributors' responses to this fundamental question elucidate the divide between developmental and social psychologists. Bowlby viewed the infant caregiver bond as the prototypical attachment relationship, and this view is reflected in developmental studies of attachment. Social psychologists introduced criteria for attachment figures that broadened this category of relationship to include adult "romantic relationships." In their commentary on these chapters, the editors emphasize the congruence among contributors in terms of the definition and purpose of attachment relationships:

> All of the authors tend to define attachment relationships as well as their basic functions similarly ... Attachments are conceptualized as a special type of relationship that serves the primary function of safe haven and secure base provision. Additionally, most adult attachment scholars emphasize proximity maintenance as a key attachment function.
>
> (Thompson et al., 2021, p. 395)

Although the development of an adult romantic attachment question-naire and the creation of the AAI have "inaugurated profound advances in attachment in adulthood," results from studies using these different assess-ments of security and related aspects of personality and functioning are not highly correlated, either concurrently or across time. For example, although the AAI and the Experiences of Close Relationships Scale are both predict "important aspects of close relationship functioning in adulthood, they do not predict the same outcomes in the same ways" (p. 396).

The Nature and Function of Internal Working Models: How do Internal Working Models Develop and how do they Influence Adult Attachment Functioning?

The concept of internal working models (IWMs) is a fundamental feature of attachment theory in both developmental and social psychology and has been described as "one of the most generative concepts of attachment theory" (Thompson et al., 2021, p. 3). As we discussed in Chapter 1, Mary Main, with the development of the AAI, operationalized the concept of internal working models and introduced a novel method for assessment that is still in use. In his own writing, Bowlby was not precise in his elaboration of the meaning of internal working models, and this lack of specificity in the use of this (and other) terms has left room for interpretation and variation in how internal working models are defined and the purpose they serve. In their respective chapters social psychologists Mikulincer and Shaver refer to IWMs as "a person's network of attachment related memories" (Shaver & Mikulincer, 2021, p. 42) that are the foundation of adult attachment patterns. For Cassidy, a developmental psychologist, IWMs develop primarily to *ensure safety* in the context of threat (Cassidy, 2021). According to Cassidy's threat model of attachment loss, bereavement triggers a fear response related to the loss of safety, which in turn reinforces cognitions that are associated with an exaggeration of threat.

Finally, Thompson (2021) also a developmental psychologist, emphasizes the importance of internal working models as a scaffolding for how individuals think about themselves, and their capacity understand and relate to others. Thompson's research documents the process through which internal working models develop, with an emphasis on the nature of interaction between children and their adult caregivers (Thompson, 2016). Mothers of securely attached children engage in conversation that is narratively and emotionally richer than the mothers of insecurely attached children. These exchanges are part of the "relational co-construction" of internal working models (Thompson, 2016). As the child matures into adulthood, these models continue to influence their expectations about other people, their assumptions about the value of social support, and their use of therapy.

The significance of how internal working models are viewed can be appreciated when we consider the implications of these perspectives for our understanding of differences in adaptation to loss, problems that arise in bereavement, and the formulation of treatment goals and strategies. Internal working models also influence how the client in grief therapy approaches the relationship with the therapist, and are relevant to how the therapist understands the client's reactions to their loss. For example, Cassidy's threat model suggests the need to focus on how the loss has triggered fears related to the loss of safety, which are in turn linked to cognitions that tend toward the exaggeration of threat. The broader view of internal working models proposed by Thompson raises questions about how the bereaved's sense of self and their expectations about other people factor into their response to significant loss, and are reflected in their seeking of social support, their use of therapy, and so on.

Thompson identifies several features of these different variations that are held in common. First, attachment researchers agree that there is consensus around the idea that different attachment orientations are associated with different developmental trajectories, different communication patterns, and differences in how people respond to loss (Mikulincer & Shaver, 2020). Attachment researchers also agree that internal working models change developmentally and with relational experience. Studies of "developmental changes in IWMs and the evolution of IWMs based on relational experience attest to this dynamic quality" (Thompson, 2021, p. 399).

Stability and Change in Attachment Security: Does Early Attachment Correlate with Adult Attachment?

Research findings concerning the persistence of attachment orientation through childhood and into adulthood demonstrate a variety of patterns of stability and change. Children, adolescents and adults can remain stable in their attachment orientations over time, can change from being secure to insecure, or from being insecure to secure. "One core principle that underlies these findings is that people tend to maintain their current attachment orientations unless they have significant attachment-relevant experiences that strongly contradict their working models, which in turn launch accommodation processes" (Arriaga et al., 2018, p. 71). Particular attention has been paid to the potential of romantic relationships to enhance attachment security, and various strategies for making the most of this potential have been proposed, including the Attachment Security Enhancement Model (Arriaga & Kumashiro, 2019).

Questions remain regarding the specific conditions under which attachment security and insecurity change. Roisman and Groh's analysis of large scale and meta-analytic studies finds only modest evidence linking early attachment security with greater social competence and fewer problematic behavioral symptoms (Roisman & Groh, 2021). Meta analyses of research on the persistence of attachment orientation from childhood to adulthood suffer from a number of limitations, the most problematic being that they rely on the "aggregation of mostly underpowered studies ... which are not informed by recent methodological advances" that allow for finer analysis of data (Roisman & Groh, 2021, p. 190).

In considering findings related to the stability of attachment orientation, researchers' definition of "attachment relationship" must be taken into account. Commenting on mixed results from longitudinal studies of attachment, Fraley and colleagues suggest that this finding may have less to do with a change in attachment orientation and more to do with the individual having established new attachment relationships in adulthood (Fraley & Dugan, 2021). The consequences of this discontinuity from one relationship to another can be positive or negative; a person may be secure in their relationship with parents but insecure in their romantic relationship, or vice versa. In short, consideration must be given to "which working models or relational schema are most active for a person in any given context" (Fraley & Dugan, p. 147). In addition, a person's attachment style in adulthood may reflect "recent interpersonal experiences rather than distal ones alone (p. 147).

This conclusion is in line with Main's description of "earned security," the ability to have a secure state of mind with respect to attachment despite recounting early experiences of unloving relationships with caregivers. Attachment security in these cases could be related to the availability of an alternative attachment figure in childhood, to a secure romantic relationship in adulthood, or as we shall discuss later, to a secure psychotherapeutic relationship after a loss.

Most research on individual differences in attachment and their links to emotion, cognition and behavior in close relationships has focused on either children or adults, Chopik, Edelstein & Grimm (2019) report on a study of adult attachment using longitudinal data that tracked 628 respondents over a 59-year period, from age 13 to 72. Focusing on differences in attachment and fluctuations in attachment features over time, they found that attachment anxiety and avoidance declined on average with age. Being in a relationship predicted lower levels of anxiety and avoidance across adulthood. Men were higher in attachment avoidance at each point in the life span. "Taken together, these findings provide much-needed insight into how attachment orientations change over long stretches of time" (Chopik et al., 2019, p. 598).

The strongest and most consistent evidence of continuity between childhood attachment and adult functioning comes from studies of adults classified as Disorganized in their attachment orientation. Consistent with Mary Main's observations in the Strange Situation, disorganized attachment in early childhood is predictive of externalizing (behavioral) symptoms of disorganized attachment in older children and adults (Allen, 2001, 2013). This finding is in line with a substantial and ever-increasing body of evidence pointing to the lasting effects of early relational trauma on biopsychosocial development and health as well as on the development of psychiatric disorders (LeBlanc et al., 2017; Ringel, 2019).

These findings must, however, be considered alongside evidence that not all disorganized attachment is related to abuse. "Disorganized attachment is more common among maltreated infants, but does not necessarily indicate maltreatment" (Granqvist et al., 2017, p. 3). Other contributing factors may include genetic and temperamental susceptibility and major or repeated separations such as are experienced by children in foster care.

EMERGING TRENDS IN RESEARCH ON EMOTION REGULATION ASSOCIATED WITH ATTACHMENT ORIENTATION

The Benefits of Attachment Security: How Does Security Support Development of Emotion Regulatory Capacity, Buffer People from Illness and Strengthen the Ability to Cope with Stress?

Over the past 20 years, the role of emotion regulation in mental and physical health has drawn increasing attention from researchers. Emotion regulation abilities and strategies have been identified as a transdiagnostic factor linked to a wide range of psychological symptoms and to psychological well-being across many studies (Mikulincer & Shaver, 2019). With the proliferation of studies has come substantial variation in terminology and assessment. As used here, emotion regulation refers to an ability to be aware of, monitor, evaluate, and change one's own emotional reactions (Gratz & Roemer 2004). The advantages of emotion regulation include emotional clarity, distress tolerance, acceptance of aversive thoughts and emotions, controlling one's emotion-driven impulses, and effective utilization of emotion regulation strategies (Naragon-Gainey et al., 2018). Emotion regulation difficulties include a lack of emotional awareness and clarity, nonacceptance of emotional responses, limited access to emotion regulation strategies, impulse control difficulties and difficulty engaging in goal-directed behavior when distressed (Cesur-Soysal & Durak-Batıgun, 2022).

Mikulincer and Shaver (2019) take Bowlby's ideas about the importance of secure attachment in the development of the capacity to manage emotion as a starting point for their review of further studies on the topic. In the review, they test hypothesized links between different forms of attachment insecurity (anxiety, avoidance) and strategies people use in relating distress and coping with threatening events. They find evidence in correlational and experimental studies of associations between cognitive and behavioral patterns of emotion regulation and individual differences in attachment orientation. Findings suggest that avoidant people are more likely to cope by relying on cognitive distancing and emotional disengagement. Anxiously attached individuals, by contrast, tend toward rumination about the loss and sustained engagement with distress eliciting stimuli (Reisz et al., 2018).

An emphasis of current models of adaptive grief, as will be discussed in Chapter 4, is the importance of behavioral and emotional flexibility, as evidenced by the griever's ability to direct their attention toward the loss, and, at intervals, toward ongoing roles and relationships (Stroebe & Schut, 1999, 2010). From an attachment standpoint, anxiously attached grievers have difficulty coping with loss because they get "stuck" on feelings about their loss, and often withdraw energy from ongoing roles and relationships, while avoidantly attached individuals get "stuck" as a result of denying or suppressing their feelings. In Chapter 4, we will have more to say about these models and evidence concerning attachment related difficulties that arise in bereavement.

The ability to manage emotion has been linked to a range of desirable outcomes including positive mood, favorable expectations about the future, higher academic and work performance and better social relations (see Mikulincer & Shaver, 2016, for a review). Deficits in emotion regulation feature in almost all mental health disorders included in the DSM V, such as depression, anxiety, substance abuse, non-lethal self-harm and suicidality, and problems related to interpersonal relationships (Ozeren, 2021; Aaron et al., 2020; Letkiewicz et al., 2021).

Emotion regulation has been identified as a factor in how people think about themselves, their beliefs and attitudes toward others, and their expectations about the future, all of which can become salient in the wake of significant loss. Several studies offer evidence of a link between the severity of emotional response to loss and negative grief related cognitions (Boelen & Lenferink, 2020; Cesur-Soysal & Durak-Batıgun 2022) which can be targets of treatment for problematic grief (Skritskaya et al., 2020).

While there is evidence concerning the advantages of certain strategies over others in managing emotion (Huh et al., 2017), it is also the case that different strategies may be most effective depending on the person and the circumstances that confront them (Bonanno & Burton 2013). Optimal emotion regulation, studies suggest, involves the flexible use of a variety of strategies, as required by the circumstances of the stressful event (Kobylinksa & Kusev, 2019).

The Benefits of Attachment Security: How Does Emotion Regulatory Capacity act as A Mediating Factor in Grief Response?

Studies of emotion regulation typically look at how people are able to manage their emotions under stressful conditions, with response to loss a frequent focus for such research in both laboratory and naturalistic settings. Attachment related differences in emotion regulatory capacity have been credited with much of the variation observed in grief response, and there is evidence that deficits in emotion regulation contribute significantly to problematic grief (Cesur-Soysal & Durak-Batigun; 2020; Gegieckaite & Kazlauskas, 2022).

Difficulty in regulating emotion is most apparent in anxious grievers, and some commentators have suggested that the suppression of emotion in avoidant grievers provides a measure of protection from the painful and prolonged grief (Bonanno et al, 1995; Bonanno, 2005). Findings from more subsequent research have identified the disadvantages of avoidance-based coping strategies. Among the most compelling of these studies are reports of the counterintuitive results of attempts at thought suppression in avoidant grievers. In a study of bereaved individuals using functional magnetic resonance imaging (fMRI), Scheneck et al. (2019) found that higher levels of avoidant grieving were associated with "activation of attentional controls" which served to "reduce the likelihood that deceased-related representations reach full conscious awareness" (p. 163). Simply put, in an effort to avoid thinking about their loss, avoidant grievers engage in what amounts to constant monitoring of their thoughts to avoid awareness of their loss. Scheneck et al. conclude that the "taxing effects of maintaining constant vigilance over ever-evolving contents of mind wandering may contribute to the poor outcomes linked to deliberate grief avoidance" (p. 163).

Studies of experiential avoidance (avoiding difficult situations and emotions rather than accepting them, even if they are aversive) suggest that avoidance is a transdiagnostic feature of anxiety, depression, and other psychological problems (Fernández-Rodríguez et al., 2018). In a review of studies focused on the role of regulatory strategies in adaptation to loss, Eisma & Stroebe (2021) found moderate to strong positive associations between experiential avoidance and complicated grief symptoms. Grief rumination was also consistently associated with complicated grief in the cross sectional and longitudinal surveys reviewed.

Exceptions to this general pattern have been identified, as in a study of parents bereaved after the loss of children in a ferry accident (Huh et al., 2018). In looking at rumination, the investigators distinguished between deliberate rumination, associated with higher levels of attachment anxiety, and intrusive rumination, which occurred in avoidantly attached parents.

> Consistent with the study hypothesis, a higher level of attachment anxiety correlated positively with post-traumatic growth via a greater level of deliberate rumination ... individuals with a high level of attachment anxiety tend to cope hyperactively with severely painful situations (and) may have more opportunity than others to deliberately ruminate about their loss as a way to overcome their painful experiences, which could lead to post-traumatic growth.
>
> (p. 642)

The authors emphasize that the participants in this study suffered from an extremely stressful situation, the loss of their children in a preventable accident, so that attempts to suppress or avoid painful emotion might not have been feasible, and intrusive rumination was likely to be prominent in a severe form.

Unlike many of the factors associated with complicated grief (e.g., the nature of the death; and the nature of the relationship) emotion regulatory capacity is amenable to change, and as discussed at length in Part III, features prominently in our approach to grief therapy. Several of those who have contributed to the presentation of data from multiple studies identify attachment as a critical factor in response to loss and urge clinicians to consider attachment orientation in the evaluation and treatment of bereaved individuals. A similar call to researchers concludes Eisma & Stroebe's review:

> We consider it critical to build on current knowledge, using diverse, more advanced methodology, to enhance our understanding of the emotion regulation

mechanisms underlying complicated grief. In our view, this is one of the most urgent aims for scientific investigation in the bereavement field for the near future.

(Eisma & Stroebe, 2020, p. 13)

SUMMARY

Attachment theory, having started life as a rebel, has long since achieved the status of a respected elder. From its beginnings as a template for understanding the impact of early relational experience on human development and functioning attachment theory has been extended to studies of relationships in adulthood, and to the investigation of how people cope under conditions of extreme stress. Some writers have suggested that the diversity of the literature on attachment, the variety of questions posed, the multiplicity of methods used, and the complexity of reported data have prevented clinicians from accessing and utilizing this information. While that may have been the case in the past, recent efforts to translate and consolidate attachment theory and research have gone far to bridge the gap that separates investigation from practice. At the same time, the field itself has become more integrated, as evidenced by the growing convergence of attachment theory and research in developmental and social psychology (Thompson et al., 2021). All in all, we have substantially more information, and more coherent and accessible information, about attachment than we did even ten years ago.

This is not to say that we have clear answers to many of the most basic questions about attachment as a factor in human development and the long-term impact of early attachment on lifelong mental health. For example, there is still much to be learned about the continuing influence of early working models on adult attachment style. While research demonstrates that the effects of early experience can be detected well into adulthood, it also indicates that there is by no means a straight-line trajectory from childhood attachment to adult attachment. Indeed, it would be surprising, and even disheartening, if we could predict with confidence that an anxiously attached child will grow up to be an anxiously attached adult.. As clinicians, we want to believe that corrective emotional experiences – including the experience of therapy – can mitigate, if not override, the negative messages transmitted to people as children. Some beliefs, bred in the bone at an early age, are harder to unlearn than others. Knowing this, we commit ourselves to finding new ways to heal old wounds and commit ourselves to doing what we can to prevent further harm. We have seen, again and again that change at any level is not easy. But it is possible.

Amid real and hoped for change, one thing that remains constant is our knowledge that the quality of early caregiving matters. Our understanding of the critical role of early caregiving has been greatly extended by research into the development and functioning of the brain. In the following chapter, we will look at evidence from neuroscience regarding the ongoing effect of early experience on the development of core capacities that affect how people form relationships, how they react to stress, and how they manage emotion. We will look at what neuroscientists are teaching us about optimal and non-optimal brain development, how the brain changes, and how this new knowledge has shaped a new way of understanding the nature and process of therapeutic change.

3

ATTACHMENT THEORY AND NEUROSCIENCE: UNDERSTANDING THE IMPACT OF EARLY EXPERIENCE AND THE NATURE OF CHANGE

The purpose of this chapter is to present neuroscience research that has given us a new understanding of attachment, loss, and the nature of change in psychotherapy. As Schore (2019) explains, the intra-brain focus used extensively in cognitive neuroscience, "the newer fields of affective neuroscience and especially social neuroscience are exploring *inter-brain connections*. An inter-brain paradigm supports current 'relational' models that emphasize the potent intersubjective influences that flow between two affectively communicating minds" (Schore, 2019).

We begin by reviewing evidence of the impact of caregiving on neurological development in the first two years of life, and from there, suggest a connection between these studies of early attachment experience and adaptation to loss in adulthood. Much of the research included here concerns the role of early caregiving in the development of parts of the brain most involved with affect regulation. The significance of what we now understand

DOI: 10.4324/9781003204183-5

to be the brain's ongoing ability to grow, and change will also be discussed, with an emphasis on implications for the practice of grief therapy.

Two caveats are in order regarding what follows. First, while the emphasis in our discussion of brain development emphasizes the role of the caregiver, and in particular, the mother, this is not to suggest that the mother-child bond is the only one that matters in terms of the child's development or their orientation to attachment (Grossman et al., 2008). Attachment related research has historically focused on the mother-child bond, but the scope of early child development research has broadened to include fathers and other significant attachment figures in the child's early life. Secondly, we recall Bowlby's pronouncement about society's responsibility for children's well-being, and the social imperative of addressing resource deficits that limit parent's ability to provide children with what they need for healthy development. Research on the impact of income inequalities, racism, and other factors that are associated with disparities in health and well-being repeatedly demonstrates the effects of chronic toxic stress on caregivers, and on the development of the brain and other biological system of children in their care (Shonkoff et al., 2021).

WHY SHOULD NEUROSCIENCE MATTER TO GRIEF THERAPISTS?

As much as their interests may diverge, researchers and clinicians in the field of death and dying share a desire to account for the variation in people's responses to loss, and questions about the source of these differences have been a major focus of study. Attachment theory suggests that the answers to these questions can often be found, at least in part, in the details of people's early environment and in particular, the quality of care they received as infants and young children.

Over the past 20 years neuroscience research has helped us understand how our earliest relational experiences, the way we're looked at, the way we're held and spoken to in the first years of life – all elements of the experience we refer to as early attachment – affect the development of the brain, and in particular, areas of the brain that are most involved with processing emotion. The more we learn about the brain and how it develops, the clearer it becomes that the quality of early caregiving has a lifelong impact on emotional health, including how we deal with significant loss and other stressful life events. The brain has many responsibilities and attends to them as the need arises. In the aftermath of significant loss, much of what occupies the brain is related to emotion.

The brain is an active participant in the process of recording and responding to what we experience internally and externally, and a principal player in how we feel, what we think and how we think about it. Beginning with the first flickers of consciousness, the brain is where data related to attachment experience is gathered, interpreted, and stored. This experiential data serves as a foundation for the individual's orientation to attachment, their capacity to build and maintain healthy relationships, and their ability to deal with major life stressors, including the stress of loss. In simple terms, the brain is what we, as clinicians, are working with when we are working with emotion. When emotions are outsized and painful, they can become too much for the brain to effectively manage.

Dan Siegel, whose model of the brain is introduced below, has been at the forefront of examining the "mind" as distinct from the brain (Siegel, 2001, 2020). He defines the mind as an "emergent, self-organizing, embodied and relational process that regulates the flow of energy" (Siegel, 2012, pp. 1–6). In Siegel's view, much of the distress that manifests in a range of psychological difficulties and problems in living arises from a breakdown of integration within the mind, a discordance of thoughts and feelings that disturbs the individual's emotional equilibrium and limits their ability to function individually and in relationship to others. Siegel's conception of psychological symptoms as the outward expression of an unsettled mind and his view of healing as a process of enhancing integration by quieting the mind and directing attention to the present moment resonates with and has influenced much of our own thinking about loss and healing.

Grief, in a manner that parallels childhood separation distress, narrows the griever's attention to what they have lost. For most, this is a temporary state, but not for all. Observable differences in people's ability to direct their attention and maintain awareness of their thoughts and feelings is one way of accounting for the range of ways that people are or are not able to manage their response to stressful events, a prime example being the experience of death of a significant attachment figure. Researchers interested in the diversity of response to loss have increasingly focused on the role of variations in regulatory capacity as a contributing factor to these differences (Boelen, 2016; Gegieckaite & Kazlauskas, 2022; Mikulincer & Shaver, 2019).

Neuroscience research has shed light on the mechanisms underlying the association between a person's early experience of care, their capacity to manage intense emotional arousal, and the nature of their grief. When grief is overwhelming and unrelenting, understanding these developmental processes enables us to provide our clients with education hat can mitigate feelings of personal failure and weakness. Here again, Siegel, and notable others mentioned throughout this chapter, offer us a framework for helping our clients understand their response to loss and why problems that seem to have come from nowhere are in fact deeply rooted in their experience and their identity.

Our encounters with grieving individuals take place in the realm of deeply felt emotions, emotions that can threaten a person's sense of self and challenge their assumptions about themselves and their ability to function. If we want to understand emotion, and grief in particular, we need to understand the brain. If we want to understand why grief becomes complicated, we need to understand something of how the brain develops, the environmental influences that shape the brain, and how neurological development can be derailed by early adverse experience. If we want to help grieving people, we need to be prepared to support them in recovering, or developing, their capacity to manage their emotions.

THE BRAIN IS OUR TERRITORY

Thanks to advances in technology, researchers have begun to gather finely grained data about this territory, much of it directly relevant to our understanding of attachment and loss. These investigations address questions that have up to now been unanswerable in any but theoretical terms. A prime example of this is the debate, elaborated in Chapter 2, about how to define and measure attachment orientation. Neuroscientists have their own way of posing these questions. Does attachment security have a neurological "signature"? Can we identify the neurological correlates of secure vs. insecure attachment? Neuroscientists have also been at work on questions that are of particular interest to clinicians - questions regarding the stability of attachment orientation and the potential for change. Can psychotherapy help insecurely attached adults shift develop a secure orientation to attachment? What is happening in the brain when therapy "works"?

BRAIN TO BRAIN: UNDERSTANDING THE NATURE OF CHANGE IN PSYCHOTHERAPY

Drawing on the work of Eric Kandel (1998), the first American psychiatrist to win the Nobel Prize in physiology or medicine Cozolino (2010) explains that the shifts we observe in the thoughts, emotions, or behavior of someone engaged in a course of psychotherapy represent the top layer of change that has occurred at a deeper level.

> When one or more neural networks necessary for optimal functioning remain underdeveloped, under regulated or under integrated with others, we experience the complaints and symptoms for which people seek therapy. We now assume that when psychotherapy results in symptom reduction or experiential change, the brain has, in some way, been altered.
>
> (Cozolino, 2010, p. 13)

The primary mechanism of this kind of change is the therapeutic relationship (Norcross & Lambert, 2018) and specifically, right-brain to right-brain emotional processes not unlike the process through which the brain develops early in life (Schore, 2009, 2019; Siegel, 2020). Effective psychotherapy engages the client's emotion focused right hemisphere as well as the language focused left hemisphere. Schore (2019) goes further and has long taken the position that the right brain to right brain communication in psychotherapy is where the magic happens.

> In "heightened affective moments" of a psychotherapy session, the intuitive therapist implicitly "surrenders" into a callosal shift from the left hemispheric posterior temporoparietal system in Wernicke's receptive language area that processes grammatical processing, semantic knowledge, and syntax in verbal conversations, to the right hemispheric posterior temporoparietal system that intersubjectively processes nonverbal emotional protoconversations. The key clinical ability of the empathic psychobiologically attuned therapist is not to intellectually understand the patient but to emotionally listen to and subjectively feel the patient.
>
> (Schore, 2019, p. 14)

The idea that it is the therapeutic relationship, rather than the particulars of theory or technique, that makes change possible is not new (Norcross, 2011b). What is new is our understanding of the mechanisms by which change occurs and the essential elements of the therapeutic relationship that make it possible. Schore (2021) cites paradigm-shifting hyperscanning research that allows for simultaneous measurement of brain activity in patient and therapist during emotion focused psychotherapy sessions These studies "document a right brain to right brain nonverbal communication system in the co-constructed therapeutic alliance" (Schore, 2021, p. 1). Interdisciplinary research and updated clinical models suggest that the right hemisphere is dominant in treatment and that therapy is not so much a "talking cure" as it is an "affect communicating and regulating cure" (Schore, 2009, p. 128; Schore, 2012, 2019). We will return to Schore's model, the research on which it is based, and its implications for psychotherapy. But first things first: to lay the foundation for this discussion, it is necessary to begin with a brief orienting review of the organization and development of the brain.

ADVANCES AND LIMITATIONS IN OUR UNDERSTANDING OF THE BRAIN

While our models of the brain, processes in the brain, and brain-body functioning have grown increasingly sophisticated, it is important to recognize that these models are supported by varying degrees of scientific evidence, and as such, are continually being challenged and revised. The enormous complexity of the brain and the highly integrative nature of brain functioning, as well as fundamental differences of opinion about research methods and the interpretation of results, make it difficult to arrive at a consensus about how the brain develops and operates (Parens & Johnston, 2014; BRAIN Initiative, 2021).

ATTACHMENT THEORY AND NEUROSCIENCE   65

One of the factors that limits our ability to make definitive statements about the location of specific activities within the brain is the sheer number of operating parts it contains. The human brain has an estimated 86 billion neurons, each of which establishes thousands (estimates range from 1,000 to 10,000) synapses or connections with neighboring cells (Azevedo et al., 2009; Nunes, 2021). Neuroscientists talk about the organization of these cells in terms of bounded segments, "regions" of the brain, much as we might discuss "regions" of a country. In reality, neurological boundaries, like governmental boundaries (for instance, state borders) are not naturally occurring, but arbitrarily established. They serve a purpose, to be sure. But particularly with respect to the brain, when we talk about the "functions" of these "regions" we do not want to lose sight of the discrepancy between our representation of the brain, and the brain as it actually exists.

The functioning of the brain is more accurately represented as being simultaneously holistic and distributed (Siegel, 2012). That is, the activity that is related to end functions (e.g., vision and hearing) occurs across many areas of the brain, including some that are very old in a phylogenetic or evolutionary sense and are typically more emotional- and action-oriented, and some relatively new parts of the brain that are involved with thinking or executive functioning. These newer parts of the brain have more to do with our capacity to make reasoned decisions and to inhibit impulses to act that arise from phylogenetically older parts of the brain. The distributed nature of information processing means that healthy functioning depends not only on the integrity of discrete areas of the brain, but on the integrity of the brain's connective circuitry. The more complex the task, the greater the need for integration and the greater the potential for compromised functioning if this circuitry is impaired or damaged (Riva et al., 2011; Siegel, 2020). The role of integration in healthy brain functioning is a basic premise of interpersonal neurobiology (Siegel, 2012b, 2020; Cozolino, 2017) and it informs our understanding of psychological and neurological integration as the goal of all psychotherapy, including grief therapy, as discussed in Part III.

Models of brain structure and functioning are regularly revised to reflect current knowledge. For example, in his preface to the third edition of *The Neuroscience of Psychotherapy*, Cozolino (2017) describes as simplistic previous descriptions of the Executive System (including this own, in previous editions) that identified the frontal-parietal network as the singular locus of executive activity. This model has given way to a much broader exploration of executive functioning that involves "a network of systems with a range of specialties" (Cozolino, 2017, p. xi), including the amygdala, a component of the limbic system that detects threat and danger, the frontal-parietal network that attends to monitoring and performing tasks in the outside world, and the default-mode network (DMN), a relatively recent introduction to models of brain connectivity and functioning. The DMN is activated when attention is turned away from the self and toward others (Mars et al., 2012). The DPN is largely involved with tasks that are of a social nature, and which require processing information about the thoughts, behaviors and lives of others (Li et al., 2014).

As explained by Cozolino, optimal executive functioning is characterized by coordinated operation of this network of systems, which allow us to "react to danger, successfully navigate the world, establish and maintain attachment, and create a sense of self and internal reality" (Cozolino, 2017, p. xii). Early attachment trauma can adversely affect any one of these systems. We will return to Cozolino's discussion of these effects and his recommendations for treatment later in this chapter.

BRAIN ORGANIZATION

As Siegel has helpfully pointed out, the major regions of the brain can be visualized by using the human hand as a physical metaphor (Siegel, 2012b).

With the hand open and the thumb folded over the palm, the tips of the fingers represent the middle prefrontal cortex, and the thumb represents the limbic system, which includes the amygdala and the hippocampus. With the fingers closed over the thumb, the top of the hand (the middle joint of the fingers) represents the cerebral cortex, which is now enclosing the limbic region. The soft, meatier part of the palm below the thumb

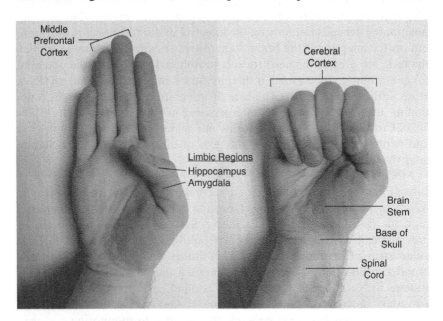

Figure 3.1. Hand Model of the Brain.
Source: Based on Siegel, 2012.

corresponds to the brainstem. The very top of the wrist corresponds to the base of the skull and the wrist corresponds to the top of the spinal column.

Staying with this model for a moment, we can say that the evolutionary development of our brains occurred from the "wrist up". The brainstem is the oldest part of the brain in terms of evolutionary development. Broadly speaking, it is concerned with mediating states of arousal and regulating automatic functions like breathing and heart rate. The brainstem also houses neurons that trigger the "fight, flight, or freeze" response when we perceive danger.

The next part of the brain to develop was the limbic system, which is involved in the generation and regulation of emotion. The limbic system also has an important role in our ability to interpret social cues and to make sense of other people's behavior. All these functions make the limbic system particularly important in mediating the response to loss and separation. Researchers interested in how early attachment affects emotional functioning have paid particular attention to the development of the limbic system, and as we will see shortly, this research is relevant to our understanding of the impact of early attachment on adaptation to loss, and to the response to trauma.

Last to develop was the cerebrum (cerebral cortex), also called the upper brain. The cerebral cortex is responsible for the cognitive skills of logic, creativity, intuition, and decision-making, and it also has a central role in the ability to understand and narrate emotional experiences. The cerebral cortex is further divided into four lobes: frontal, parietal, occipital, and temporal. The frontal lobe is necessary for higher level functions, including thinking, planning, and emotional reflection. The parietal lobe is broadly associated with motor control, the occipital lobe with visual processing, and the temporal lobe with memory formation and sensory processing. The temporal lobe of the left hemisphere is particularly important for speech recognition.

As a researcher, clinician, and educator, Siegel has been at the forefront of efforts to bring knowledge of the brain to the practice of psychotherapy (Siegel, 2012, 2020). But his belief in the importance of understanding how our brains work well extends beyond psychotherapy. Brain health and brain functioning influence how we parent, how we form relationships, how we understand our own emotions and behavior. When we understand how the brainstem operates, for example, we can be more forgiving of our automatic responses in situations that threaten or upset us. This knowledge, shared with clients who have blamed themselves for actions taken under extreme circumstances, can help alleviate ruminative guilt and self-criticism. One of the most important and life enhancing impacts of providing psychoeducation about the brain, Siegel proposes, is that it supports a more compassionate view of the self: "This may not be my fault because my brain did this, but it is my responsibility to make a change' is a common response from those who are taught about the brain" (Siegel, 2012b, pp. 2–3).

This same principle – that there will be situations in which more evolved systems for decision making and action are overridden by more primitive neurological functioning – is also a feature of the triune model of the brain introduced in the 1960s by the neuroscientist Paul MacLean (MacLean, 1990) In concordance with the tripartite "hand metaphor" model presented above, MacLean argued that our brain is actually three brains in one, and incorporates structures found in reptiles (the reptilian brain), in mammals (the paleomammalian brain), and uniquely, in humans (the neo-mammalian brain). As a result, we have various and sometimes conflicting ways of responding to environmental stimuli – in particular, our response may come from an older part of our brain when we feel threatened or angry. The triune brain model has been criticized by some writers who find it to be an over-simplification of brain structure and functioning (Reiner, 1990; Cesario et al., 2020). Others see it as a useful metaphor, one that can be introduced to clients to help them understand the range of human behavior, from the lowest forms of "mindless" aggression to the upper reaches of creativity and concern for others. (Gilbert, 2022; Hanson, 2013).

The development of an individual's brain over the course of his or her life is isomorphic with the evolutionary development of the human brain over many thousands of years, beginning first with regions involved in simple survival functions (respiration, digestion, movement), moving on to emotional processing, particularly of danger (e.g. a predator) or possible reward (e.g. a food source or sexual partner), and continuing on with those involved in higher order cognitive functions, such as thinking, reflecting, deciding and planning, At birth, the reptilian brain is fully functional and the paleomammalian brain is coming online. The cortex, however, is only just beginning to form. As a result, much of what we learn early in life is "organized and controlled by reflexes, behaviors, and emotions outside of our awareness and distorted by our immature brains" (Cozolino, 2010, p. 9). Regardless of the quality of our early experience, we carry with us into adulthood implicit (unconscious) memories of feelings, interactions, and events from personal experiences before our brains were fully developed. This includes positive emotions of pleasure and security, and negative emotions of pain and/or threat. Also significant is the fact that these very early experiences occur before our brain's capacity for language comes online. Without language, our ability to process what is going on inside us and to communicate our inner states to others is limited.

BRAIN FUNCTION AND FUNCTIONAL SYSTEMS

The brain is comprised of a left and a right hemisphere, and most parts of the brain come in twos: two amygdalae, two hippocampi, etc. This is to be kept in mind in the discussion below, in which we refer to these parts in the singular (e.g., "the amygdala") when describing their function. Despite their essential structural symmetry, we now understand that the two hemispheres diverge considerably with respect to their primary functions. The left side of the brain generally controls conscious, cognitive, and verbal mental states while the right side has the lead role with regard to emotion and non-verbal cues, mostly below the level of consciousness. In the simplest (and unavoidably over-simplified) terms, the left brain deals primarily with words and thoughts, the right brain with form and feelings. Evidence of the right brain's involvement in emotion processing, and the discovery that this part of the brain becomes operational earlier in a child's development than many left hemispheric language and reasoning functions, has fueled a major shift in the focus of psychotherapy from left to right brain processes (Schore & Schore, 2014; Schore, 2021) Although the two halves of the brain are specialized, optimal brain functioning requires integration through communication between that the left and right hemispheres of the brain. The corpus callosum, a thick bundle of neural fibers that connects the two hemispheres, is the structural foundation for the flow of information between the two halves of the brain. As the brain matures, the corpus callosum becomes increasingly efficient, allowing for a more fluid integration of the two hemispheres.

The brain can be further divided by visible tissue markers, functional boundaries, or a combination of the two. Many systems for subdividing the brain have been proposed, and each of them is useful within particular contexts. Some of these systems, for example, the limbic system, are more widely accepted within the field of neuroscience than others of more recent origin. These newer systems, for example, the social engagement system (Porges, 2011) and the primal emotional systems (Panksepp & Biven, 2012) are essentially models about the operation of various complex brain functions that as we noted previously, involve multiple regions of the brain acting in concert.

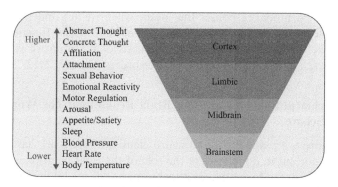

Figure 3.2. Functions of the Brain Regions.
Source: Kosminsky, 2023.

The Limbic System

The limbic system is a group of structures in the brain that play a major role in our experience of emotions, particularly the management of distressing emotions such as anger, fear, separation distress, and shame (Cozolino, 2014). The limbic system is usually described as including the prefrontal cortex, which along with the amygdala and hippocampus is crucial to the process of creating meaning and emotion. The major functions of these structures are summarized in the table below.

Major Functions of the Limbic System

Amygdala: The amygdala is composed of two almond shaped masses, one on either side of the thalamus. Often referred to as the brain's "fear hub", the amygdala activates the brain's fight or flight response and is also involved in emotions and memory.

Hippocampus: Involved in creating and filing new memories. If the hippocampus is damaged a person cannot build or store new memories.

Prefrontal Cortex: Closely linked to the limbic system, the prefrontal cortex appears to be involved in thinking about the future, making plans, and taking action.

Given its involvement in emotional processing and the interpretation of interpersonal cues, the limbic system is a key player in the attachment system. The limbic system is what we rely on to interpret the facial expressions, moods, and intentions of other people. The signals we receive from this area of the brain are crucial for making us aware of danger and triggering an appropriate, self-protective behavioral response (Braun, 2011; Rigon et al., 2016). The limbic system is also tightly linked to the autonomic nervous system and, via the hypothalamus, regulates certain endocrine functions, such as the hormonal responses that occur when we are under stress. The central role of the limbic system in emotional and social functioning has made it the focus of research into the genesis of maladaptive patterns of development and the etiology of mental disorders (Schore, 2012, 2021).

The Attachment System and Right Brain Regulation: The Work of Allan Schore

Allan Schore is a psychiatrist and neuroscientist whose work has been singularly important in documenting the role of the right hemisphere and the limbic system in the formation of attachment bonds in childhood. As Allan and Judith Schore have reported (Schore, 2012, 2013, 2021; Schore & Schore, 2008, 2014), research has substantiated the role of the right brain in affect regulation, and has also demonstrated how right brain development is affected by the quality of early care. In the best case, the process of dyadic, mutual regulation between child and caregivers fuels positive emotions, promotes mutual understanding, and fosters psychological intimacy, all elements of what Bowlby defined as a secure base (Bowlby, 2008). The child comes to depend on the parent as a source of comfort and safety; that is, he develops an internal model of the caregiver as responsive and protective, and a positive image of themselves as worthy of affection and protection from their caregiver(s). Thus supported, the child gradually develops an independent capacity for self-regulation (Schore, 1994, 1996, 2021).

Like Bowlby, Schore emphasizes the positive impact of a secure bond, and the influence of quality of caring on identity formation, emotional functioning, and ultimately, on the ability to establish and maintain healthy relationships with others. Schore has also brought attention to the physiological consequences of early caregiving, and the advantages of moderate stress. Life itself is unavoidably stressful. Episodic exposure to manageable levels of stress, accompanied by responsive caregiving from engaged and loving attachment figures, not only teaches the child that difficult feelings can be managed, it also enhances that capacity by stimulating the development of a healthy and stress resistant brain (Schore, 2009). For example, moderate stress increases the production of myelin, an insulator that enhances communication efficiency between neurons, in the orbitofrontal cortex, a region of the brain that controls arousal regulation and resilience (Katz et al., 2009). While studies support the benefits of moderate stress, there is substantial evidence of the harmful impact of excessive stress, the kind to which infants are exposed in situations involving neglect, abuse, and trauma (Herzog & Schmah, 2018; Hanson & Nacewicz, 2021; Shonkoff et al., 2021).

Recurrent traumatizing interactions between caregiver and child (including traumatizing separations in which the caregiver is unavailable when they are needed by the child) leave the child's stress response system (primarily the sympathetic nervous system and HPA axis response) in a persistent state of hyper-activation. When this state persists over time, there is, in effect, a system overload, and the hyper-aroused state gives way to a hypo-aroused state, reflected in low energy and flattened affect. This "shutdown and withdraw" behavior is what mammals engage in when they are trapped in a threatening or stressful situation from which they cannot escape (Porges, 2011). Psychologically, this shut down involves defensive dissociation to protect the person from a deeply distressing affective arousal that cannot be externally controlled. Schore maintains that this dissociative response, which he calls the "bottom line defense" (Schore, 2012, p. 60), is the foundation of most forms of severe psychopathology.

Schore is one of several researchers whose contributions to the field of affective neuroscience cross disciplinary lines, bringing together biology, psychology, and physiology. Another contributor is Stephen Porges (2009, 2011, 2021) whose work has provided a compelling explanation of how humans evolved a capacity for social engagement and how that capacity is impacted by early relational experience.

The Social Engagement System and Polyvagal Theory: The Work of Stephen Porges

Porges' Polyvagal Theory refers to the vagus nerve, the tenth cranial nerve. The vagus nerve plays a crucial role in regulating activation and deactivation within the central nervous system, which is composed of the brain, spinal column, and 12 cranial nerves (Figure 3.3).

The rest of the nervous system is known as the peripheral nervous system and is classically divided into the somatic or voluntary nervous system and the autonomic or involuntary nervous system. Note that the "voluntary" vs. "involuntary" divide is arguably less clear than it was once, since it has been demonstrated that people can be taught, through techniques like biofeedback or meditation, to regulate brain/body functions which were previously seen as involuntary (Baumann et al., 2011). The autonomic nervous system has two branches: the sympathetic nervous system (SNS), which activates the "fight or flight" response, and the parasympathetic

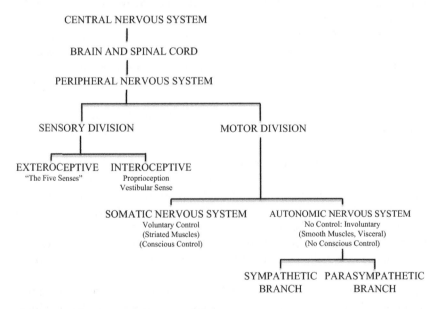

Figure 3.3. The Central Nervous System.
Source: Montgomery, 2013. Used by permission of W.W. Norton & Company, Inc.

nervous system (PNS), which inhibits this arousal and triggers the "rest and digest" response. The vagus nerve has a central role in regulating the balance between the sympathetic and parasympathetic systems. It also links the brain to other key organs, including the heart, brain, lungs, throat, and digestive system.

Of particular interest here is the fact that the vagal system is centrally involved in our response to threat. This system, shared by all mammals, originally evolved to allow an organism to respond to predators. Although most people in the developed world no longer have to deal with life-threatening encounters with predators, this system continues to serve us (and potentially cause problems for us) whenever we are faced with a challenge or danger of any kind. This includes both physical and psychological threats, such as the threat inherent in the loss of a loved one to whom we are attached, or towards whom we feel caregiving responsibilities.

When we are faced with a sufficient amount of perceived threat, the SNS is activated, and our bodies prepare to attack the threat, or to flee from it. For example, blood is shunted from the digestive organs to large muscles in the arms and legs, so that we can make a more effective attack or a faster escape. When threat is present but neither fight nor flight will work, a third option is the "freeze" response. In its most primitive (and phylogenetically oldest) form, the freeze response involves feigning death so as to "trick" the predator into leaving us alone, and instead pursuing "live" prey. It is illuminating to realize that all of these responses have corresponding subjective feelings associated with them. Thus, "fight" is usually associated with angry, hostile feelings, and the desire to attack physically or verbally. "Flight" is associated with anxiety, fear, and a desire to hide or run-away. "Freeze" is connected with psychological dissociation and numbness, as described above (Montgomery, 2013; Schore, 2012). Lastly, recent theorizing about the trauma responses of " fight, flight, or freeze" has also included a fourth trauma response of "fawning". This can be thought of as a "submission" response that involves pacifying and soothing the attacker and signaling that the animal being attacked is unlikely to fight back. This fawning response can have the effect of "switching off" the aggressive response of the predator (Walker, 2018).

As Porges explains, the vagal system in humans evolved to allow for two different approaches to deactivation, or down-regulation of the sympathetic nervous system. These two vagal circuits, one "old" and one "new", correspond to the dorsal and ventral portions of the vagus nerve respectively. This differentiation of the vagal system provides for a more nuanced response from our peripheral nervous system to perceived threat in the environment - what is in effect a middle ground between SNS activation (all out fight or flight) and PNS activation (which leads to passive shut-down and withdrawal). Rather than running away, fighting, or becoming immobilized (what Porges calls "immobilization with fear") we have the ability to stay present when threatened by something without attacking or shutting down. Porges suggests that this *ability to stay put without shutting down is essential for social engagement.* The dorsal vagal circuit, which is not myelinated and which we share with more primitive species (e.g., reptiles), is involved with adaptive reactions characterized by immobilization and decreases in arousal and metabolic output (the "freeze" response of a mouse trapped in the mouth of a cat). In contrast, the myelinated ventral circuit down-regulates activation of the SNS. Thus, the newer ventral circuit is involved in producing the calm but alert state that allows for social engagement by balancing sympathetic and parasympathetic activation. Porges introduces the term "vagal tone" to identify this capacity to modulate our response to threat (particularly interpersonal threat) and to respond in a nuanced, rather than blunt manner to the threat or the safety of our social environment (Porges, 2009, 2021).

How does our nervous system "know" whether or not we are safe? According to Porges, we make this determination based on cues received through *neuroception,* "a neural process that is distinct from perception and that is capable of distinguishing environmental features and visceral reactions that are safe, dangerous, or life threatening" (Porges, 2009, p. 45). Foremost among these cues are the signals read from another person's non-verbal behavior, such as facial expressions and tone of voice. This explains why Porges calls this sophisticated vagal circuit the "social engagement system". This system also provides us with feedback about our own, internal physiological state, particularly our heart rate, lung functioning, and digestive processes. Neuroceptive cues from the body are implicitly or unconsciously processed by the brain and result in the "gut feeling" we have about their relative emotional safety or threat when we meet someone new or who, in the past, has represented a threat.

We can link these ideas to attachment theory by noting that our earliest experiences serve as the basis for our learned ability to interpret all manner of interpersonal signals, including information about safety vs. danger (including social acceptance vs. rejection and curiosity/exploration vs. fear/ avoidance). Put differently, our earliest experiences shape our vagal tone, which is also likely related to our evolved attachment styles and strategies. We have all worked with, or known, people who have overactive "threat detectors". These people are hyper-vigilant for and reactive to the smallest sign of interpersonal rejection and see danger in every social situation. This is often an indication of early relational trauma (van der Kolk, 2014). According to Porges, the persistent or frequent experience of too much stimulation (hyperarousal) or too much inhibition (hypo-arousal or dissociation) that results from abuse or neglect in early life sets our vagal tone, compromises the brain/ body communication system, leads to faulty neuroception, and has an overall negative effect on social and emotional functioning in adult life.

Let us summarize the contributions of Porges's model. The peripheral nervous system is classically divided into the voluntary somatic nervous system and the involuntary autonomic nervous system, which is further divided into the sympathetic and parasympathetic branches. The sympathetic system excites, triggering the "fight or flight" response, while the parasympathetic system inhibits, triggering the "rest and digest" (or in extreme form, the freeze) response. Ideally, these two systems operate to maintain a state of balanced physiological arousal. Porges proposed that this balanced state of arousal can be disrupted, with the result being either too much excitement (hyperarousal) or too much inhibition (hypo-arousal or dissociation). *If this state of imbalance persists or occurs frequently, as in the case of early relational trauma, the normative interplay of the two branches may be compromised* (Porges, 2011). The significance of Porges' theory as it relates to grief therapy will become clear below in the chapters to follow, where we will elaborate on the neurobiology of the stress response (Chapter 6), and the role of grief therapy in helping the bereaved person return to a regulated state (Chapters 7–10).

THE IMPACT OF EARLY CAREGIVING ON BRAIN DEVELOPMENT

"Parenting" Feldman proposes "is the process most critically implicated in the survival and continuity of life on Earth" (Feldman, 2015b, p. 387) could argue this point, but let's take it at face value for a moment and consider that what Feldman is getting at here is that parents are the chief architects of their children's brains in the first years of life, and as such play a unique role in determining what kinds of people end up populating the planet. What is clear is that although the brain is functional upon birth, its full potential for growth is only realized when we come into contact with other people. It is not only that people need other people, but that brains need other brains, to survive and flourish (Trevarthen, 1993; Schore, 2016). Co-construction of the infant brain involves a process of co-regulation that is actuated through what Feldman describes as *biobehavioral synchrony*, an attunement between parent and child that is the "neural substrate of what Ainsworth described as maternal sensitivity" (Holmes & Slade, 2018).

Similarly, Atzil et al. (2018) describe humans as "social animals" who "cannot survive alone and rely on members from their group to regulate their ongoing physiology (or allostasis")" (p. 624). Like other social animals, we are not born with "social brains" but rather, must "grow" the neurological networks that equip us to become social, a developmental sequence that depends on attuned parental care. Lack of support in the first years of life inhibits growth of the social brain and can lead to an accumulation of psychological stress sometimes referred to as "allostatic load". This term, first coined by McEwan & Stellar (1993) has been defined by Siegel as the "current sum of stresses experienced by an individual" (Siegel, 2020). In sum, child development is optimized through the provision of care that meets the child's allostatic needs and supports development of the social brain which, Atzil et al. conclude, "is at the basis of every human's wellbeing" (Atzil et al., p. 633).

Development in the First Year

While brain development continues throughout life, the first year after birth is a *critical period* with respect to the development of the right brain, and consequently, a critical period with respect to the development of affect regulation and attachment (McEwen &Akil, 2020). For optimal functioning, the neural networks involved in balancing emotional arousal, and particularly the management of negative affect, need to develop and integrate, and the first year after birth is the critical beginning of this process. Optimal affect regulation, in turn, promotes neurological (and psychological) growth (Cozolino, 2010, 2014; Siegel, 2012a). In other words, brain development supports the development of affect regulation, the capacity for which then allows for further cortical development. As affect regulation increases, the growing child gradually comes to rely more on their own capacity for internal modulation of emotion, and less on external regulation from their caregiver – a process that is central to physical, emotional, psychological maturation and differentiation.

Arousal that disrupts this balancing act between the sympathetic and parasympathetic systems is necessary for an infant to learn to regulate his or her affect – in a sense, a child needs "practice sessions" to learn how to handle emotional distress. However, it is essential that the infant's growing brain not be subjected to an overload of emotional arousal, particularly negative stimulation, since stress results in an internal biochemical environment (reduced levels of endorphins and dopamine and increased stress hormones) that inhibits brain development and learning (Schore, 2001, McEwen & Akil, 2020) . Early chronic exposure to negative emotional arousal (primarily fear or separation distress) can affect neurological development, influencing psychological functioning throughout the rest of life (McEwan & Akil, 2020). These changes have been linked to the development of many psychiatric disorders in adulthood (Lanius et al., 2010; Shonkoff et al., 2021). To summarize, repeated experiences of moderate, *regulated* arousal stimulate the development of neural circuits that support an increased capacity for emotion regulation. In Part III, we will return to this principle of titrated emotional arousal, which is also central to the skillful conduct of psychotherapy, including grief therapy.

Development in the Second Year

During the second year of life, a growth spurt in the left hemisphere is announced by the emergence of language skills and increased locomotion.

More than ever, the child is able to move about and interact with her environment. Given the extravagant growth in neural integration occurring during this time, the quality of care the infant receives is critical, not only for the infant's physical and emotional health, but also for the child's long-term development and functioning. The development of budding language skills, the ability to interact with peers and teachers – these and other rudimentary abilities are coming online, establishing a foundation for neurological and personality development to come. Research over the last three decades has demonstrated that development in any or all of these areas can be compromised not only by outright abuse, but also by a lack of responsive and attuned nurturing (Trevarthen, 2009; Cozolino, 2017). More severe adverse early childhood experiences produce an increased vulnerability to psychiatric disorders in adulthood (Siegel, 2020). It seems reasonable to suppose that this vulnerability might extend to development of complicated grief after the loss of an attachment figure in adulthood. This possibility will be further explored in Chapter 4.

THE ROLE OF ATTACHMENT IN BRAIN DEVELOPMENT: EMPATHIC ATTUNEMENT, NEURAL INTEGRATION, AND AFFECT REGULATION

Motherhood, as many women have long suspected, changes the brain. The release of oxytocin and other endogenous brain chemicals increase the mother's sensitivity to her infant's emotions and affect her behavior, including how she looks at her infant and her tone of her voice (Ammaniti & Gallese, 2014).

These features of maternal caregiving in turn have an impact on development of the infant's brain. In discussing the fundamentals of attachment theory, writers often observe that human beings are predisposed in mind and body to connect to other humans. In describing the behavior of neurons, Cozolino explains that they are similarly predisposed to connect to one another: "Just as we survive and thrive through our relationships with others, neurons survive and grow as a function of how 'well connected' they are" (Cozolino, 2010, p. 67). When these connections are used, neurons synthesize new proteins that strengthen them – a process cogently captured in the well-known phrase "neurons that fire together wire together" (Keyser & Perrett, 2004, p. 504).

In the first few years of life, much of how this process unfolds depends on non-verbal, "right brain to right brain" communication between child and caregiver (Schore, 2003b, 2009, 2020). A critical element of this process is the mother's capacity to empathically attune to the infant's inner state, and to convey this attunement to the infant through her actions through non-verbal communication and eventually through spoken words. Repeated experiences of "empathic accuracy" give the child the experience of "feeling felt" (Siegel, 2010, p. 11). This caretaking ability, part of what Siegel refers to as "mindsight" (Siegel, 2010) also actively fosters mentalizing capacity in the growing child (Fonagy et al., 2014).

A related concept, coming from psychodynamic psychotherapy, is the "intersubjective field", which is created through the synchronization of two embodied minds into one transactional therapeutic field during the course of psychotherapy (Ammaniti & Gallese, 2014), which can also be applied to the connection between caregiver and child. Attunement promotes empathy by providing the caregiver with a felt sense of the child's thoughts and emotions, which in turn enhances the caregiver's sensitivity and responsiveness. The net effect of consistent and responsive caregiving is a strengthening of the attachment bond. As elaborated in Part III, relational attunement is also the foundation of effective grief therapy.

Mirror Neurons: What are they, and what do they do?

Mirror neurons were first described by researchers conducting studies of monkeys, who noticed incidentally that when they (the researchers) performed certain actions (picking up a peanut; putting the peanut in their mouth), parts of the monkeys' brains lit up that were the same as the regions of their brain that were engaged when the monkey itself was picking up or eating the peanut (Rizzolatti et al., 1996). This discovery was received with considerable excitement in the scientific community and led to a number of theories about the role of mirror neurons in communication, learning, social interaction, and empathy. Others in the scientific community have reported on research results that do not support these claims (Hickok, 2014; Albertini et al., 2021).

Daniel Siegel has consistently argued in favor of the existence of mirror neurons, the discovery of which "gives us a window into the profoundly social nature of our nervous systems" (2020, p. 251). Acknowledging the controversy that has been generated by this discovery, what is clear is that "a human's brain is able to detect the internal states of others and to alter both behavior and the human's own internal state in response."

> How we come to know who we are is shaped by the communication we've had with others. If that communication has been filled with confusion and unpredictable actions - or filled with hostile intention - than our internal sense of a coherent inner self will be compromised. In contrast, being around caregivers early in life who are attuned to our young internal worlds in a reliable way will provide us with the mirror experiences that enable us to have a coherent and flexible sense of both our inner and interpersonal selves in the world. This coherence nay be the integrative heart of a resilient mind.
>
> (Siegel, 2020, p. 252)

Positive attuned caregiving and secure attachment

Before discussing the quality of caregiving and its impact on brain development in greater detail, a comment is in order regarding our emphasis on maternal care. This emphasis reflects the fact that most attachment research has focused on the bond between mothers and infants. Researchers have reported that fathers also undergo neurological and hormonal changes when they are involved in care giving (Grossmann et al., 2005; Swain et al., 2014). Based on an analysis of MRI data, Swain and his colleagues reported that these changes, which begin to appear about four months after the birth of the child, are more pronounced in fathers who stay home to care for their children (Swain et al., 2007). Attention to the nature and impact of the paternal/child bond has increased over the past 15 years, as has the share of fathers caring for children at home (Livingston, 2018). Longitudinal parenting studies have found that paternal involvement from the prenatal stage through a child's lifetime benefits the psychosocial and behavioral development of their children, often in ways different from and complementary to maternal involvement (Yogman & Garfield 2016). Other research has focused on the biological and epigenetic influence of fathers on their children identified differences in the biological mechanisms of male vs. female caregivers (Rajhans et al., 2019).

As Schore and other researchers have reported, attuned interactions between caregiver and child trigger the release of endogenous opioids that have an important role in sculpting the developing architecture of the infant's brain and producing subjective feelings of pleasure and well-being in both parent and child (Martínez-García et al., 2022; Schore, 2019). One of these endogenous opioids is oxytocin, a hormone and neurotransmitter that induces a sense of well-being. When a mother holds and comforts her child, oxytocin is released in both the infant and the mother, producing pleasurable sensations that promote further contact, which releases more oxytocin, and so on. And since neurons that fire together wire together, the result is the growth of areas of the brain associated with social recognition and bonding. At the same time, the experience of responsive maternal care and the resulting neuronal growth lay the foundation for internal working models that contribute to attachment security.

Drawing on the attachment literature and neuroscience studies of social cognitive development, Fitter et al. (2022) examined the link between mothers' attachment representations and neural development in children. In evaluating mother's attachment representations, the researchers assessed the role of the mother's "secure base script'. "Secure base script knowledge" refers to the extent to which individuals' internal model of attachment is organized around, a sense of security, based on what they have experienced, and reflected in how they interact with their own children. "The secure base script – like cognitive scripts more generally - has been claimed to be acquired through repeated experiences of a similar kind, in this case secure base support and sensitive care from primary caregivers and other attachment figures" (Waters et al., 2017, p. 185).

The study included 52 mothers whose attachment were assessed with the Attachment Script Assessment (Mikulincer et al., 2009) and the Experiences in Close Relationships scale. Assessment of the mother's 'secure base script" knowledge refers to the hypothesis involved an assessment of the relationship between "Secure base script Mothers' secure base script knowledge was significantly related to children's smaller left amygdala volume and also a significant influence on the mother's capacity to co-regulate the emotions of her child. Based on these results the researchers "cautiously suggest that mothers' secure base script knowledge is a more relevant attachment representation than attachment style for predicting brain structure in early childhood (Fitter et al., 2020, p. 13).

ABUSE OR NEGLECT: THE NEUROBIOLOGY OF INSECURE ATTACHMENT, AND VULNERABILITY TO STRESS

Decades of research devoted to understanding the impact of early adverse experience on brain development, structure and functioning have identified a range of factors linked to neurological deficits that manifest in a range of psychological symptoms (Davis et al., 2018; Herzog & Schmahl, 2018; Schore, 2003b, 2011, 2012a, 2019b). These symptoms include delayed cognitive development (Teicher et al., 2016); emotion regulatory deficits (Hanson & Nacewicz 2021); and difficulty coping with stress (Holmes & Slade, 2018). Schore (2001) emphasizes the "cumulative nature" of stress related to ongoing relational trauma:

> Because attachment status is the product of the infant's genetically encoded psychobiological predisposition and the caregiver experience, and attachment mechanisms are expressed throughout later stages of life, early relational trauma has both immediate and long-term effects.
>
> (Schore, 2001, p. 206)

A word about terminology in what follows is in order. Adverse early experiences have been described under a number of different umbrella terms, including as "early life stress" "child trauma," "early relational trauma" "toxic stress," "early life adversity "(also referred to as ELA) and "adverse childhood experiences (also referred to as ACEs)". Early Life Adversity is assessed with a variety of measures, one of which is the ACESs Questionnaire. The ACEs Questionnaire (Felitti et al., 1998) is a ten-item measure which assesses ten types of childhood trauma identified by the ACEs study conducted by the Centers for Disease Control and Prevention (Nelson & Gabard-Durnam, 2020).

Much of the research on the neurological impact of early relational experience has focused on the impact of maternal caregiving on the development of emotional circuitry and cortical functioning and on the release of hormones, especially oxytocin. Some studies have looked at the brain as a whole, but particular attention has been directed to the brain region that includes the amygdala and the hypothalamic pituitary axis (HPA). Hanson and Nacewicz observe that the basic functions of this region make it a "strong candidate for understanding the multiple mental health issues common after Early Life Adversity (ELA)". However, in contrast to the consistency of findings concerning the impact of attuned caregiving and secure attachment, reports of the adverse effects of adverse early experience are markedly inconsistent, with reports of larger, smaller, and no differences in the effect of suboptimal care on differences in regional volumes of this area of the brain (Hanson & Nacewicz, 2021). To resolve these inconsistencies in research findings Hanson and Nacewicz propose an "integrative model of stress neuro-development grounded in 'allostatic load', the clinical usefulness of which is suggested in the case example presented later in this chapter. Examples of findings relating early stress to developmental abnormalities are presented in Table 3.1.

Table 3.1 Effects of Maltreatment on Brain Structure and Activity

Researcher(s)	Findings	Developmental Deficit(s)
Shonkoff (2012)	Reduced volume in grey matter in the hippocampus can limit the hippocampus's capacity to bring cortisol levels back to normal after stress events	Impaired affect regulation
Teicher et al. (2012)	Reduced grey matter in the left hippocampus	Impaired executive functioning and affect regulation
Gorka et al. (2014)	Reduced gray matter in the medial prefrontal cortex and left hippocampus.	Impaired affect regulation, increased trait anxiety in adulthood
Teicher et al. (2016)	Abnormal development of affect sensory systems, network architecture and circuits involved in threat detection, emotional regulation and reward anticipation.	Impaired affect regulation, overactive (?) stress detection

(Continued)

Table 3.1 (Continued)

Researcher(s)	Findings	Developmental Deficit(s)
Herzog & Schmahl (2018)	ACE and ACE related disorders are associated with enduring effects on the structure and function of neural stress-regulatory circuits such as for example the hippocampus, the amygdala or the Anterior Cingulate Cortex (ACC)	Increased stress sensitivity and impaired emotion regulation
Hanson & Nacewicz (2021)	Grey matter abnormalities in the amygdala	Impaired affect regulation, enhanced or diminished fear activation

NEURODEVELOPMENTAL EFFECTS OF VARIOUS FORMS OF EARLY TRAUMA

Other reviewers of research concerning the specific effects of maltreatment on brain development and functioning have also commented on the divergence of findings. These reviewers have emphasized the need for greater consistency in definitions of key concepts and research methods employed (Teicher et al., 2020). Despite the divergence in findings, Hanson and Nacewicz conclude that taken as a whole, "these different bodies of research underscore the amygdala as central to emotion, with aberrant structure and activity in multiple forms of psychopathology" (Hanson & Nacewicz, 2021).

In his account of the impact of early adversity on brain development, Cozolino describes a range of problems, including deficits in affect regulation, relational difficulties, and a fragmented sense of self (Cozolino, 2017). Many of these problems involve the interaction of the amygdala, which has a central role in emotional processing (particularly of fear or threat-inducing stimuli) and somatic organization of experience, and the hippocampus, which is vital for logical thought and discrimination. The amygdala is specialized to identify specific areas of the environment, particularly those which pose a threat; the hippocampus inhibits responses. In this sense

> the amygdala is involved with generalization, while the hippocampus is involved with discrimination ... In other words, the amygdala will make us jump at the sight of a spider, while the hippocampus will help us to remember that this particular spider is not poisonous, so we shouldn't worry.
>
> (Cozolino, 2017, p. 85)

Applying this metaphor to human interaction, an individual with an early abandonment experience, for example "reacts to the perception of abandonment when little or none exists in reality" (p. 85). This response is an indication that the amygdala has assumed a dominant role in directing memory, emotion, and behavior, and suggests underdevelopment of the hippocampus which, being late to develop and establish connectivity with the cortex, is subject to prolonged sensitivity to developmental disruption and trauma. Although it can occur at any time in life, damage to the hippocampus is a particular threat during the critical period of development in infancy (Cisneros-Franco et al., 2020).

Taking a different approach to understanding how early adverse experience affects health and development throughout the lifespan, Neves, Dinis-Oliveira and Magalhães (2021) propose that abuse may alter the "genetic predisposition of the cellular response to the environment" with resulting "changes in the regulation of multiple organ systems" (p. 103). Based on their meta-analysis of findings from 28 studies, they report that adverse childhood experiences appear to be associated with genetic changes that have long term physiological and psychological effects. They conclude that these changes in specific gene sites "appear to be involved in the development of psychiatric illness in adulthood" (p. 103).

Clinical observations align with scientific neurobiological research concerning the long-term impact of adverse early life experience and other environmental stressors on brain development in infancy (Lanius et al., 2010; Shonkoff et al., 2021). The persistent effects of chronic childhood stress are evident in this comment from a client, now in his forties, as he attempts to describe to the therapist (PK) the insecurity and fear he experienced as a child.

Vince

My mother wasn't just an alcoholic, she was a rageaholic. When you're a kid and your mother is a really scary person, you just freeze ... I realize that I'm still that way, I realize I still do that.

Another client describes her relationship with her father as a 25-year ordeal. Six years after his death, he remains an unwelcome presence in her life.

Margaret

I can remember being eight and thinking that all I wanted to do was to disappear. I would think: I'm nothing to my father but something to be used. But the worst part was knowing I wouldn't get it right and the fear that he was going to hurt me. That feeling is still so deep in my gut, that I'm going to get hurt. My sister says it's like he's still hurting us from the grave.

We should not be surprised to find that many people who have difficulty coping with loss did not have the kind of attuned caregiving that supports the development of a child's capacity to understand their emotions, reflect on what they are feeling, and reregulate from a state of distress. Gunnar (2017) explains these negative effects in terms of an absence of "social buffering" of the hypothalamic-pituitary-adrenocortical (HPA) system during critical periods of neurological development. Drawing on attachment theory, Gunnar argues that infant's experience of stress and arousal regulation "lays the foundation out of which individual differences in the capacity to gain stress relief from social partners emerges."

Neuronal Pruning

Another way of understanding how adverse early experience compromises function is through the process of "neuronal pruning" (Cozolino, 2010, p. 67). As we have said, neurons must be connected to one another to survive. Neurons that are not wired to other neurons lose their inactive branches or die completely. In the absence of opportunities to be reregulated with the help of the mother's mature nervous system, the neural networks that would build self-regulatory capacity in the infant's brain are not activated, do not connect with other neurons, and fail to develop. This means that important opportunities for learning are lost, critical areas of the brain do not develop, incentives for bonding are diminished, and what could be a process of expanding social engagement and growth is short circuited. The negative effects of neural pruning are not limited to severe mistreatment. In fact, severe neglect may result in even greater harm:

> When a child is physically abused the brain is challenged to adapt, which stimulates growth and connectivity. But with extreme neglect, the result is neural atrophy...Victims of severe neglect consistently show ongoing deficits in sensory, cognitive and social functioning.
>
> (Cozolino, 2017)

It has become increasingly clear that the effects of early trauma are the most damaging and difficult to undo, a finding that is not unexpected given the vulnerability of young children and their immature neurological development. Early relational trauma is a "double whammy" of painful experience and impaired capacity to regulate the emotions elicited by those experiences. Schore, van der Kolk, and others have described the impact of chronic deprivation of contingent, attuned care on neurological development, and the tendency toward dissociative states that is observed in many children subjected to these conditions (Hart & Rubia, 2012; Luecken, 2008; Schore, 2003a; Solomon & Heide, 2005; Van der Hart et al., 2006;

Van der Kolk, 2015). When a child feels unsettled, she looks to her caregivers for comfort and reassurance. If she cannot manage her response to this expressed need, then instead of providing comfort, the parent may become angry or rejecting. This response from the caregiver leads first to hyper-arousal in the child. That is, the child initially tries harder to get her parent's attention. During this phase, the child's heart rate, blood pressure, and respiration all speed up. If the needed response is repeatedly not elicited, however, the child will eventually enter a state of psychological hopelessness and neurological hypoarousal or down regulation, at which point a second cascade of internal events will be triggered. In this phase, the child appears to shut down or freeze, almost as though she is trying to avoid attention and become "unseen". This is viewed as a strategy of last resort, employed when the child feels terrified and helpless, and can only hope to survive by avoiding notice. As previously discussed, this pattern of freezing and psychological numbing when confronted with distressing feelings can become a lifelong strategy for managing unbearable affect. As an adult, such an individual is more likely to freeze, shut down, and dissociate when confronted by painful feelings. Dissociation becomes the *primary way a person learns to regulate their emotion,* or as Schore concludes, in these cases the "dissociative metabolic shutdown state is a primary regulatory process used throughout the lifespan" (Schore, 2009, p. 120). This, in turn, lays the foundation of many young adult and adult psychiatric disorders that involve difficulty with affect management and a maladaptive coping style that centers on dissoci-ation as a psycho-biological defense (Schore, 2003a).

Marta

Marta, 42, has come for therapy following the death of her father. She cannot remember much of her childhood. When the therapist gently asks a series of questions about what her family was like when she was growing up, Marta becomes quiet and her gaze drifts over the therapist's shoulder to the opposite wall. Within moments she has dissociated, and it takes several minutes to reestablish contact with her. Even then, she appears stunned, avoids eye contact, and is unable to speak.

No matter how attuned and compassionate the therapist is, recalling early abuse is painful and frightening. *Given that grief is also painful and frigh-tening, it is not surprising that bereaved clients who have experienced early abuse, neglect, or loss may become overwhelmed, emotionally numb, and psychologically dissociated.* This kind of response seems to be related both to a client's limited recall of painful events and his or her limited capacity to tolerate the affective arousal that remembering these events provokes. We now understand that both of these responses are more likely to affect people whose early environment did not support brain development that would facilitate affect regulation, cognitive control, and memory recall.

ADULT DEVELOPMENT AND THE LASTING EFFECTS OF EARLY ATTACHMENT: IS ATTACHMENT ORIENTATION ETCHED ON THE BRAIN?

Investigators have increasingly directed their efforts to answering questions about the specific neural structures and pathways that are impacted and to what extent it is possible to effect change in the adult brain in the service of improved health and functioning.

In related research, investigators have looked into the brain to see if they can identify the neural correlates of secure vs. insecure attachment. Early results, reviewed by Perlini et al. (2019) suggest that different attachment styles correlate with volumetric differences in brain structure and to different patterns of activity during the processing of social and attachment related stimuli. Studies have used a variety of methods but have in particular relied on magnetic resonance imaging (fMRI). In their review of 11 studies conducted between 2008 and 2018, Perlini's group found consistent findings of augmented amygdala response to threatening stimuli in anxiously attached individuals. "The correlation between amygdala hyperactivity and anxious attachment style suggests increased vigilance to emotional stimuli in these individuals" and supports the role of the amygdala in regulation of anxiety and social behavior. "Overall," the authors note "different attachment styles have been correlated with volumetric alterations" and differences in patterns of activation in different brain regions (Perlini et al., 2019, p. 371).

Researchers have also employed mixed methods approaches to study the stability of attachment orientation and its long-term influence on emotional processing. Moutsiana et al. (2014) collected data on infants' attachments to their mothers at 18 months old. In an MRI based study with these subjects 22 years later, the researchers found an association between secure vs. insecure attachment at 18 months and neural processing during regulation of positive affect in young adulthood.

> Specifically, while attempting to up-regulate positive emotions, adults who had been insecurely versus securely attached as infants showed greater activation in prefrontal regions associated with cognitive control" and other responses "consistent with relative inefficiency in the neural regulation of positive affect.
> (Moutsiana et al., 2014, p. 999)

In other words, subjects previously classified as insecure had to make a greater effort to feel positive than the securely attached subjects. These results are among the first to provide empiric support for the proposition that "disturbances in the mother-infant relationship may persistently alter the neural circuitry of emotion regulation" (p. 1001).

The overarching conclusion reached by researchers is that childhood maltreatment and neglect constitute a major risk factor for adult psychopathology (Teicher, Gordon & Nemeroff, 2022). Chronic activation of the stress response system "can result in a brain stuck in a maladaptive state" making it difficult or impossible to recover "even after the source of stress is eliminated or reduced" (Shonkoff et al., 2021, p. 117). Individuals thus affected "may require behavioral and/or pharmacological intervention for later depression or an anxiety disorder" (Shonkoff et al., 2021, p. 117).

Significant loss, it should be noted is not simply a "stressful event" but an ongoing experience. Given that the source of stress in these cases cannot in any meaningful way be "eliminated", the capacity to manage stress is particularly important, and limitations in this capacity are likely to emerge. In introducing interventions, clinicians must be mindful of clients' sensitivity to stress and the potential to overwhelm their regulatory capacity. Approaches that involve a re-experiencing of traumatic events, for example, activate the amygdala and inhibit frontal-hippocampal neural networks that could help put them into context, and can result in a cascade of unmanageable emotion.

SOCIAL FACTORS RELATED TO CHILDHOOD HEALTH AND MALTREATMENT

Research on the negative developmental consequences of childhood stress has increasingly emphasized the impact of socioeconomic and other environmental factors that can undermine the foundations of healthy development, many of them beyond the control of caregivers.

> Potential precipitants include the socioeconomic hardships of poverty and racism; the psychosocial threats of child maltreatment and community violence; the interpersonal challenges of maternal depression and parental addictions; the physiological disruptions of . . . environmental toxins; and the metabolic consequences of poor nutrition.
>
> (Shonkoff et al., 2021, p. 127)

These factors also impact the mental and physical health of parents and their ability to care for their children (Hunter & Flores, 2020). In a review of 33 studies relating to the role of social determinants of health (SDH) in relation to child maltreatment, Hunter & Flores (2020) found that poverty, parental educational attainment, housing instability, food insecurity and lack of insurance were all associated with child maltreatment.

Shonkoff, Slopen, and Williams note that studies of early childhood adversity have largely focused on the implications of early adversity for later educational achievement, and that "most interventions are driven by an enrichment model that focuses on providing enhanced learning

opportunities for young children combined with information on child de
development for their primary caregivers. . .

> Advances in the biology of adversity and resilience point to the need for a
> complementary protection model that focuses on shielding the developing brain
> and other biological systems from the physiological disruption of toxic stress
> that can lead to disparities in both school achievement and lifelong health.
>
> (Shonkoff, Slopen, & Williams, 2021, p. 127)

Another growing area of interest is brain research is *epigenetics,* the
process by which early experiences alter the expression of our genetic code.

> An *epigenetic* modification occurs when chemical 'signatures' attach themselves
> to genes, which, in turn helps determine how the genes are expressed (i.e.,
> whether they are turned on or off).
>
> (Child Welfare Information Gateway, 2023)

Epigenetic change is one of the mechanisms by which our brains adapt to
our environment. These adaptations, while they may be of service in
the short term, may or may not support healthy functioning over time.
Neural pathways that are developed under negative conditions "prepare
children to cope in that negative environment, and their ability to respond
to nurturing and kindness may be impaired (Shonkoff & Phillips,
2000). Hardships linked to poverty and racism are "potent predisposing
factors" for lifelong impairments of physical and mental health (Shonkoff
et al., 2021).

Neuroplasticity and Neurogenesis

Schore (2019, 2021) cites several studies that support his assertions regarding the fundamental contribution of *right brain to right brain communication* between caregiver and infant in neurological development and
in the development of attachment security. Some of this evidence comes
from studies demonstrating that it is the right brain that is most involved in
communication between mothers and infants. This finding is in accord
with what we most often observe in these interactions, namely that both
mothers and infants rely less on words than on a combination of facial
expressions, sounds, and other emotion laden cues that are the domain of
the right brain.

The caregiver's ability to communicate in an empathic, attuned manner to
the infant's bids for attention and care is essential to building a secure orientation to attachment in the child. The flow of brain-to-brain communication is what allows the child to move from dependence on the caregiver for
emotional regulation, to the development of self-regulatory capacity. And

the effects of this flow of communication can be observed not only in the infant's brain, but also in the brain of the mother.

Contrary to what was earlier thought to be the unchanging nature of the brain past a childhood, we now know that the brain continues to morph in structure and capacity throughout the life cycle. Well into adulthood, new neurons grow in areas of the brain involved with learning and memory, including the hippocampus, the amygdala, and the cerebral cortex. Synaptic connections between neurons also increase with age. As in infancy, what promotes continued development in adulthood is a level of arousal that stimulates but does not overwhelm the brain. New learning builds the brain, while excessive stress or trauma inhibits growth and interferes with the integration of experience.

Schore has also expanded his narrative of how the brain changes in psychotherapy, through a right brain to right brain process of communication that supports brain development and builds emotion regulatory capacity. The effectiveness of therapy depends upon this link between therapist and client, and on the willingness of both participants to set aside interpretations and recommendations coming from the left brain, in favor of insights coming from a deeper level of consciousness:

> Neuroscience has legitimized subjectivity in psychology and in therapy. Both science and clinical theory agree that psychotherapy is basically relational and emotional, and so we now think that emotionally and intersubjectively being with the patient is more important than rationally explaining the patient's behavior to himself.
>
> (Schore, 2019, p. 256)

Regarding his view of psychotherapy, and psychiatry in particular, Schore has come to believe that "we've overvalued the analytic mind."

> I now see the change mechanism acting beneath the words – in process more than content. We now have a better idea what this process is about, and how relational interactions literally can change that process and thereby change character structure.
>
> (Schore, 2019, p. 258)

With regard to early relational trauma, Schore emphasizes that it is not just the trauma itself that leads to the "traumatic disposition":

> It's also the lack of repair, and that repair and interactive regulation requires a very personal authentic response on the part of the therapist. Attachment trauma was originally relational, and so the healing must be relational, a mutual process.
>
> (Schore, 2019, p. 268)

"Healing Must Be Relational": A Client's Perspective

"I've been in therapy most of my adult life, with a variety of therapists.

Following my mother's death I was overwhelmed with grief, joined a group that was run by (the first author) and later began seeing her individually. While my mother's death has been a theme throughout my time with Phyllis we've also discussed my work, relationships, etc. I suppose it's all connected.

For a very long time when I first started seeing Phyllis. I hardly looked her in the eye. Her office was small, and I remember being comforted by the fact that I was closer to the door than she was. I'm not sure why. I never felt physically threatened by her but it's something I definitely scoped out.

I'm quite sure that I've now spent more time talking to her about my feelings (or as close to that as I can get) than I have with anyone else in my life. Phyllis. shared some things about herself. . . I feel certain that knowing these things about her allowed me to bond with her in a way that I would not have had she presented herself as a "blank slate".

Realizing where I am at this age makes me sad, but the only consolation is that I have arrived at a point where I can begin to recognize what's lacking. I credit Phyllis with getting me to this place - it must mean that I feel a level of safety that I haven't before, and I'm hoping that it will allow me to bond with others in a way I previously didn't even know existed."

Maturation and Neural Integration

As adults, we generally have more control than we did as children over the circumstances of our lives. As a result, we usually have more ability to directly influence what becomes wired into our brains (Hanson, 2013). Nevertheless, it remains true that much of what happens in life is unpredictable and beyond our control. Certain events, like the kinds of traumatic losses that are discussed in Chapter 6, can disable even the strongest and most resilient among us. Still, we know that some people seem more capable than others of integrating the effects of adverse experience into their identity and moving on with their lives.

We might suppose that these people are among the lucky ones who were raised in a good environment, by caregivers who supported their emotional and physical growth, and to a significant degree, we would be right. But as we have seen, adverse experience early in life is not a definitive predictor of compromised functioning. According to attachment theory, and in line with studies using the Adult Attachment Interview, the effects of early experience, particularly early traumatic experiences, are mediated by the extent to which a person has been able to process and make sense of those experiences (Bakermans-Kranenburg & van IJzendoorn, 2009). If our emotional foundation has been subject to assaults that have not been addressed and repaired, whatever we build on it may be fragile. But if, with the support of others, we have identified and attended to our emotional injuries, and integrated our experiences into a coherent life narrative, then this need not be the case (Cozolino, 2010; Hesse, 2008; Holmes, 2010). Integration has two separate meanings that can both be used in discussions of how experience shapes the brain. In infancy, interaction with an attuned caregiver promotes the development of neural networks and the integration of functional areas of the brain, resulting in increased self-regulatory capacity. Over the course of a person's life, the integration of experience on a neuronal/psychological level occurs when a person has been able to address the experiences rather than dissociate from them, make sense of the feelings, memories, and thoughts associated with those experiences, and ideally grow from them. Sense making allows the individual to integrate his experiences into a larger and more adaptive worldview. In cases of traumatic experiences, integration becomes a more challenging enterprise, since people typically develop unconscious protective stances towards those experiences (i.e., psychological defenses) that serve to dissociate them from the distressing emotional and physiological arousal triggered by the events.

Viewed this way, many of the problems that cause people to seek therapy, including grief therapy, can be understood as a lack of integration. A prominent proponent of this view is Siegel (2012, 2020) who identifies difficulties in emotion regulation, as well as a range of psychiatric symptoms, as related to adverse early experiences of care lacking in attuned communication and interaction.

> We can view these situations as being the inadequate development of a coherent sense of another's mind within the mind of the child. Such interactions are "incoherent," and fail to facilitate the child's own integrative processes. The fundamental outcome of such non-integrative states can be seen as impairment in self-regulation.
>
> (Siegel, 2020, p. 87)

This perspective suggests that the work of psychotherapy is about supporting development of capacities that have not been fully developed. Here Siegel introduces the idea of "mindsight", to describe the ability to perceive the mind of the self and others.

> Mindsight is a kind of focused attention that allows us to see the internal workings of our own minds. It helps us get ourselves off of the autopilot of ingrained behaviors and habitual responses. It lets us "name and tame" the emotions we are experiencing, rather than being overwhelmed by them.
>
> (Siegel, 2011, p. xi)

We note the parallel between the concept of mindsight and that of mentalizing discussed in the previous chapter. Like mentalizing, mindsight is a learnable skill. Siegel takes the further step of identifying the development of mindsight as work that changes the brain.

> When we develop the skill of mindsight, we actually change the physical structure of the brain. This revelation is based on one of the most exciting scientific discoveries of the last twenty years: How we focus our attention shapes the structure of the brain. Neuroscience has also definitively shown that we can grow these new connections throughout our lives, not just in childhood.
>
> (Siegel, 2011, p. xi)

Applying Neuroscience Findings in Clinical Work with the Bereaved

One of the objectives of Hanson & Nacewicz's 2021 review was to assess the relative impact of unpredictability in maternal behavior as a risk factor for compromised neurological development, as compared to the impact of a factor identified in their report as "entrapment", the sense of being powerless to find a way out of a painful environment From Main on, researchers have cited the erratic nature of maternal behavior as a significant factor in the development of insecure attachment and disorganized attachment in particular (Davis et al., 2017; Main & Solomon, 1990). Based on their review of the current state of knowledge in the research literature, Hanson & Nacewicz report that the cumulative effect of feeling trapped, which increases the child's allostatic load, is as much or more of a threat to stress related neurological developmental deficits as unpredictability on the part of the mother.

Having come across this research as she was preparing this chapter, the first author thought to share it with a bereaved spouse who has struggled with unremitting grief. The metaphor of entrapment seemed apt as a description of this client's mental state. As soon as she finished explaining entrapment to her the client burst out with: "That's exactly how I feel! There's no escape!" This opened up a discussion about how for a child, there really is no esc ape. But for this client, the trap – the inescapable pain of grief – was *not something over which she had no control*. There were things she could do to ease her suffering; she knew this.

The explanation and subsequent discussion served as an incentive for the client to continue her efforts to see friends, exercise, and travel. But these activities, she insisted, were really just temporary diversions: they did not give her relief from the pain of her grief. Here, the clinician brought up another concept from neuroscience, this one suggested by Dan Siegel, a researcher whose work was familiar to the client. After first acknowledging the truth that her pain was real, and that no activity would relieve it, the clinician said "You know Dan Siegel, right? Well, he says that where we focus our attention can change our brain. So, when we focus our attention on something other than grief, we're actually doing something that over time helps us suffer less." Here again, the purpose of sharing this insight from neuroscience was to provide the client with a sense of agency and an incentive to take steps toward adaptation to her loss.

The lack of integration can also be understood as a fragmentation or dissociation of the psychological self into different parts (Schore, 2003a; Van der Hart et al., 2006). This brings us back to the quote from Cozolino that opened this chapter. Cozolino asserts that many complaints and symptoms are related to sub-optimal functioning of neural networks that are underdeveloped, under-regulated, over-taxed, or poorly integrated (Cozolino, 2010). "Applying this model" he writes, "therapy is a means of creating or restoring coordination among various neural networks" (p. 24). The therapeutic environment is a *learning environment* designed to *enhance the growth of neurons and the integration of neural networks*.

Cozolino's prescription for a therapeutic environment that supports these goals is worth noting here. As we will see, his recommendations have much in common with what Wallin, Holmes, and others have described as attachment informed approach to psychotherapy (Wallin, 2007; Holmes, 2013). Cozolino cites the following as the characteristics of an environment that enhances neural plasticity, growth and integration in psychotherapy:

- The establishment of a safe and trusting relationship
- Arousal of mild to moderate levels of stress
- Activating both emotion and cognition in the service of integration
- The co-construction of new personal narratives through the encounter between therapist and client.

(Cozolino, 2010, 2017)

In the third edition of *The Neuroscience of Psychotherapy* (2017), Cozolino's explanation of the therapeutic environment and the process of change reflects a revised model of executive functioning. Remember that this model includes:

- the amygdala, a component of the *limbic system* that *detects threat and danger*
- the frontal-parietal network that attends to *monitoring and performing tasks in the outside world*
- the default-mode network (DMN) that is activated *when attention is turned to the self and others*

These systems generally operate one at a time, so that when one is active, the other is inhibited. In addition, there is a "salience network centered in the insula and anterior cingulate cortices that signals the frontal parietal system to become active in situations of novelty and danger, which also serves to inhibit the DMN" (Cozolino, 2017). This insight about the functioning of the executive system, Cozolino explains, helps us understand the fragmentation of self and difficulty in social relationships seen in individuals who have experienced early stress and trauma. Under conditions of sustained stress, the executive network centered in the amygdala activates the salience system and inhibits the default-mode network.

> From an early age, victims of trauma and stress will be more stressed both at rest and when challenged, have overactive salience networks, more active frontal-parietal networks, and inhibited DMNs.
>
> (Cozolino, 2017)

All in all, inhibition of the default mode network deprives the individual of the ability to manage their emotions, maintain a coherent sense of self, and feel compassion for themselves or empathy for others. These findings concerning the consequences of prolonged periods of DMN inhibition, especially early in life, "require separate and specific interventions" that can help restore regulatory function and repair fragmentation in relation to the self and others (Cozolino, 2017).

Cozolino's recommendations in this edition include "meditation, yoga, dance, or any other way they can simultaneously soothe their anxiety and explore all corners of their minds and bodies." These activities, and other interventions proposed by Cozolino to help with emotion regulation and stress management are offered not as a universal prescription, but as options to be considered in developing a treatment plan that moves the client in the direction of balanced, integrated executive functioning.

Porges, in his continuing development of polyvagal theory, has also made substantial contributions to the clinical literature. In *Polyvagal Safety: Attachment Communication, Self-Regulation* (2021), which was written during a period of world-wide illness and death, Porges reminds us

once again of our fundamental need for safety and human connection and
sets out the consequences of the prolonged fear and isolation brought on
by the COVID-19 pandemic. Porges reminds us of the importance of the
body in emotion regulation and offers a collection of the interventions
designed to assist in recovery from painful emotional states grounded in a
view of regulation as a process of internal integration achieved in an environment that offers safety and engagement with others. Therapy, when it
is provided in a way that is attuned and sensitive to the individual client,
can be such an environment.

A study by Kalia & Knauft (2020) offers another finding with clinical
implications. Noting that the chronic stress associated with adverse
childhood experiences "debilitates activity in the prefrontal cortex" the
authors began by investigating whether adult's perceptions of their adverse
childhood experiences mediated the effects of ACEs on cognitive flexibility.
Their initial finding confirmed a relationship between perceived ACEs and
a decrease in cognitive flexibility. However, "stress is a subjective experience" and the researchers hypothesized that effective use of emotion regulation strategies could affect the individual's perception and stress
response. To test this hypothesis the researchers also examined differences
in subjects' emotion regulation strategies and found that that individual
differences in use of emotion regulation strategies

> moderated the influence of ACEs on chronic stress, specifically, habitual use of
> cognitive reappraisal attenuated stress levels whereas habitual use of expressive
> suppression exacerbated stress levels. Overall, our study highlights the impor-
> tance of examining emotion regulation in individuals who have experienced early
> life adversity.
>
> (Kalia & Knauft, 2020)

The significance of this finding with respect to the importance of emotion
regulation as a moderating influence on the effects of early adverse experience is amplified by research demonstrating the role of cognitive
inflexibility in problematic grief, as we will discuss further in the following
chapter.

GOALS OF PSYCHOTHERAPY

When emotions and thoughts cannot be tolerated, the mind finds ways to
circumvent or suppress them, a point elaborated by Vaillant in his classic
work *The Wisdom of the Ego* (Vaillant, 1995). The defensive coping
strategies that are mounted distort reality to varying degrees, but the goal
is always the same: to reduce the painful anxiety that accompanies the
underlying affect. As the research cited throughout this chapter suggests,
once the neural connections that make up these defensive strategies are

wired in, they shape our lives, influencing what we approach and what we avoid. The work of therapy, in this regard, is to help clients become curious about what causes them distress, and in a controlled way, to move toward rather than away from this distress. By bringing up the source of the anxiety in a safe context and by allowing the person to experience the anxiety in a titrated fashion, the person gradually builds up their ability to tolerate the seemingly intolerable, to confront their thoughts and feelings, and ultimately to reexamine and put into perspective the experiences that engendered these feelings. The result is that therapist and client work together to create a narrative of the person's life that is both honest and balanced, at once emotionally resonant and tolerable.

The direct applicability of this perspective to bereavement therapy becomes clear when we consider how frequently clients' narratives of relationships or losses seem to us to be incomplete or distorted. An adult child who cannot understand why they grieve for a parent who abused them; a spouse who cannot let go of the belief that they "should have known" that their husband was going to take his life - these come to mind as examples of narratives that omit or distort factual details, and that fall far short of capturing the complexity of attachment or of grief. Persistent feelings of shame, of weakness, of not being "enough", fear that one doesn't have the resources to survive the death of a loved - these are feelings that complicate grief and that become a focus of bereavement work.

When a person has latched on to a perspective that is unfair or illogical, and which the clinician's efforts (as well as those of family and friends) have done nothing to modify, it is time to give the language based left brain a rest and try a different approach. By attending to the client's facial expressions, posture, and other non-verbal cues, and by identifying the emotional correlates of experience, the therapist can help a client to develop a narrative of the relationship and the loss that is more inclusive, balanced, reality based, and often times, forgiving of self and others. This kind of therapeutic process has much in common with the repeated positive interactions that ideally occur between parents and children, particularly those that take place when a child is upset, and the parent helps them regain emotional balance (Kosminsky, 2014; Cozolino, 2017, Siegel, 2020).

Thus, a consensus is emerging around the proposition that the work of psychotherapy is to change the brain through sustained empathic and directed interaction. The process by which change occurs in the adult brain is both similar to and different from the kind of brain sculpting that occurs in childhood. In both cases, learning is a process of making new neural connections, particularly in areas of the brain that support emotional processing and meaning making. However, while parenting is mostly about construction, psychotherapy is more about reconstruction and revision. Children are at a disadvantage with regard to making sense of experience because their brains are still developing. They do the best they can to process incoming data, but distortions inevitably creep in: they feel responsible for things that are not their fault and draw conclusions about themselves based on the sometimes unfair and harsh words they hear from others. The remnants of these lessons from childhood carry on into adulthood and may constitute much of the material that people end up addressing in therapy.

Whatever childhood fears and feelings linger beneath the surface of an apparently well- functioning adult, they are most likely to emerge when the person is under stress (Van der Hart et al., 2006). Faced with the stress that accompanies significant loss, many people find themselves flooded with memories about old hurts, imagined failures, and fears about their ability to function as adults. Thus, the loss of a significant person is an event that for many people triggers a painful re-experiencing of old and unprocessed hurts, and also one that offers an opportunity for new learning and growth.

REBUILDING THE BRAIN IN WORK WITH THE BEREAVED

When people are afraid, when they have reached a point where they feel they cannot possibly manage one more emotional hurdle, the idea of shutting down or running away can hold great appeal. What grief therapy can provide in these circumstances is the support a person needs to stay put, psychologically speaking, so that they can develop the capacity to tolerate their feelings, make sense of their thoughts, and accommodate to the changed reality of their life. One way of understanding complicated grief is that it represents a breakdown in the processing of information related to the loss (Shear & Shair, 2005). According to this view, such a breakdown occurs when the reality of the loss cannot be tolerated, as in the case of sudden violent death, or when the bereaved was highly dependent on the person who died. Under these circumstances, defenses can be triggered that allow the mourner to delay confrontation with reality, but which can also interfere with the integration of the loss. An important aspect of therapy in these cases is to provide an environment in which the bereaved can learn to tolerate feelings associated with the loss, as well as gain perspective on the meaning of the relationship and its absence for the individual. This occurs through a process of support, skill development, activation and integration of memories, and the co-construction of new personal narratives (Hollinger, 2020; Shear et al., 2011). As with all new learning, this psychological strengthening process is associated with enriched synaptic connections between existing neuronal networks, and even the creation of new neural networks in the brain (Siegel, 2012, 2012b, 2020).

SUMMARY

Neuroscience research in the new millennium has further enhanced our understanding of how the brain develops in early childhood and of how it continues to grow and change throughout life. Research evidence, much of it relying on cutting edge technologies that have enabled researchers to observe the development and functioning of the brain, has contributed to a surge of interest in attachment theory as a framework for understanding how the quality of a child's first bonding experience exerts a continuing influence on psychological and physical well-being. This work has also substantiated the view of therapeutic change proposed by Kandel (2013) and the preeminent importance of the quality of the therapeutic relationship in effecting that change (Norcross, 2018).

A great deal has been learned over the past twenty years about how the brain processes information and the role that temperament and experience play in people's capacity to integrate the situations that they encounter. The investigation of the neurological basis of thought and behavior is in its early stages, but it has already generated findings that help us understand what factors support healthy development, and how development is adversely affected when this support is unavailable or severely deficient.

Reports of the impact of early adverse experience on lifelong mental and physical health have fueled advocacy efforts on behalf of children and families, and have led to a range of intervention efforts, including the expansion of programs designed to help caregivers develop secure attachment relationships with their children. Other investigators have emphasized the need for public health interventions that address environmental stressors related to racism and poverty. In recent years the problem of "food insecurity" has been a talking point in discussions of social and economic inequities impacting families. References to "food insecurity" cannot help but make us aware of the implicit irony of expecting caregivers to instill a sense of security in their children when access to basic resources is uncertain. There is much we have to learn about the brain and how it develops, but we know more than enough to recognize the social imperative of ensuring that all families have access to the material resources that are prerequisites to physical and emotional health.

We humans are a curious lot. We want to understand how things work, ourselves included, and we design progressively more sophisticated operating systems to find answers to progressively more complex questions. The human brain is both the ultimate operating system and the tool we use to understand that system. In the next chapter, we will look at how what we have learned so far about the brain, together with insights from attachment theory, can enrich our understanding of bereavement and the process of healing after loss.

Part II

BEREAVEMENT THROUGH THE LENS OF ATTACHMENT: ADVANCES IN RESEARCH, THEORY AND PRACTICE

Research on the nature and course of grief over the past twenty years has consistently identified people's attachment orientation as a significant factor in their adaptation to loss (Burke & Neimeyer, 2013; Mikulincer and Shaver, 2016; Lopez, 2019). Contemporary models of bereavement draw heavily on attachment theory, particularly Bowlby's views regarding the association between insecure attachment and complications in grief (Mikulincer & Shaver, 2013, 2021). Also in the past two decades, concepts from attachment theory have been integrated into a growing number of models of general psychotherapy practice (Costello, 2013; Danqueth & Berry, 2014; Holmes & Slade, 2018). Much of the literature detailing attachment informed approaches has direct applicability to work with the bereaved, and in Part II, we bring together emerging insights from attachment theory and contemporary models of grief and bereavement. and introduce an attachment informed approach to grief therapy. In Chapter 4, we review contemporary models of bereavement, highlight the ways in which attachment orientation interacts with and expands upon these models, and illustrate the application

DOI: 10.4324/9781003204183-6

of these expanded models in clinical work with the bereaved. The specific contribution of attachment theory to our understanding of loss in different kinship relationships will be examined in Chapter 5, and Chapter 6 will focus on how attachment history and mode of death intersect, with an emphasis on traumatic loss.

4

INSECURE ATTACHMENT AND PROBLEMATIC GRIEF: CONTEMPORARY MODELS AND THEIR IMPLICATIONS FOR PRACTICE

There is a reason that the words "love and loss" are so frequently linked in literature and in writing about bereavement. Love and loss are part of the same experience; in choosing one, we invite the possibility of the other, as Nicholson poignantly observes in his film adaptation of *A Grief Observed* by C. S. Lewis. Love is a risky business, but it's a risk he has chosen to take in loving his wife:

> Why love if losing hurts so much? I have no answers any more ...
>
> Twice in (my) life I've been given the choice: as a boy and as a man.
> The boy chose safety, the man chooses suffering. The pain now is
> part of the happiness then. That's the deal.
>
> Shadowlands, William Nicholson (1993)

Lewis's account of his wife's death expresses what many would consider the inescapable connection between deep love and deep grief. But although someone who has loved deeply may also grieve deeply, one is not a measure

DOI: 10.4324/9781003204183-7

of the other, and there is more to understanding the connection between love and loss than the intensity of the attachment.

How, then, do we make sense of the variations in peoples' response to loss? What factors play a part in influencing the duration and intensity of grief? Researchers and clinicians have their own distinct ways of evaluating relationships and predicting how someone will react and cope in the aftermath of significant loss. What has emerged as a common theme in both the research and clinical literature concerning bereavement is that understanding the nature of a person's orientation to attachment – in particular, the extent to which they have learned to trust and depend on others and their willingness to be depended upon - provides a good deal of insight into how they grieve, and this perspective is evident in current models of grief and grief therapy. In this chapter, following a brief review of the evolution of models of grief therapy, we will look at two of these contemporary models, the Two-Track Model of Bereavement (Rubin, 1981) and the Dual Process Model of Bereavement (Stroebe & Schut, 1992). From there we will use case examples to illustrate how attachment orientation influences response to loss, with an eye to showing how understanding the nature of a person's attachment can help us understand the nature of their grief and guide us in providing attuned and effective grief support.

MODELS OF GRIEF AND GRIEF RESOLUTION

Stage and Task Models

The literature on death and dying remained of little interest outside of a small cadre of professionals until 1970, with the publication of Kubler-Ross' seminal work, *On Death and Dying* (Kübler-Ross, 1997). Although she intended the book to be a description of the five stages (denial, anger, bargaining, depression, acceptance) that a terminally ill patient goes through in gradually coming to terms with their own impending death, Kubler-Ross's model was popularized as a description of the course of grief (Hall, 2014).

In the first edition of his hugely influential book *Grief Counseling and Grief Therapy*, Worden (1992) introduced an alternative model that depicts the process of healing from loss as involving a series of tasks, including accepting the reality of the loss, processing the pain of the loss, and adapting to the new life circumstances imposed by the loss (Worden, 1982, 2009, 2018). Similarly, Rando (1993) has described grief as a series of six "r" processes, including reacting to the loss, readjusting and reinvesting. Both Rando and Worden emphasized the active work involved in grieving, a view described as the "grief work hypothesis" (Stroebe, 1992) and both models have been widely utilized by practicing grief therapists (Worden et al., 2021).

A MOVE AWAY FROM STAGE MODELS OF GRIEF AND MOURNING

In the late 1980s, several reports were released that raised questions about the efficacy of grief interventions, and by extension the models of grief and grief resolution on which they were based (Wortman & Silver, 1989). Much of what was written in the aftermath of these reports challenged the assumption that all bereaved people need to move through the "stages" of mourning by engaging in "grief work" (Allumbaugh & Hoyt, 1999; Jordan & Neimeyer, 2003; Kato & Mann, 1999). While stage models and the grief work approach are appealingly straight-forward, the idea that people recover from loss by completing a set of tasks or progressing through a series of stages has been challenged by researchers (Stroebe et al., 2017) and educators in the field (Corr, 2022).

Another challenge to traditional grief models concerns the shift from an emphasis on the bereaved's release of psychic energy from the deceased (decathexis) as the desired end point of mourning, to an assumption that many grievers will maintain a "continuing bond" with the deceased (Klass et al., 1996; Rubin, 1999). While initial accounts of continuing bonds theory emphasized the advantages of continuing bonds with respect to adaptation to loss, subsequent research has shown that the bonds people maintain with the deceased, like the relationships they have with the living, are sometimes healthy and adaptive, and sometimes self-destructive and problematic (Field & Friederichs, 2004; Kosminsky, 2017). Chapter 5 includes a fuller discussion of continuing bonds in bereavement viewed through the lens of attachment theory.

Whatever differences they may have as to the nature and course of grief, the consensus view among theoreticians, researchers and clinicians engaged in work related to grief is that people's response to loss is influenced by multiple factors, the effects of which range in intensity from short term and manageable to severe and persistent. We suggest that a corollary to this view of the heterogeneity of grief is that therapists' approach to providing grief support must be sensitive to the nature of the griever, the relationship with the deceased, and the circumstances of the death: in other words, their approach must be multidimensional and fluid (Harris & Winokuer, 2019; Neimeyer, 2016; Rubin et al., 2012). This appreciation of the diversity of factors that influence grief response, in particular the significance of the nature of the griever's continuing bond with the deceased, is a key aspect of Rubin's Two- Track Model of Bereavement.

The Two-Track Model of Bereavement (TTM)

In reviewing the state of bereavement research in the 1970s and 1980s, Rubin (1989) observed that researchers appeared to have set off on two different paths. In one line of research, significant loss was viewed as a life stressor, and studies were designed to assess the impact of this stressor on the bereaved's biopsychosocial functioning, including their mental and physical health, their relationships, and their work performance. The other research group was focused on the nature of the bereaved individual's ongoing emotional attachment and relationship to the deceased. These investigators, for example, asked: how is grief affected by the griever's memories of the deceased? When are memories a source of comfort, and under what circumstances are they a source of distress?

With the introduction of the Two-Track Model of Bereavement, Rubin advocated a more integrated and comprehensive approach to grief research and to the practice of grief therapy. According to the Two-Track Model, the loss of a significant person presents the mourner with two distinct and complex sets of challenges. The first concerns their biopsychosocial functioning (Track I) and the second concerns the nature of their continuing relationship with the deceased (Track II). In contrast to earlier characterizations of grief and loss, the Two-Track Model combines the psychodynamic and interpersonal view of loss, which emphasizes the loss of the relationship with the living person (Track II) with the perspective that identifies loss as first and foremost a stressful event, the outcome of which can be evaluated in terms of "biological, behavioral, cognitive and emotional processes similar to the response of individuals to any other situation of crisis, trauma and stress" (Track I) (Rubin et al., 2012).

In his conceptualization of Track II, Rubin draws on continuing bonds theory (Klass et al., 1996) and treats the connection to the deceased as a relationship that does not end with death. That said, and in keeping with the view that continuing bonds are not always of benefit to the griever, Rubin and colleagues emphasize the need to consider the quality of this relationship and its effect on how the griever is managing their response to loss. Consideration of this relationship "deserves attention well beyond the coping associated with the initial grief and mourning" (Rubin et al., 2012, p. 26).

To understand and intervene in grief, we must remember that loss occurs at the interface of the individual, and their relationship with another person. "Once the significance of the interpersonal has been grasped, the nature of the relationship to the deceased rightfully takes its place as a major domain of interest" (Rubin et al., 2012, p. 23).

Applying the Two-Track Model in Cases of Traumatic Loss

The authors illustrate their approach with a case example of a client whose husband died by suicide. Suicide survivors often display signs of ongoing trauma (Track I, biopsychosocial functioning) along with waves of emotion evoked by relational aspects of the loss (Track II) including unresolved conflicts, guilt, anger, and preoccupation with the deceased's decision to end their life (Track II). The client in this case had significant distress on both tracks: evidence of trauma including intrusive thoughts, avoidance, and hyperarousal (Track I) and significant difficulty in accessing positive memories of her relationship with her husband (Track II). In line with the Two-Track Model, treatment included components to address traumatic symptoms as well as instruction in techniques that the client could use to modulate her affect. With the creation of a strong therapeutic bond, and some reduction in her trauma symptoms, the client was able to think about her husband and their relationship in a more balanced way and could recall positive aspects of her husband and happy memories of their years together.

The Two-Track Model has served as the basis for a substantial body of research and practice literature over the past 30 years. The fact that it has remained salient and useful is due, certainly, to its descriptive and explanatory power, but it may also be seen as a measure of its flexibility and eclecticism. Rubin and colleagues are not advocating a protocol for grief therapy so much as they are suggesting a way of *viewing the client*, with the program of therapy to be determined based on the client's strengths, difficulties, and needs. When treatment interventions fail, it may well be because some aspect of the grief experience not been considered. Rubin and colleagues observe that assessment and intervention paradigms used with traumatic bereavement have in many cases focused on the trauma and ignored the centrality of the loss of relationship. The "bifocal approach" represented by the Two-Track Model "rebalances" clinical attention by incorporating the story of the death and the nature of the bereaved's continuing bond with the deceased (Rubin et al., 2020).

The Two-Track Model focuses less on the *process* of bereavement and more on the *factors* that influence its course. A second model, The Dual Process Model, has more to say about the dynamic process of both normal and problematic grief.

The Dual Process Model (DPM)

The Dual Process Model (Stroebe & Schut, 1999a, 2010) posits that healthy grief involves a process of oscillation of attention on the part of the bereaved. Feelings and behaviors related to the loss, such as crying and yearning (the *Loss Orientation*), alternate with periods in which attention is directed toward changing roles and responsibilities in the mourner's life (the *Restoration Orientation* (Figure 4.1). The balance between loss and restoration will shift over time and will be influenced by factors related to the griever, the relationship, and the circumstances of the death.

The DPM builds upon Bowlby's assertions regarding the importance of "flexible attention". In childhood, flexible attention is evidenced by the

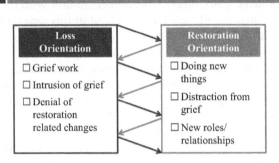

Figure 4.1 The Dual Process Model: Flexible Attention.
Source: Adapted from Stroebe & Schut (1999).

child's movement between exploratory activity and attachment or "reunion" behavior with caregivers, with whom the child has established a secure attachment. Bowlby regarded bereavement in adulthood as a parallel to the child's response to separation from their caregiver and proposed that adults' response to loss would also vary with their orientation to attachment (Bowlby, 1977). Bowlby suggested that anxiously attached individuals, whose emotional dependence would have been apparent when their loved one was alive, could be expected to have an extended and highly disruptive response to the person's death. Avoidantly attached individuals, those who are resistant to forming close attachments and generally downplay the importance of emotions and their own need for emotional support, would tend to suppress conscious grief.

With the Dual Process Model, Strobe and Schut expand on Bowlby's framework and propose that in anxious and avoidantly attached grievers, flexibility in response to the loss is compromised by the overuse of a limited repertoire of attachment related strategies. Stroebe and Schut propose that anxious, avoidant, and disorganized attachment patterns contribute to specific types of disturbances in oscillation, which in turn are associated with predictable problems in adaptation to loss (Stroebe et al., 2005). These predictions have been the subject of dozens of studies, and a substantial amount of this work has been done by Mario Mikulincer and Philip Shaver.

AN ATTACHMENT PERSPECTIVE ON DISORDERED GRIEF: MARIO MIKULINCER AND PHILIP SHAVER

Mikulincer and Shaver's model of attachment system functioning focuses on its interaction with other behavioral systems, including exploration and caregiving (Mikulincer & Shaver, 2007, 2017, 2019, 2022). According to this model, which the authors describe as an "extension and refinement of previous control systems models of attachment dynamics" (Mikulincer & Shaver, 2007, p. 30), once a person's attachment system is activated, they will initiate strategies to regain a sense of felt security, and will not engage in activities governed by other behavioral systems until this goal is attained. The behavioral patterns proposed by Bowlby as insecure/anxious and insecure/avoidant and incorporated into the DPM by Stroebe and Schut parallel the *hyperactivating* and *deactivating* strategies described by Shaver and Mikulincer (Shaver & Mikulincer, 2009, p. 23).

Research by Mikulincer and Shaver and others supports the proposition that attachment style moderates the choice of proximity or support seeking as an emotion regulation strategy (Kim et al., 2014; Mikulincer & Shaver, 2019) That is, children who are secure in their attachment style are more likely to seek contact when they feel separation distress, a response that reflects their expectation that their attachment figures will be available and responsive to their needs. Insecurely attached children, having different expectations, will tend to employ one of two secondary attachment strategies: *hyperactivation* (for the preoccupied/anxious) or *deactivation* (for the fearful/avoidant). The child adopts these strategies as a way of managing their relationship with an unavailable, unreliable, or rejecting attachment figure.

While they may be functional for the child in the context of their caregiving environment, these strategies can become problematic in adulthood. Anxiously attached adults risk alienating potential friends and partners with their excessive neediness and clinging behavior (hyperactivation of the attachment system). Avoidantly attached adults, in contrast, may alienate potential friends and partners with their excessive independence and their apparent lack of interest in intimacy (deactivation of the attachment system). These problems in relationship also affect the trajectory of bereavement in the insecurely attached (Mikulincer & Shaver, 2013, Sekowski & Prigerson, 2021).

While secure attachment confers an advantage in managing separation distress, it does not prevent people from experiencing emotional pain when a significant relationship ends. In the absence of the attachment figure, the primary strategy for seeking comfort is no longer relevant, and secondary strategies come into play. Bereavement, being the response to an irreversible loss of connection, "provides an excellent, if saddening, research laboratory in which to study secondary attachment strategies" (Mikulincer & Shaver, 2007, p. 72).

In the months following significant loss, securely as well as insecurely attached people are likely to experience days in which they cannot think of anything but the person who has died, and days in which their energy and attention are unaccountably taken up with other things. *This is the nature of grief,* and even healthy grief involves alternation between confrontation of the loss and periods of compartmentalization, avoidance, and psychological distancing from the reality and implications of the loss.

> By driving people to experience the deep pain of loss, repeatedly reactivate memories of the deceased alongside the realization that the person is gone, and yearn for his or her proximity and love, attachment system hyperactivation allows mourners to explore the meaning and significance of their lost relationships, and find ways of maintaining reorganized, mainly symbolic bonds with loved partners. Deactivating strategies can also contribute productively to the reorganization process by enabling momentary detachment from the deceased and inhibition or suppression of painful feelings and thoughts.
>
> (Mikulincer & Shaver, 2008b, p. 95)

What Mikulincer and Shaver are describing here is a process of oscillation represented by the Dual Process Model. We can now begin to see the usefulness of this model as a guide for therapeutic intervention.

The Dual Process Model in Practice

According to the DPM, an individual who is overly focused on the loss side of the loss/restoration process will not be helped by interventions that actively and consistently direct their attention to the details of the loss (Stroebe & Schut, 1999; Stroebe & Schut, 2010; Wijngaards-de Meij et al., 2007b). Clinicians who use these strategies with loss-focused clients run the risk of deepening the bereaved's feelings of distress and amplifying their tendency to ruminate about the deceased, with the potential result being a downward spiral of decreased energy, increasing isolation, and hopelessness. Techniques that move the individual towards a restoration orientation will be more important in these cases. For example, if an individual has become socially isolated, reconnecting with friends may become a major focus of grief therapy. Conversely, for a client who avoids any confrontation with the loss, the clinical task becomes one of helping the bereaved person to gradually expose themselves to the reality of the death, with all of its attendant thoughts and feelings. In summary, as the name of the model suggests, bereavement is a process of alternately moving "towards" and "away from" the loss, and the role of a grief therapist is to help the client engage in that part of the process that they seem unwilling or unable to engage in themselves.

The process of alternating attention represented by the dual process model is straightforward, and easily explained to clients. The terminology introduced by Stroebe and Schut is likely to require some explanation. Reporting on their study of the dual process model, Caserta and Lund note that their respondents found it hard to understand the concept of "restoration-oriented" coping, and had difficulty knowing if, and when, they had engaged in it (Caserta & Lund, 2007). Caserta and Lund observe that clear identification of the concept is needed to help bereaved individuals understand and ultimately engage in restoration-oriented coping.

In the following exchange, the clinician (PK), who has previously discussed the Dual Process model with this client, brings the client's attention to her use of restoration-oriented coping. The client, whose husband of 45 years had died two months ago, was tearful, afraid, and convinced that she would never be able to stop crying. When would she ever feel like doing anything? How would she ever settle her husband's estate? In a gentle tone the clinician acknowledged that

> right now, it's very hard for you to think about anything but how much you miss your husband ... But even now, you mentioned that you spent the weekend with friends and worked in your garden. And you felt well enough to organize the papers you need to go through to settle your husband's estate, even though you didn't feel up to looking at them.

These activities, the clinician explained, were hopeful signs of the client's ability to take a break from her grief, even though her loss was very new.

Since its introduction, Stroebe and Schut have continued to modify and expand the Dual Process Model. One such addition is the concept of Grief Overload, which they define as *the bereaved person's perception of having more than they feel able to deal with* – too much or too many activities, events, experiences, and other stimuli (Stroebe & Schut, 2016, p. 96). (Note the overlap here with the concept of *allostatic load* introduced in Chapter 3.) Although the original DPM emphasizes the need for balance between restoration and loss-oriented coping, in developing the model Stroebe and Schut found that they had not considered the possibility that oscillation could be beyond the capacity of someone whose "burdens are too over-whelming" (p. 101). Overload can occur due to the number of deaths a person has had to face, but it can also arise from the combined weight of loss and restoration-oriented stressors. We observe overload in many of our bereaved clients, people whose grief is compounded by worries about the health of family members, conflict with siblings, alienation between parents and adult children, financial difficulties, to name a few. The problems that loss may bring with it can have their origins in ongoing issues that were active before the death that have become more intensified (e.g, conflict between two family members), and/or, there may be problems that are a direct result of the absence of the deceased (e.g., if the deceased was the "breadwinner", and the survivors now face financial problems that are new). In addition, stress over and above the stress of grief can contribute to the incidence of physical symptoms and accidental injuries, adding to the griever's sense that "the universe is against me."

Sophie, a recent widow who fractured her shoulder and has now received a frightening medical diagnosis, begins her session by asking:

> Why is all of this happening to me? Isn't it enough that my husband died? What is the matter with me that the world is so determined to keep knocking me down? Sometimes I feel like just staying in bed and giving up.

Interpersonal difficulties may also contribute to a feeling of overload. The loss of a parent who kept conflict among family members under control can result in an eruption of suppressed anger and resentment. Estrangement from adult children and restricted access to grandchildren has left another client, an older widow, feeling alone and hopeless:

> It's like they feel that the wrong parent died – that it should have been me. I don't know what I'm living for anymore.

The concept of grief overload as an extension of the dual process model draws attention to the potential for breakdown of oscillation under conditions of excessive stress and raises the possibility that for clients who feel overwhelmed by one or more stressors arising from their loss, interventions designed to promote oscillation may not be effective. In these cases, "what is essential is control over the stressors – *efforts need to be made to reduce their impact*" (Strobe & Schut, 2016, p. 203). This can take the form of encouraging the client to ask friends or family members for help, setting boundaries with people whose demands increase the bereaved's level of stress, and letting go of expectations about what their deceased loved one "would have wanted" them to do.

DOES THE DUAL PROCESS MODEL OF COPING WITH BEREAVEMENT ACCURATELY REPRESENT THE BEREAVEMENT EXPERIENCE?

Research on Oscillation

To answer this question, Fiore (2021) conducted a systematic review of research on the Dual Process Model. Of the 474 articles initially identified, 86 underwent full-text review, with 22 quantitative or mixed-methods studies included. The author reports that the bulk of the studies identified focused on loss- or restoration-oriented strategies, but no specific study results could be related to the process of oscillation. Nevertheless, the research reviewed suggests that "the DPM provides a realistic framework to illustrate the bereavement experience as it accounts for multiple bereavement stressors occurring simultaneously, and the use of confrontation and avoidance behaviors as part of the bereavement experience" (p. 415). Further research should address the oscillation process, how to incorporate research on the model into practice, and how to develop a variety of clinical approaches that address the varied needs of bereaved individuals.

Several studies based on small clinical samples have reported evidence that supports the oscillation described by the DPM. In a study of mothers coping with the loss of their children in the 2008 China earthquake, in-depth interviews were conducted with six bereaved mothers over a two-year period. (Chen et al., 2017). Immediately after the earthquake the mothers suffered intense grief. Over the course of the study, they "began to focus on restoration-oriented stressors to face changes in life" (p. 69). Citing what they described as a "dynamic process" of oscillation between loss and restoration-oriented stressors, the authors conclude that the study supports what the DPM characterizes as the course of normal grief.

Although the DPM was developed as a bereavement model, Stroebe and Schut propose that it is applicable to any grieving experience (Stroebe & Schut, 2010). In a sample of 29 parents whose child had a rare and life-threatening heart defect Cantwell-Bartell (2018) found that parents experienced intense feelings of loss upon diagnosis but shifted to a focus on restoration-oriented tasks to support their child. "Over time most parents employed a healthy oscillation between loss- and restoration-oriented coping."

> Parents' grief was not a constant, but when it was aroused it could involve intense suffering.: "We go on like a normal couple and then the grief hits us like a sledgehammer." [father of a 13-year-old boy]
>
> (Cantwell-Bartell, 2018, p. 573)

Parents continued to experience periods of intense grief interwoven with restoration-oriented coping. The father of a chronically ill 8-year-old girl said, "There is a dark cloud that hangs over us all the time, but you have to enjoy her as she is" (Cantwell-Bartell, p. 574).

Research on the Role of Attachment Orientation in Response to Loss

Bowlby regarded adult bereavement as a parallel of childhood attachment related distress, and proposed that in both cases, the nature the individual's orientation toward attachment would be reflected in their ability to cope with and recover from episodes of separation. The Dual Process Model draws on this view of the role of attachment in response to loss, while recognizing that secondary strategies of hyperactivation and deactivation, which in children are seen as problematic, occur as part of normal grief in adults.

Attachment orientation has been identified as a significant factor in response to loss in a large number of studies (Burke & Neimeyer, 2013;

MacCallum, 2021; Parkes, 1972; Smigelsky et al., 2020; Zech & Arnold, 2011, 2016), with consistent findings that anxiously attached grievers experience more intense and more persistent grief than those who are securely attached (Mikulincer & Shaver, 2022; Sekowski & Prigerson, 2021). The picture concerning avoidantly attached grievers is less clear, with researchers finding positive, negative, and little or no association between avoidance and problematic grief. Black et al. (2022) found that avoidant attachment was associated with more intense grief in samples of people mourning their romantic partner or spouse, with similar findings reported in relation to loss of a friend (Jerga et al., 2011); child (Wijengaards-de Meij et al., 2007a) and a violently deceased family member or close friend (Meier et al., 2013).

Other researchers have reported a negative association between avoidance and more severe grief symptomatology. In a study based on the DPM, Delspaux and colleagues investigated the mediating impact of an individual's negative vs. positive self-appraisal of bereavement stressors on subject's flexible coping, that is, their use of both loss-oriented and restoration-oriented coping strategies (Delespaux et al., 2013). They predicted that individuals with anxious attachment would exhibit more negative appraisals of stressors, would use primarily LO coping strategies, and would show more intense grief reactions, while individuals with higher attachment avoidance would have lower negative appraisal of stressors, use primarily RO strategies, and have less pronounced grief responses. Their findings confirmed these assumptions, suggesting that avoidant individuals, despite their primary use of only one type of coping strategy, manage their grief more successfully than those who are anxiously attached. The authors urge caution in this interpretation of their findings, most importantly, because none of their subjects made exclusive use of either RO or LO strategies.

A study by LeRoy et al. (2020) was designed to assess the association of anxious vs. avoidant attachment in bereaved spouses with a range of physical and emotional symptoms. The researchers hypothesized that attachment anxiety would be associated with poorer loss adjustment, operationalized by higher levels of physical inflammation (assessed by measuring inflammation related markers in participants' blood), poorer self-reported mental and physical health, and other grief related symptoms. Noting the inconsistencies in the literature regarding avoidant attachment as a risk factor for grief related complications, their expectations for this group were open ended. In line with expected results, attachment anxiety was associated with greater grief symptoms as well as poorer mental and physical health. In contrast, attachment avoidance was not associated with inflammation. The avoidant group also evidenced better self-reported physical and mental health.

These findings should be considered in light of the sample drawn in this study. All participants had lost a spouse three months or less prior to the study, hence the researchers' conclusion that attachment avoidance may be adaptive for recently bereaved spouses and their acknowledgement that the scope of their study does not fully capture the potentially deleterious longer term effects of avoidant strategies for dealing with bereavement, such as a lack of support seeking and a reluctance to fully process the loss. This conclusion is in line with studies suggesting that while the suffering of anxious grievers may be more apparent, particularly in early grief, avoidance as a defense can collapse under the weight of high stress, particularly in cases of traumatic bereavement (Mikulincer & Shaver, 2019).

Much of the grief related attachment research conducted over the past twenty years has been aimed at clarifying disparate findings related to attachment orientation. Fraley and Bonanno (Fraley & Bonanno, 2004) studied attachment style in 59 participants, who were assessed for grief, anxiety, and depression 4 and 18 months after the first measurement. The authors used the categorization introduced by Bartholomew and Horowitz (1991), which differentiates fearful avoidance, "characterized by a fear of being hurt or rejected," from "dismissing avoidance," characterized by the minimization of emotion and an emphasis on self-reliance and independence. Fraley and Bonanno hypothesized that fearfully avoidant attached individuals would have a significantly more problematic response to bereavement than dismissingly avoidant attached individuals. The results of their study substantiated this hypothesis, leading them to suggest that in assessing the impact of avoidant strategies, researchers and clinicians need to consider the underlying dynamic driving the individual's avoidance.

In a subsequent study, researchers assessed the psychological adjustment of people who were close to the World Trade Center in New York City at the time of the terrorist attacks in 2001 (Fraley et al., 2006). This study confirmed the researchers' hypotheses regarding the response of fearfully avoidant individuals, but findings with regard to dismissively avoidant individuals were mixed. While reports from friends and family regarding the adaptation of these individuals indicated that they were doing well, the respondents themselves reported a high level of PTSD symptoms and depression. These findings make sense when we consider the tendency of avoidantly attached individuals to downplay their need for support from others, a denial that stems both from the desire not to draw attention to their distress, and from their belief that there is little to be gained from reaching out to others, as there is nothing that anyone can do to help them (Parkes, 2013; Parkes & Prigerson, 2010). In short, despite external evidence suggesting that they are doing well, people with an avoidant coping style may continue to experience considerable internal distress. In line with this view, Mikulincer & Shaver (2022) emphasize that depending upon the circumstances, avoidance can create problems in bereavement, particularly in cases of traumatic loss, and should not be confused with resilience.

In another effort to clarify the role of attachment anxiety and avoidance in coping with bereavement, Meier, Carr, Currier and Neimeyer (2013) collected data on 656 recently bereaved young adults. In the first of two studies using this data, the authors looked at the differing impact of anxious and avoidant attachment, and found that higher levels of attachment related anxiety, but not avoidance, were associated with more problematic bereavement. The second study focused on the response of anxiously and avoidantly attached individuals to violent loss (accident, suicide, homicide). Results from this study showed that avoidance was associated with problems in physical and mental health, a finding that is consistent with the study of World Trade Center survivors cited above (Fraley et al., 2006). Also consistent with that earlier study, the authors emphasize the role of trauma in the collapse of avoidant defenses and argue that this finding challenges the "illusion of coping in avoidant attachment" (Meier et al., 2013).

> This study highlighted the illusion of coping in avoidant attachment, as grief appears to manifest in general health symptoms and even poorer mental health functioning ... Those violent loss survivors attempting to cope with the loss through avoidance may have been unable to integrate the loss as part of their life narrative, rendering them more susceptible to prolonged grief disorder.
>
> (p. 331)

Findings from a study by Yu, He, Xu, Wang and Prigerson (2016) offer some clarification of the impact of anxiety and avoidance on the severity and long-term effects of grief. Based on a sample of bereaved mainland Chinese participants, the researchers found that anxious attachment was associated with more intense grief. However, the process of confronting their loss enabled these grievers to

> ... reconstruct their relationship to the deceased and in so doing to establish a connection to the deceased as an ongoing source of security ... Thus, the (anxiously attached) bereaved person may experience grief and obtain post-traumatic growth through the loss.
>
> (p. 98)

In contrast, attachment avoidance "prevents the bereaved person from reestablishing psychological proximity to the deceased ...

> Thus, the individual misses an opportunity to relearn the world through grief or revise his or her schema to new realities of post-loss life. In short, attachment avoidance presents a heightened risk of maladaptive bereavement adjustment.
>
> (p. 98)

In line with the Dual Process Model, the authors propose that without needed processing of the loss, the avoidantly attached bereaved person "may not recover from grieving process or experience posttraumatic growth following the loss", and as a result, will be apt to experience problematic grief (p. 98).

Other researchers have looked at variables that may mediate the effects of attachment orientation on bereavement. In their study of bereavement after pregnancy loss, Scheidt and colleagues found that social support correlated inversely with grief, symptoms of anxiety and depression, and overall psychological distress and PTSD symptoms (Scheidt et al., 2012). This finding is consistent with studies demonstrating the importance of social support in coping with bereavement (Mancini & Bonanno, 2009; Mikulincer & Shaver, 2019; McCallum, 2021). Whatever benefits accrue from the availability of social support, these may well be less available to avoidantly attached individuals, who, in comparison to those who are securely attached, tend to have lower numbers of individuals they can turn to for support and are less satisfied with whatever support they receive (Wallin, 2007; MacCallum, 2021).

The role of attachment in the decision to seek professional counseling has also been studied. As predicted by attachment theory, the available evidence suggests that avoidantly attached individuals are less likely than anxiously attached individuals to seek counseling (Cheng et al., 2015; Mccallum & Bryan, 2018). They are less likely to believe in the value of therapy relative to the potential risks of self-disclosure as compared to anxiously attached individuals, who, in keeping with the observation that the anxiously attached devalue their ability to manage without the help of others, are more inclined to seek help from a therapist, more willing to self-disclose, and more positive in their appraisal of the potential benefits of therapy (Vogel et al., 2008).

The question of whether an individual's attachment orientation is consistent across relationships was the subject of a study by Smigelsky et al. (2019) that highlighted the asymmetry between global attachment style and attachment to particular individuals. A sample of 385 bereaved college students completed measures retrospectively assessing relationship quality, attachment to the deceased, and grief symptomatology. The study adapted an existing measure of attachment and employed a novel instrument of relationship quality to examine specific attachment to and relationship quality with the deceased as contributors to grief symptom severity. Results support the view that specific attachment to the deceased can differ significantly from global attachment style, a finding that the researchers emphasize should inform the selection of interventions for bereaved clients. In short, interventions should be suited to the quality of the bereaved's relationship with the deceased. For example, relationship-enhancing interventions such as directed journaling (Lichtenthal & Neimeyer, 2012), and facilitation of a continuing bond (Klass & Steffan, 2018; Kosminsky, 2018) may be appropriate for some, but not all grievers.

Sekowski and Prigerson (2019, 2022a, 2022b) have addressed what they identify as a missing piece in the puzzle of attachment orientation and grief severity. They note that while the role of relational anxiety and avoidance in response to loss have been studied extensively, with attachment anxiety being consistently associated with intensity of grief, the results from studies of attachment avoidance have been highly inconsistent. Their study was designed to shed light on factors underlying these disparities in the research literature. In detailing the rationale for their study Sekowski and Prigerson present a novel integration of aspects of disorganized attachment that relate to grief. A summary of their findings follows.

Disorganized attachment and prolonged grief disorder (the list below is a summary)

- Bahm et al. (2017) have theorized that feelings of *fear and confusion* experienced in the context of disorganized attachment and loss have been identified in unresolved loss.
- These feelings of fear and confusion "activate the mechanism of dissociation, used in the context of disorganized attachment relationships to separate the conflicting aspects of the relationship (distressing fright and soothing safety" (Sekowski & Prigerson, 2021, p. 1810).
- Dissociation is also evident in AAI interviews in which the subject's responses suggest an intermittent lack of awareness that the deceased person is permanently gone (as explained in Chapter 3, these are described in the language of the AAI as "lapses in discourse and reasoning").
- Bowlby proposed a similar mechanism of dissociation, which he called "segregation" as an explanation for pathological chronic grief (Bowlby, 1980).
- Unresolved loss, which is an attachment status, and prolonged grief disorder "may not only have similar hypothetical dynamics" (Bahm et al., 2017; Bowlby, 1980) but may also share common characteristics such as prolonged lack of acceptance of the loss, disbelief in the death of the loved one, and preoccupation with loss Sekowski & Prigerson, 2021; Thomson, 2010).
- A study of 18 inpatients (Gander, 2018) showed that out of 18 patients meeting PGD criteria, all were all were classified as unresolved with respect to loss, suggesting PGD overlaps with unresolved loss. Thus, fear and confusion in attachment relationships can be positively associated not only with unresolved loss – as was theorized by Bahm et al. (2017) – but also with PGD symptoms.

Sekowski & Prigerson, 2022b.

In their assessment of the significance of this analysis Sekowski and Prigerson propose that the association between disorganized attachment and PGD involves a *different mechanism* than either attachment anxiety or avoidance. Attachment anxiety excessively activates the attachment system and avoidance effectively or ineffectively deactivates the attachment system. In contrast, disorganized attachment can be positively related to PGD symptom severity mainly based on

> dissociative mechanisms that enable the coexistence of incoherent states of mind in the attachment relationship: one which knows that a close person has died, and the second which cultivates disbelief in the ultimate nature of loss, constantly activating attachment behavior in the form of longing, searching, and despair, which is manifested by the symptoms of PGD.
>
> (Sekowski & Prigerson, 2022b, p. 1809)

Results from their study confirmed the relationship between disorganized attachment and PGD symptom severity. Their findings also help to explain the disparity in results concerning avoidant attachment.

> Attachment avoidance leads to effective or ineffective deactivation of the attachment system in the face of loss, so the strength and direction of the relationship between this attachment style and PGD symptom severity may vary ...*Thus, the mechanism of the positive relationship between disorganized attachment and prolonged grief can be not only effective but also different from the mechanisms of association of attachment anxiety or avoidance with PGD symptoms.* (emphasis added). This would justify not only further explanation of PGD symptoms through disorganized attachment, relative to attachment anxiety and avoidance but also the uniqueness of this effect. Future research into the relationship between attachment and PGD should consider disorganized attachment in addition to attachment anxiety and avoidance ...
>
> (Sekowski & Prigerson, 2022b, p. 1809)

Sekowski & Prigerson's closing remarks concerning the implications of their study are understandably of particular interest to Kosminsky and Jordan:

> If future studies confirm our results, this would suggest that disorganized attachment and attachment anxiety, and in some cases, attachment avoidance could be a possible target for interventions for bereaved persons who experience PGD symptoms. The attachment-informed grief therapy (Kosminsky, 2018; Kosminsky & Jordan, 2016) suggests a number of such interventions aimed at working with individuals with specific attachment styles in the context of loss.
>
> (Sekowski & Prigerson, 2022b, p. 1818)

We believe that researchers studying the relationship between attachment and PGD should consider disorganized attachment alongside attachment anxiety and avoidance. Finally, future research should focus on verifying the effectiveness of attachment-informed grief therapy in the treatment of symptoms of PGD.

(Sekowski & Prigerson, 2022b, p. 1820)

HIERARCHICAL RANKING OF ATTACHMENT FIGURES AS A FACTOR IN RESPONSE TO LOSS

The bond between infants and mothers has been a focus of much of the research and theory related to attachment, because in most cultures, mothers tend to be the primary source of comfort and security during early childhood years (Ainsworth et al., 1978). However, by adolescence and adulthood, other relationships, including relationships with fathers, extended family members, and friends and romantic partners, generally assume greater importance as a source of support and care (Doherty & Feeney, 2004). This reassignment of roles occurs at various points throughout life and is described as the *reorganization of the attachment hierarchy* (Girme et al., 2021). According to this model, the intensity of grief a person feels when attachment figures die will be directly related to the deceased's position in the griever's attachment hierarchy. The bereaved's distress will compounded by the unavailability of the very person to whom they would be most inclined to turn to when faced with a stressful event.

The concept of an attachment hierarchy, as suggested by Girme et al. (2021), provides another way of understanding variations in grief response, as well as the necessary conditions for adjustment to significant loss. When faced with the loss of someone at the "top" of their hierarchy, recovery will depend on the griever's ability to revise their attachment hierarchy. That is, they will need to transfer some of the support and care needs previously met by the deceased to others in the griever's social network. As is true with so many aspects of response to loss, some people will be better equipped than others to do this. The more secure the individual is, the more likely it will be that they will be able to identify others in their network from whom they can draw support.

We have found that introducing the concept of an attachment hierarchy to a bereaved client can help them understand the magnitude of their grief. Recognizing that the person they have lost was "at the top of their hierarchy" can help the bereaved individual understand the intensity of their response to loss as well as normalizing feelings of fear and vulnerability.

Neurological Evidence of the Role of Attachment in Coping with Attachment Related Stress

While most studies of the role of attachment in coping with emotionally stressful events rely on self-report measures or interviews, over the past 20 years inquiries into how people manage emotion have taken advantage of advances in brain imaging to address questions about how people manage emotion at a neurological level. In one of the first such studies, Gillath and colleagues used functional magnetic resonance imaging (fMRI) to identify differences in the neural processes underlying the emotion regulation strategies of avoidantly and anxiously attached individuals (Gillath et al., 2005). Given the instruction to think about negative relationship scenarios (conflict, breakups or death of a partner) subjects with an anxious attachment orientation showed more activation in areas of the brain related to emotion and less activation in areas related to the down regulation of emotion than non-anxious people, suggesting they "react more strongly to thoughts of loss while under-recruiting brain regions normally used to down-regulate negative emotions" (Gillath et al., 2005, p. 835).

In another study using fMRI, Vrticka, Bondolfi, Sander and Vuillemier identified distinct patterns in brain activation as a function of attachment anxiety or avoidance (Vrtička et al., 2012). For example, when exposed to strongly negative emotional scenes, avoidantly attached individuals were found to have less activation in areas of the brain associated with the reappraisal of negative stimuli and higher activation in areas of the brain associated with the suppression of emotion. These results " ... .reveal that reappraisal may not work for these individuals, leading to impaired down regulation of amygdal reactivity" (Vrtička et al., 2012, p. 473). This pattern may help explain "... ..why avoidantly attached individuals become highly emotional when their preferred regulation strategies fail or cannot be employed" (Vrtička & Vuilleumier, 2012, p.12). More recently, research on the impact of early adverse experience (see Chapter 3) has sharpened our understanding of brain structure as a factor in emotion regulation. A consistent finding has been increased reactivity in the amygdala, and a blunted response in the reward system, in individuals with a history of adverse early life experiences (Teicher et al., 2020).

BRIDGING RESEARCH AND PRACTICE

Along with the research presented in Chapter 3 concerning the impact of early attachment on development, and in particular the negative effects of early relational trauma, the findings reported above have implications for every aspect of service delivery for problematic grief, from program development to diagnosis and treatment. Shaffer, Vogel and Wei assert that the most important limitation of counseling is that it can only help people who seek treatment (Shaffer et al., 2006). The research cited here suggests that many people who are bereaved are lacking in social support, and that within this group, the subgroup of avoidantly attached individuals are among the least likely to seek the help of a professional counselor (Shaffer et al., 2006; Vogel et al., 2008). If a bereaved person does make it into a grief therapist's office, research suggests that the therapist will be more likely to build a strong alliance and to develop an appropriate strategy for treatment if the client's attachment orientation is taken into account (Levy et al., 2011). Levy, Ellison and Scott recommend that clinicians "titrate their interpersonal styles so as not to overwhelm dismissingly avoidant patients or to appear disengaged, aloof or uninterested" to patients who have a pre-occupied/anxious attachment style (Levy et al., 2011, p. 396).

The loss of someone who is loved and trusted is a wrenching blow, but it is all the more difficult for people who are lacking in internal coping resources and external support. These resource deficits are among the factors that complicate the grief of people who are insecurely attached. The defensive strategies that insecurely attached individuals employ are, in addition, frequently obstacles to treatment. Establishing a strong therapeutic bond with a bereaved person who is insecurely attached is both essential and challenging and depends very much on the clinician's ability to gain the client's trust. Trust is what allows the avoidant client to risk an encounter with feelings that are usually pushed away or denied. Trust is what makes the anxious client willing to try to do things that they don't want to do, whether it is to go more deeply into their experience of their grief, or conversely, to let go of it and to begin to adapt to the new and changed world. As we will discuss more fully in Chapter 8, *trust in the therapist* promotes behavioral flexibility and a willingness to experiment with a broader range of coping behaviors.

In the following section we provide examples from our own work and from the clinical literature on the integration of an attachment perspective into work with the bereaved. Several of the clients introduced here will reappear in Chapter 7, where we will focus on how to help people develop the resources they need to integrate significant loss.

INSECURE ATTACHMENT AND COMPLICATED GRIEF

The Anxious Client

Ruth

Ruth, 48, admits to her therapist that she always worried about something happening to her mother or father. An only child, she stayed close to her parents after graduation from college and saw them regularly. Now that her parents have both died, she talks about having "lost her footing." Unmarried and with only one close friend, Ruth admits that she has never felt entirely comfortable being on her own. She depended on her parents for help in making all life decisions and does not know how she will go on without them. Asked to speak about her childhood, Ruth describes a father who continually accused her of being too provocative in her dress and too free in stating her opinions. Although they were frequently in conflict about Ruth's choice of friends, career, and views, she never gave up on the idea that she could "win his love" by being a dutiful daughter

Gloria

Gloria, 52, is a wife and mother of two teenage children. Her own mother is in a nursing home and is not expected to live for more than six months. Gloria visits her several times a week. Her mother is extremely critical of Gloria, complains her daughter does not spend more time with her, and is never pleased with Gloria's efforts to bring her things she thinks her mother would like. Gloria feels tormented by the need to visit her mother and by her persistent feeling that she is a failure as a daughter. She weeps throughout the session,, stopping only briefly when the therapist asks her a question or encourages her to pause and breathe. With all this, what terrifies Gloria the most is that her mother will die, and that without her, she will not be able to live. She sees her future as a period of torment while her mother lives, to be followed by a collapse into complete desperation when she dies.

Many people experience the fear and dislocation described by Gloria in the early stages of grief, but for the anxiously attached person, this fear is pervasive and unrelenting. What is different about the grief of a person who is anxiously attached, and why is it so often difficult for them to believe that they can go on with their lives?

In the parlance of the Dual Process and Two-Track models, this anxiously attached client has become entrenched in a loss orientation, and their biopsychosocial functioning is compromised. Gloria is afraid of how she will manage without her deceased, or soon to be deceased mother, and her fear is amplified by a tendency toward negative expectations concerning the future, and a lack of faith in her capacity to deal with the uncertainties and stresses of everyday life on her own. Another client who was seen by the first author five years after the death of her husband was similarly doubtful of her ability to manage without him.

Trudy

Trudy, a 55-year-old widow, has been in a support group for five years, but continues to feel that her life is out of control. Trudy describes her husband as a caring and responsible husband and father who earned a steady income, paid all the bills, and generally managed all the details of their lives. Prior to her husband's death Trudy had never worked or lived on her own; she moved in with her husband directly from her parents' home at the time of her marriage. Trudy recalls her parents as having been very loving. She was an only child and they treated her, in her words "like a china doll." There was never any question when Trudy was growing up that her future would be in a marriage exactly like the one she eventually found, with a husband who would take care of her in much the same way that she had been cared for by her parents.

Not surprisingly, the illness and death of her husband threw Trudy into a panic. In addition to having to take on all domestic and financial responsibilities, she was faced with the need to find a placement for her adolescent son, who was diagnosed with autism, and whose periodic outbursts were disruptive and frightening. She despaired of being able to make plans for her son without her husband's help.

Trudy was extremely tearful in her sessions and frequently expressed the fear that she would never be able to get her life back on track. She felt alone and overwhelmed. Her sadness about her husband's death was layered with anger for his having deserted her by dying.

Anxiously attached clients can be some of the easiest people with whom to establish a therapeutic bond, because they are desperate for connection. Their desperation is fueled by the need to stay close to someone who will supply the strength and insight they find lacking within themselves, and they typically look to the therapist to fill this role. These clients also tend to have a pervasive fear of being criticized, rejected, or abandoned by the clinician. Their already shaky sense of self-esteem and self-efficacy has been compromised by the loss, and they find the world without the deceased to be mostly devoid of pleasure, meaning, or hope. They are pessimistic about their ability to survive the loss, and many report that others around them do not understand the extent of their grief and despair. Their memories of the deceased are often idealized, and they report significant distress at the thought of losing those memories of and connection with their loved one.

The individual who is anxiously attached will generally be relieved to have someone really listen to them, and may seek extra contact with the therapist, either by trying to prolong a session, or by requesting more frequent sessions or additional contact (phone or e-mail) between sessions. Anxiously attached clients usually have ready access to their feelings about the loss, themselves, and their future, particularly their negative feelings. They will typically be open to any suggestions that the therapist makes that involve self-care but will often insist that they have no energy for exercise or social activities. In addition, their pessimism about being able to feel better with time and effort on their part may sometimes interfere with a willingness to put effort into the therapeutic process.

An important consideration in understanding the dynamic of bereavement in people who are anxiously attached, and one with noteworthy implications for their treatment, is that these individuals tend to operate on the assumption that sadness, yearning and other painful emotions are "congruent with attachment goals, and they may seek to sustain and even exaggerate them" (Mikulincer & Shaver, 2014, p. 241). In other words, anxiously attached individuals have learned that holding onto painful feeling states, and making their distress known to others, increases the likelihood that they will have their attachment needs met. They sustain this state of hyperactivation through an appraisal process in which the threatening aspects of events are magnified, their inability to manage their distress is exaggerated, and attention is focused on recalling past painful experiences and anticipating those that may occur in the future (Mikulincer et al, 2010; Shaver & Mikulincer, 2010). While anxiously attached clients may have some insight into their distress, their ability to reflect on the loss, reflect on its meaning and construct a coherent narrative will often be compromised by the intensity of their affect.

The Avoidant Client

Margaret

Recalling the deaths of her mother and then her father in the preceding two years, Margaret sat on the edge of her chair, expressionless, her checkbook in one hand and her keys in the other. She looked around the room and her eyes settled on the office clock. With a tentative smile, the clinician said, "You look like you're going to bolt at any minute. The feeling I'm getting is that you think this is a waste of your time." "Oh, no," Margaret replied. "It's not that you're wasting my time; it's that I don't want to waste your time. Me talking about my feelings – why would anyone want to listen to that?"

The therapist said: "Hmm, well that's an interesting question - it makes me wonder where you got the idea that no one could possibly be interested in hearing about your feelings. Have you always felt that way? What about when you were a child? What did you do when you were say, five or six and you were upset, crying?"

Margaret replied: "I don't remember ever crying as a child. I guess I was a very stoic child."

The nature and course of bereavement among avoidantly attached people, who do not present with what is typically considered the "picture" of a grief stricken individual, has been a source of ongoing disagreement among researchers and clinicians (Parkes, 2013). The question that has consistently been raised about people who profess no particular emotional distress following a loss is whether these people are coping effectively with the loss, or are employing a strategy of suppressing uncomfortable or intolerable feelings. Clinical experience suggests that what brings avoidantly attached individuals into treatment is the breakdown of this strategy, signaled by the emergence of feelings that they are not equipped to manage, and often accompanied by a range of physical symptoms or dysfunctional behaviors, such as substance abuse or irritability in relationships. An additional motivation for treatment can be social pressure, typically from family members or friends, to seek professional help for their problems, and sometimes for their apparent lack of any response to the loss. As the following narrative suggests, these clients can be quite straightforward when it comes to their personal boundaries and the rules by which they want the clinician to abide.

Hannah

Hannah sought grief counseling six months after the death of her husband, who had been living with chronic heart disease for six years. Hannah made it clear from the outset that she had only come for counseling because her husband's hospice nurse told her that she should. When Hannah seemed about to tear up and the clinician made her usual gesture of offering her a tissue, Hannah balked, assuring her that she would not be crying, that she did not "cry in front of anyone, and what's the point of crying anyway." Asked about where she had learned that crying is pointless, Hannah waved away the question, adding that she was "not here to talk about my family, and don't expect me to do that." Hannah was determined to get through her bereavement as she had gotten through life until that point – with fierce determination and the resolute forward movement of a soldier in battle.

Despite her skepticism, Hannah continued to come to therapy, and after two months began to talk about the guilt she felt about not having taken better care of her husband. She also consented to disclose some details of her childhood. Hannah's parents ran their own business and traveled a great deal, during which time Hannah was left in the care of a series of nannies. She dismissed the idea that this was a problem for her in any way because she was "very independent."

After two months and six sessions, Hannah cancelled several appointments, eventually leaving a brief message saying that she was doing much better and that she was very busy and would call to reschedule when she had more time. She returned three months later at the urging of a friend who was aware that Hannah was not sleeping, had lost a great deal of weight, and had suffered several minor physical injuries. When she arrived, Hannah reported that in addition to her physical symptoms, which were beginning to concern her, she had little interest in doing anything or seeing anyone and little hope that things would get better for her in the future.

Avoidantly attached clients, particularly those who, as Muller (2010) has suggested, developed this orientation in response to early experiences of abuse or neglect, are likely to be guarded in relation to the grief therapist. They often display a reluctance to self-disclose, and their tone may at times become hostile. The avoidantly attached client will frequently minimize any need for help with their grief. Within the sessions, they will appear wary of losing control of their emotions or making themselves vulnerable in the clinical encounter. Moreover, they often appear to be out of touch with or dissociated from their own thoughts and feelings about their loss, tending to minimize its impact on themselves and their life or showing an inability to articulate their feelings (Deno et al., 2013).

Avoidant clients may show little interest in cultivating on-going psychological connection with the deceased, since they will see this as either not possible, or not necessary. The clinician may find themselves wondering "Is this all you feel?" or "Why don't you seem upset about this?" In response to questions about past losses or early experiences with caregivers, avoidant clients will typically state that "everything was fine," or "it was no big deal," or they may say that they are unable to recall memories and associated feelings about childhood. They may have an initially impressive ability to intellectualize about their experience, but their story will often lack a sense of the deep feeling that loss usually elicits in people. They will usually want practical answers, advice, and tools for coping – particularly about quickly restoring their functioning and "getting on" with their lives. In terms of the Dual Process Model, these clients often present with a premature and exclusionary Restoration Orientation, one which allows them to avoid going deeply into a Loss Orientation.

The likelihood of ruptures in the therapeutic relationship with avoidant clients will be reduced if the clinician is respectful of the boundaries that the avoidant client has so assiduously constructed, both in respect to their response to the loss, and their engagement in the therapeutic process itself. The overarching goal in working with an avoidant client is to help them, gradually and at their own pace, develop access to and tolerance for their negative emotions about the loss, while supporting their ability to explore, and then extract themselves from, the depths of their grief.

Michael

A father seeks grief support six months after losing his 17-year-old son to cancer. A successful lawyer with one younger son, the client reports that he copes by staying very busy, and for the most part is able to keep his emotions in check. However, at least once or twice a day, usually without warning, he starts to cry. This is very disturbing to him, and he is very self-critical about his crying. The clinician introduces him to the idea that if he makes some time and space for his feelings – if he allows them to be there without judgement – they will be less overwhelming. She briefly explains the rationale for this suggestion and the research on which her recommendation is based.

Finally, while early trauma is most often associated with disorganized attachment (see below), Muller proposes that it is also a factor in the development of an avoidant attachment orientation (Muller, 2010). Avoidantly attached individuals, he writes, remember and report traumatic events, but tend to minimize their meaning or negative impact. Referencing Bowlby's concept of *defensive exclusion*, Muller describes avoidant attachment as a strategy developed to keep hurtful attachment experiences out of awareness:

> Having developed a worldview that others cannot be depended on, the individual tends toward a pattern of self-reliance and a view of self as independent, strong, and normal. Along with this pattern, there is a tendency to dismiss and devalue experiences of closeness, intimacy and vulnerability.
>
> (p. 2)

The Disorganized Client

Vince

> Vince first sought help following the death of his best friend in a house fire. In the course of his sessions with the therapist it became apparent that Vince had significant problems with anxiety. He used alcohol to self-medicate, mostly on weekends, and was able to function at work. In gathering information about Vince's history before the loss, it emerged that his mother had died two years earlier. He did not at first have much to say about his mother, but what soon became clear to both the therapist and client was that Vince's anxiety had begun in childhood, a time in his life when he often felt alone and afraid. Vince also admitted that he felt very alone, doubted his capacity for intimacy, and feared that now that his friend was gone he would be completely alone.
>
> As a fuller picture of Vince's early life emerged, the traumatic nature of his childhood and extent of unresolved feelings about his mother came more clearly into focus. Speaking of her, Vince became quite agitated, and his sentences became disjointed and contradictory, reflecting the nature of the relationship with a woman who was alternately nurturing and (usually after several cocktails) terrifying. Vince described his mother as "two people … and you never knew which person you were going to get. Even now, I can't tell you if she was a good mother or a bad mother, a sober, responsible person or just a raging alcoholic".

In our experience, many people who seek help in dealing with complications in their bereavement have the kind of early relational trauma reported by Vince. The observation that early trauma is prevalent in people who present in treatment with bereavement issues has been widely reported and contextualized by Sekowski and Prigerson (2022b). In Vince's case, problems with emotion regulation that could be traced back to a chaotic and frightening childhood became overwhelming in the aftermath of his friend's death. The flood of feelings, and the sudden traumatic loss of the one person he had been able to turn to for support, set off a secondary wave of painful memories about his childhood, many of which involved a similar sense of being alone and unsafe.

Vince's description of his mother as "two people", one safe and comforting, and the other frightening and hurtful, brings to mind Main's accounts of the mothers of infants classified as disorganized with respect to attachment (Main & Solomon, 1986). Main observed that the behavior of infants whose mothers exhibited this kind of erratic and unpredictable behavior was likewise, unpredictable and contradictory, as though the infants were never sure about whether they should approach, or avoid, their caregiver. In the most extreme cases, these infants lapsed into a state of dissociation, immobilization and feigned death (Main & Hesse, 1990). These responses can persist into adulthood, and are often evident in the behavior of bereaved adults who, in the language of the AAI, have unresolved losses or trauma (Thomson, 2010). In the following example, a bereaved client exhibits the shutdown and dissociation described by Main, a response that as discussed in Chapter 3, may be a reprise of her first and best strategy for coping with emotional pain.

Marta

Marta, 42, sought grief counseling after the death of her father. It seemed difficult for Marta to settle in the therapist's office, and she spoke of her father in a halting manner, stopping often to look down at the floor until she was prompted by the therapist to continue. Marta had no long-term relationships and few friends. Her relationship with her mother and siblings was strained, and she spent much of her time alone. Marta explained that health problems had prevented her from living a fuller life, but she was not able to clearly describe the nature of her symptoms or why she had not been able to find any relief from them.

In discussing Marta's history, it emerged that her father had been a "difficult" man, and that her mother frequently had angry outbursts that included physically attacking her children. Questions about the extent of the abuse and her father's involvement in it were met either with silence or with fragmented accounts of violence between various family members, some of it directed at Marta.

Soon after beginning treatment Marta indicated that she wanted to understand more about her childhood and why she was so reluctant to go anywhere near the neighborhood where she had grown up. Several attempts were made to help Marta assemble memories of her childhood, but on each occasion, her narrative would become fragmented and dreamlike, until she stopped talking and sat staring into space. On some occasions these episodes were preceded by Marta reporting that she felt a tingling in her legs, followed by loss of feeling in her lower extremities.

Retelling the story of a painful and frightening childhood is a difficult, but critical component of treatment for many survivors of early attachment trauma (Allen, 2001, 2013). However, when this memory work results in a dissociative, shut down response, it is our practice to reconsider and adjust the course of treatment (Rothschild, 2000). This type of response in a client signals the need for work on building internal resources and external sources of support, as detailed in Part III. Once these resources are in place it may be possible to resume building the narrative and to move the client, one step at a time, toward whatever reconstitution of memory helps them to make sense of their current functioning. For example, a client who goes through life convinced that other people cannot be trusted, and who looks for the insult in every comment directed their way, may not relate these attitudes to early relational trauma. By providing an explanation of the effects of early trauma, the clinician can help the client begin to modify their appraisal of the intentions of others, which may be the first step in helping the client reduce interpersonal conflict and build social support.

Audrey

Although her father had died two years before, Audrey, 51, still felt his presence every day. The emotional abuse that she and her siblings had suffered as children continued to affect all of them, but in different ways, and it was hard for her to talk to either of them about her childhood, or about what they had been through growing up. Her relationship with her mother was even more problematic, largely because of her mother's refusal to acknowledge that theirs had been anything but a "perfect" family.

In the two years since her father's death Audrey's life had "collapsed"; she had lost her (good) job and had a series of brief, unsuccessful relationships. Her poor health was also a matter of serious concern. She did not have the energy to look for a new job and was about to lose her condo. She was afraid that if that happened she would then have no alternative but to move in with her mother.

The intensity of Audrey's account of her relationship with her father and her tendency to periodically lapse into the present tense in talking about him were evidence of the lack of resolution concerning Audrey's early trauma and her father's death. She felt that the residual effects of her father's unrelenting verbal attacks had left her crippled, depriving her of the energy, direction and will needed to establish a "normal relationship and a normal life."

Audrey was able to access many memories of her childhood; but these memories only fueled her anger, frustration, and sense of powerlessness. Financial difficulties that arose while Audrey was being seen in therapy led to her moving in with her elderly mother, with whom Audrey had a relationship precariously balanced between love and hate. Within a few weeks of moving in with her mother, Audrey reported that she was "mad all the time." Her anger was frequently triggered by comments from her mother that she interpreted as expressions of her mother's belief that Audrey was incompetent and would never be able to live independently, even though she had been doing so for more than two decades. Perhaps the hardest to bear, Audrey heard in her mother's criticism the voice of her father, who could emotionally flatten any member of the family with his furious contempt.

As these examples illustrate, survivors of abusive and/or neglectful early caregiving, many of whom have features of disorganized attachment, face a number of difficulties in dealing with grief, including impaired emotion regulation, mistrust of others and difficulties finding a comfortable balance between being dependent on and independent of others, problems with cognitive and executive functioning, and low self-esteem (Allen, 2013). The reluctance to let down their guard reflects the experience of being mistreated by, and consequently being afraid of, their caregiver. The negative view of self is a holdover from childhood when most of what they heard and internalized was criticism and accusation. Given the deeply embedded nature of their low self-regard, these clients tend to reject positive comments regarding their strengths or competencies. The more hopeful and positive the clinician, the greater the likelihood that the clinician's opinions will be dismissed, resulting, paradoxically, in an empathic failure in the therapeutic relationship.

In keeping with their need to protect themselves from others, people with a disorganized attachment orientation shaped by early trauma tend to attribute hostile or critical intent to others, and the speed and intensity with which they rise to their own defense makes it difficult for them to establish or sustain healthy relationships, even though they may yearn for such attachments. Like Marta, they may not have a clear memory of specific incidents of abuse, but over time, a sense of the danger and dysfunction of their early family life may come into focus. When the memories and emotions do come back, the person is then confronted with a whole new set of questions, the biggest one being, "Why"? This is a question that Vince confronted again and again as he tried to make sense of his mother's frighteningly erratic behavior. Like Audrey, he despaired of ever being able to understand the behavior and intentions of other people well enough to risk letting them get close. The ability to hold another person's mind in mind – to mentalize – is something that, ideally, children develop in the context of an attuned, caregiving relationship. A child who has not had the opportunity to develop this capacity is at a disadvantage in forming and sustaining close relationships. Lacking in the ability to mentalize, they may feel as if their encounters with other people are forever taking place in a dark room, without the benefit of any clues as to other peoples' mood or intentions.

As a senior staff psychologist and later Director of Psychology at the Menninger Institute, Jon Allen has observed and written about the lasting effects of trauma for over 40 years. The focus of his recent work has been on the concept of mentalizing: what it is, why it is important, the adverse impact of early trauma on mentalizing capacity, and the role of psychotherapy in restoring mentalizing capacity in work with trauma survivors. (Allen, 2013). He proposes that

> mentalizing – attending to mental states in oneself and others – is the most fundamental common factor among psychotherapeutic treatments ... To be effective – in establishing a therapeutic alliance, for example – we clinicians must mentalize skillfully; concomitantly, we must engage our patients in mentalizing.
>
> (Allen et al., 2008, p. 1)

THE RESTORATION OF MENTALIZING: A COMMON FACTOR IN ATTACHMENT INFORMED GRIEF THERAPY

Allen has written extensively on the impact and lasting adverse effects of early abuse and neglect (Allen 1995, 2001, 2003). Young children have emotional and physical needs that they cannot fulfill on their own, and they become distressed if an attuned caregiver is not present to satisfy them. An attuned caregiver understands well enough the child's thoughts and feelings, mirrors back these aspects of the child's experience, and responds to the child's needs based on that understanding. Part of what Peter Fonagy refers to as mentalizing, this process is at the heart of healthy emotional development, a premise we have examined in previous chapters. The engaged presence of a caregiver who can mentalize accurately about the child's experience and then reflect that back to the child is central to what enables a child to become aware that they are an independent being who has the capacity to understand themselves and to expect that others will understand them. Put differently, the empathic attunement involved in mentalizing on the part of the caregiver supports the development of mentalizing in the child. In Allen's view, mentalizing is the "psychological glue that bonds attachment relationships" as well as the foundation of emotion regulation (Allen, 2013, p. 31). In the absence of mentalizing on the part of the parent, the child is "left psychologically alone in unbearable emotional states repeatedly" (Allen, 2013, p. 31). Allen proposes that treatment in these cases begins with the creation of a safe therapeutic environment, which promotes the development of mentalizing and with it, increased capacity for emotion regulation. A key element of our approach to attachment informed grief therapy is that the therapist, performs the fundamental function of an attachment figure in a secure bond, supporting reregulation in the short term and promoting the growth of internal self-regulation over the longer term, by virtue of strengthening the individual's capacity for mentalization.

In childhood, secure attachment enables a child to move flexibly between seeking safety and engaging in learning and exploration. In adulthood, the goal is much the same. In grief therapy, this flexibility is what enables the bereaved person to move between a loss and restoration orientation, between abject grief and emotional equanimity. Supporting emotional and behavioral flexibility, as we have seen, is a goal not just for grief therapy with survivors of early relational trauma, but for grief therapy as a whole.

Vince

Over the course of a year, Vince began to identify the roots of his anxiety in the frightening and unpredictable conditions of his childhood environment. It was difficult for Vince to acknowledge just how out of control his mother had been on many occasions because he felt that talking about these memories was a kind of betrayal. He eventually came to realize that what was at issue was not a need to blame his mother, but to assign responsibility for events in his life that had resulted in a negative sense of himself, a view bound up with shame about his own drinking. It was important for Vince to realize that he did not have to vilify his mother, but neither did he have to totally absolve her of responsibility for her behavior. What he needed to do instead was see her behavior for what it was, and then to consider some of the factors in her own life that had led her to behave as she had – in other words, to mentalize about his mother. As the intensity of Vince's feelings about his mother decreased, he was able to talk about her, and ultimately about the loss of his friend, without becoming overwhelmed. While he continued to periodically refer back to his childhood experience, Vince became increasingly interested in talking about his present life and his goals for the future.

These cases illustrate the connection between attachment experience and bereavement, and accord with research that has identified attachment as a significant factor in a range of life transitions and stressors, including significant loss (Burke & Neimeyer, 2013). In the remainder of this chapter, we will expand upon the role of attachment status as a factor in response to loss. Specifically, we will consider the implications of viewing attachment as a neurobiological system helping to maintain physical and psychological homeostasis, and the dysregulation that inevitably results from the death of a loved one – an event that permanently removes from a person's life an object of attachment or who in some way was critical to system functioning. Finally, we will place insecure attachment within a broader context of complicated grief and look at how it relates to and interacts with other factors – specifically traumatic death and kinship – that are also known to intensify and prolong the dysregulation resulting from the death of a loved one (Parkes, 2013; Parkes & Prigerson, 2008).

ATTACHMENT, LOSS, AND DYSREGULATION: INSIGHTS FROM NEUROSCIENCE RESEARCH

As discussed in Chapter 3, findings from neuroscience research have demonstrated the lasting impact of the quality of early caregiving and the persistence of regulatory deficits in children and adults who do not receive adequate physical and emotional nurturance. These deficits are associated with a range of emotional problems and with difficulties in coping with a variety of life stressors. While many life events can impact a person's psychological functioning and physical well-being, several writers have suggested that significant interpersonal loss imposes a uniquely significant strain on coping capacity and biological regulation (Sbarra & Hazan, 2008; Rubin, Malkinson & Witztum, 2020; Shear & Shair, 2005). Shear and Shair offer a model of the mourning process that is informed by attachment theory and by Hofer's (Hofer, 1996) animal research on the role of attachment relationships as "biobehavioral regulators." According to Hofer, in mature adults, many of the mutual regulatory functions of relationships are maintained by an internal representation of the relationship when the attachment figure is not available. Thus, adults do not need the continual physical presence of an attachment figure to feel secure and to keep their attachment system deactivated. Instead, the internal representation of the person largely serves that function, as long as the psychological availability of the attachment figure is not threatened. However, as Shear and Shair observe, and as we have noted above, the death of an attachment figure is a different matter. Responding to this kind of loss requires the mourner to confront the *permanent absence* of the deceased both as a real and present attachment figure and as a representational attachment figure in the individual's internal working model of the relationship.

Another important contribution to our understanding of interpersonal loss as a uniquely significant stressor is Sbarra and Hazan's analysis of research concerning the physiological and emotional impact of bereavement (Sbarra & Hazan, 2008). Consistent with the position taken by Shear and Shair (2005), as well as by Mikulincer and Shaver (2008), Sbarra and Hazan argue that the grief triggered by the loss of an attachment figure is fundamentally different than the response to other types of (non-relational) loss.

> When long term mate relationships end, many adults lose the person who helps them maintain psychological and physiological homeostasis ... Accordingly, when relationships dissolve, it is this state of security that must be regained as individuals recover from separation and loss experiences.
>
> (Sbarra & Hazan, 2008, p. 142)

This understanding of the impact of partner loss, which is supported by research concerning the neurobiology of adult attachment, the functional elements of human co-regulation, and the particulars of biobehavioral response to attachment figure loss (Shear & Shair, 2005; Pietromonaco, Barrett, & Powers, 2006; Mikulincer & Shaver, 2008b) accords with Schore and Schore's assertion that the primary function of attachment relationships is to *interpersonally regulate multiple biological and psychological systems within the individuals involved in the relationship* (Schore & Schore, 2008, 2014). It is also consistent with Mikulincer and Shaver's discussion of grief as a *dysregulation of these systems* (Mikulincer & Shaver, 2008a). Citing Mikulincer and Shaver, Sbarra and Hazan explain that the loss of a significant attachment figure deprives us of the felt sense of safety that enables us to engage in exploratory activity. Sbarra and Hazan integrate this view of dysregulation into a two-stage model of grief in response to relational loss. The first stage is dysregulation, a consequence of the disruption of homeostasis described above. The transition from dysregulation to the "organized stress response," represented by the Dual Process Model, comes second.

The authors suggest that we can better understand how the DPM process of oscillation breaks down in complicated grief by understanding *the role of attachment relationships in regulation of biological systems*, and the dysregulation that results from loss of the attachment figure. In Sbarra and Hazan's model, the sleep disruption, loss of appetite, and decreased energy associated with acute grief result from the loss of a person who served a "homeostasis maintaining function" (Sbarra & Hazan, 2008, p. 149). In the immediate aftermath of loss, these admittedly distressing symptoms can have an adaptive function. Like the weakness and fatigue that accompany physical illness, these symptoms are arguably "part of a state that aids in physiological reorganization and recuperation during times of stress" (Sbarra & Hazan, 2008, p.153). In other words, grief depletes our energy and makes it hard for us to focus on the things that usually occupy our attention, facilitating increased attention to the reality of the loss and the feelings associated with it. Grief forces us to slow down, so that we can adjust to the changes presented by the loss.

However, when this acute phase of mourning does not abate, the result is a continued flow of stress hormones and compromised immune functioning, along with a number of other negative biological events that adversely affect mental and physical health (Kiecolt-Glaser et al., 2002; Thoits, 2010). Sbarra and Hazen conclude that managing the biological dysregulation associated with the loss of an attachment figure is "the chief task in coping with loss" (Sbarra & Hazan, 2008, p.161). Lacking this support, the mourner may default to maladaptive regulatory strategies and relationship behaviors that adversely affect their physical health and their relationships with others.

O'Connor (2019) has reviewed research on the physical and psychological impact of grief, including multiple epidemiological studies that have identified increased morbidity and mortality during bereavement.

> The increased risk is for all-cause mortality, including cardiovascular disease, acute health events, chronic disease, and cancer.
>
> (Elwert & Christakis, 2008)

> This increased risk from bereavement is higher than well-established cardiovascular risk factors, such as smoking.
>
> (O'Connor, 2019, p. 735)

In a further examination of neuroscience findings related to grief and loss, O'Connor & Seeley (2020) propose that the dysregulation that characterizes grief arises from a conflict between the bereaved's expectations regarding the "everlasting nature" of the attachment figure, and "episodic memories of the death" (p. 317).

> Our gone-but also-everlasting model emphasizes that grieving may be a form of learning, requiring time and experiential feedback. Difficulties before the loss, such as spousal dependency or pre-existing hippocampal volume, can prolong learning and predict PGD.
>
> (p. 317)

Prolonged stress and inflammation, O'Connor suggests, may signal that the individual is developing complicated grief. These findings also highlight the fact that grief affects people in different ways and manifests in varying degrees of intensity. Support for of this conclusion also comes from fMRI studies reported in Chapter 3. In all, adverse neurological and physical effects reported in response to loss seem to predominate in those with the most severe grief reactions. In light of these findings O'Connor recommends that future research "should assess grief severity and not lump those with complicated and noncomplicated grief together" (O'Connor, 2019, p. 736).

These themes – of dysregulation, from mild to severe, in response to loss, and of the role of attachment figures, including the grief therapist, in facilitating reregulation – are ones that we will return to throughout the remaining chapters of this book.

FROM REREGULATION TO INTEGRATION

Taken together, these observations from Cozolino (2010) make an interesting point about recovery from bereavement:

When all is well and we are in a state of calm, there is no reason to learn anything new. At the other extreme, states of high arousal and danger are not the time to learn anything new ...

(Cozolino, 2010, p. 231)

We need to always keep in mind that as primates, attachment equals survival and abandonment equals death.

(Cozolino, 2010, p. 285)

First, Cozolino tells us that human beings tend to learn new things when there is a *need* for them to learn new things, i.e., when there is a disconnect between what we know, and the knowledge we need to survive and succeed in a changing world. In this sense, a certain amount of discomfort is good. But too much arousal, too much discomfort, and we are not able to learn. And if, as Cozolino succinctly puts it, the loss of key relationship triggers terror in a person, then as long as that state continues, it is unlikely that the person will be able to learn anything new. With respect to grief therapy, this would suggest that the dysregulation brought on by acute grief must be brought within manageable limits before the integration of experience can occur. Before the therapist can help a grieving client to explore their relationship with the deceased, and with the new world they face in the absence of their loved one, the immediate, acute physical and psychological impact of the loss must be addressed. Once a certain amount of reregulation and system "settling" has taken place, then the client can begin to learn, and to rebuild an internal and external world in congruence with their changed circumstance.

Even mourners with a secure attachment orientation will for a time be dysregulated by the loss of a loved one. For these individuals, intervention may be more on the order of "grief counseling" than "grief therapy" (Worden, 2009, 2018). While dysregulated by their loss, helping mourners to re-regulate and begin to adjust to life without their loved one may primarily be a matter of being a good listener, helping to normalize what they are going through, and offering a cognitive scaffolding for understanding their reactions to the loss. For individuals with insecure attachment, the process is likely to be more complicated, and treatment more nuanced and tailored to the client's specific attachment orientation. Yet even in these cases, as we already have seen, the attuned therapist can help a client reregulate and begin to focus flexibly, openly, and honestly, on the work of establishing a continuing bond with the deceased, while attending to the demands of their new life, and the relationships that remain a part of it.

For many bereaved people, living with grief is a daily hardship that feels unbearable, until they bear it, and discover that there are still things in life that can surprise and delight them. The opportunity to be a witness as people discover their own strengths, to be there when the flicker of light in their eyes signals the beginning of renewed hope for a future in which happiness is once again a possibility, is part of what makes counseling the bereaved such fulfilling work. In Part III we will describe and illustrate how this process unfolds.

SUMMARY

Our goal in this chapter has been to demonstrate the role of attachment in grief and to illustrate the variety of ways in which factors related to attachment can contribute to complications in grief. A further goal has been to suggest that sensitivity to attachment orientation or style can help the therapist develop and strengthen the therapeutic bond with the client and avoid errors that may compromise that bond over the course of treatment.

We began with an overview of bereavement models and noted that as grief professionals' understanding of grief has deepened, these models have undergone significant revision. Both the Two-Track Model and the Dual Process Model depart from the earlier idea of a fixed grief trajectory and instead draw attention to the range of grief responses and the multiple factors that affect the course of bereavement. Both models recognize the importance of attachment orientation, and the Dual Process Model, in particular, draws upon Bowlby's views regarding the role of attachment security in enabling a person to respond to loss in a manner that promotes healthy adaptation.

Mikulincer and Shaver make explicit use of Bowlby's theory in their explanation of how insecure attachment compromises the ability to flexibly attend to thoughts and feelings related to the loss and those related to ongoing relationships and responsibilities. Further research conducted by Mikulincer and Shaver and others supports these theoretical assumptions about the importance of attachment in how people respond to significant loss. Additional support for the importance of early attachment experience on grief comes from neurological studies that provide evidence of the lasting effects of childhood trauma and neglect on people's ability to manage stress and recover from events that disrupt and dysregulate their emotional equilibrium.

With case illustrations from our own practices, we then began to address some of the implications for practitioners of an attachment informed approach to bereavement therapy. We concluded with a brief examination of attachment relationships as a co-regulated biobehavioral system that becomes dysregulated by loss, bringing attention to the imperative for the therapist to bring the system back within tolerable bounds before the real work of reintegration and restoration can begin.

We come into the world primed for connection, knowing instinctively that our very survival is at stake. Our complex brains have a long way to go, developmentally speaking, and our bodies (irresistible as they may be to our parents) are not fit for much beyond the consumption and extrusion of essential nutrients. Our needs at this juncture are simple but nonnegotiable, and our dependence on others is absolute. But our dependence in infancy goes beyond the need to have our physical needs attended to. Our caregivers' ways of responding to our arrival will influence how we feel about ourselves and will factor into our assessment of the risks and rewards of connecting with others.

The multiplicity of variables that influence early development and the potential for developmental derailment is, as we have seen, cause for concern for many reasons, only one of which is our concern for people's capacity to cope with loss. Our concern is amplified when we consider the role of early attachment experience in neurological development, in particular the limitations in regulatory capacity that are associated with early relational neglect and trauma.

Life, it seems, involves increasing complexity and increasing risk. At the outset we have little to do and little to worry about. Life happens *to* us when we are young; with age comes the understanding that to a large extent life is what we make of it. This realization can be difficult to come to terms with, especially for people whose early relationships did not prepare them for dealing with stressful events and the painful emotions that accompany them.

In these first chapters we have followed in the tracks of attachment theorists, touched on the work of neuroscientists, and considered the utility of contemporary models of grief. In the next two chapters we will direct our attention to variations in bereavement response and bereavement treatment that are attributable to two related sets of factors: those having to do with the kinship relationship with the deceased, and with trauma in the mode of death.

5

THE IMPACT OF THE RELATIONSHIP WITH THE DECEASED

To begin to understand the nature of a person's grief we need to understand what it is that they have lost, which we can only do if we understand what it is that they *had*. The loss of a significant attachment figure, in many cases, deprives the griever of access to the very person they have been used to depending on for help in managing painful emotions.

Self-sufficiency, it seems fair to say, is regarded as a virtue in our culture. But there are limits to self-sufficiency. In his book *A General Theory of Love*, psychiatrist Thomas Lewis tells us in no uncertain terms that the mammalian nervous system does not do well in isolation. Total self-sufficiency, he tells us, is a myth. "Stability" Lewis writes "means finding people who regulate you well and staying near them" (Lewis et al., 2020, p. 83).

Relationships serve different functions and fulfill different needs in people, and these differences are reflected in the diversity of responses to loss. In this chapter, we will examine the impact of a variety of relational factors on adjustment to loss, including kinship relationship to the deceased, the nature of the relationship with respect to dependency, emotional distance or proximity, and other psychological factors. We will also look at findings concerning how these factors affect the quality of the attachment bond with the deceased *after* the death has occurred, a relationship that has been described as the continuing bond with the dead

DOI: 10.4324/9781003204183-8

(Klass et al., 1996; Klass & Steffen, 2017). We will then explore the implications of these findings when viewed through the lens of modern attachment theory.

The grief that follows attachment loss leaves the bereaved with an empty space inside, and in this chapter we will consider factors that contribute to the size and shape of that space, including the position of the relationship in the griever's relationship hierarchy (LeRoy et al., 2019).

KINSHIP RELATIONSHIP WITH THE DECEASED

Death of a Spouse/Partner

> Your absence has gone through me
> like thread through a needle.
> Everything I do is stitched with its color.

Separation, W. S. Merton[1]

In most western cultures adulthood is a time when, sooner or later, a person's primary attachment relationship is transferred from parents to a spouse or partner (Holm et al., 2019; Walsh & McGoldrick, 2013). Ideally, the relationship a person builds with their life partner provides an emotional safe haven in times of distress, and a secure base for dealing with the larger worlds of work and social relationships.

Thanatology researchers have focused a great deal of attention on the impact of partner loss, with many of these studies concentrated on the loss of a married spouse among the elderly (Carr & Jeffreys, 20011; Carr et al., 2006; Meichsner et al., 2020). These studies have identified a number of negative sequelae of partner loss, including elevated rates of depression, anxiety, complicated grief, financial difficulties (particularly for women), loss of social connections, and excess mortality, including suicide (particularly for elderly males) (Hybholt, 2020; Innamorati, et al., 2011). Among the elderly, the emotional burden of loss often comes at the end of an extended period in which the survivor has cared for their partner through a long and debilitating illness, and is already stressed and exhausted (Holm et al., 2019). However, these negative outcomes are by no means universal or inevitable after the death of a long-term partner. Instead, researchers have identified several different loss trajectories after the death of a partner, which range in intensity and duration from a relatively minor and short-lived disturbance in the surviving partner's functioning, to chronic depression and/or complicated grief in other mourners (Meichsner et al., 2020).

Fewer studies have been conducted of the grief of younger widows and widowers, with the cutoff being age 45 (Taylor & Robinson, 2016). Available evidence suggests that younger spouses generally experience more psychological distress, a finding that in many cases appears to be related to increased difficulties of single-parenting and economic hardship that may accompany the loss of a partner in the child-rearing years (Chami & Pooley, 2021; Taylor & Robinson, 2016). Young people who have lost a partner, and who also have children by that partner, may worry that their deceased spouse will be forgotten, particularly by children too young to have clear memories of the parent. In effort to shield their children and maintain a sense of "life going on" parents often suppress outward signs of sadness. Bereaved spouses also express a determination not to put their children in the position of having to provide care or comfort. This suppression of grief contributes to an atmosphere in which in which grief cannot be shared by all family members.

Many of the challenges that accompany partner loss are related to the long-term nature of the relationship, and the functional and emotional interdependency that marriage and other long term intimate relationships entail. Life partners provide economic benefits, sexual and psychological companionship, reciprocal affect regulation, emotional support for coping with stressful events, the opportunity for shared parenting if children are involved, labor sharing around domestic responsibilities, and mutual caregiving in times of illness. Loss of a person who is relied upon to fill these role functions amplifies the responses that are characteristic of partner loss: yearning, loneliness, anxiety about coping in the world without the partner, and a sense of disorientation about how to proceed in life (Meichsner et al., 2020).

This is particularly true in cases where the marriage was a source of love, comfort, and safety previously absent in the survivor's life. The importance of such a relationship is suggested by Popova and illustrated in the case that follows.

> Some loves can unseal, irradiate, and heal those small dark old places in us where joy has been compacted into a hard dense loneliness.
>
> (Popova, 2021)

Jane is a woman in her early seventies whose husband died two months ago. His death came at the end of a three-year period of progressive decline, during which time Jane was his primary caregiver. In the following exchange with the first author, Jane reflects on her years of caring for a mother whose mental instability and erratic behavior kept Jane in a constant state of hypervigilance.

> J: *With my mother there was no point having feelings, she was never going to see or care about my feelings. Since Richie died, with a lot of people I know, I feel the same way I did then: people don't want to know how I feel ...*
>
> *I understand now how I spent my life trying to get out of the line of fire. Trying to avoid the attack, even if the attack wasn't directed at me. And you know what - this is*

how I got onto this track. When my mother died, I didn't shed a tear. I couldn't wait for my mother to die. I truly felt that way. I had a therapist who said: she couldn't help it. And there were a lot of things that my parents did for me. But that doesn't make up for all of the craziness. I didn't feel anything when she died.

PK: *You didn't get the kind of love and nurture that children need, and that connects them to their mother. When people grieve the loss of their mother, that's what they're grieving -the feeling of being seen, and valued, and loved. What they're grieving is the loss of all of that. The feeling that no one else is going to love them the way their mother loved them.*

J: *Absolutely.*

PK: *When you don't have that as a child, what happens is that everything you know, everything you feel, gets suppressed. Your feelings don't matter so you just shut them down. So that you don't even know at a certain point what your feelings are.*

With Richie, there was such a depth of love, and understanding and compassion that he drew you out of yourself.

J: *It was the first time in my life that I didn't have to perform to have someone have my back. And I didn't have to worry that all of a sudden the peace would just explode.*

The way I grew up - I realize that it impacts you for life. Even though you may go on and live your life.

Anyway, I guess I lost my security blanket.

PK: *Yes, I understand. I get all of that.*

Attachment and Partner Loss

A growing body of research suggests that one of the most robust predictors of complicated grief following partner loss is the attachment style of the bereaved partner (Parkes, 2013; Fávero et al., 2021). This includes both the bereaved individual's attachment style in the relationship with the deceased partner and the attachment style developed by the individual in their family of origin. For example, numerous studies have shown that high levels of dependency in the marital relationship are usually associated with poorer bereavement outcomes following the death of the spouse (Campbell & Stanton, 2019; Mikulincer & Shaver, 2019). Dependency appears to be a marker for an anxious or preoccupied attachment style in both the relationship with the deceased, and in the mourner's general attachment style (Johnson et al., 2008). In these instances, the marriage may have helped the spouse by offsetting earlier attachment deficits, including difficulties with emotional self-regulation. Without the partner's support, these difficulties may reemerge, leading the mourner to transfer their dependency to family members and friends. The strain placed on these relationships can lead to a further loss of support and an increasing feeling of isolation on the part of the mourner.

Referencing research findings that link difficulties in emotion regulation with insecure attachment, Fávero et al. (2021) reviewed studies designed to assess the role of emotion regulatory capacity in the quality of romantic relationships. In a dyadic relationship, emotion regulation is a "bi-directional co-regulatory process that enhances the couple's emotional satisfaction and stability and strengthens emotional connectedness" (p. 2). The quality of romantic relationships is enhanced when partners are able to effectively regulate their emotional responses. In contrast, difficulties in the co-regulation of emotion regulation within relationships can be destructive to the partners' bond. Based on their review the authors conclude that a partner's limited ability to regulate their emotions creates "excessive demand of the partner's attention and motivates intense emotional reactions that tend to produce the opposite effect, driving the partner away". Problems also result when there is emotional deactivation and suppression of emotion (Fávero et al., 2021, p. 4). When the partner of someone with an anxious or avoidant attachment style dies, the surviving partner may experience difficulty in managing their emotional response, as illustrated by the two case examples that follow.

Jennifer

Jennifer is a 68-year-old woman whose husband has been diagnosed with ALS. She has two adult children. She has had a long and happy marriage and is extremely tearful as she talks about her husband's diagnosis and her fears about what is to come. "It's like I'm in building where there's an active shooter, and I'm hiding, but I know it's only a matter of time until he finds me". The prospect of living without her husband is terrifying for Jennifer. "When I think about living without him I just start shaking. I can barely breathe."

(She begins to cry). "He's not going to be there. And I won't want to do anything or go anywhere. I'll be locked inside of myself. And nothing will matter. I can't go on without him."

Anne

Anne is 73 and lost her husband after an extended illness, during which time he became bedridden and required round the clock at home nursing care. She has come for counseling at the suggestion of her daughter, who cannot understand her mother's absence of grief. At our first meeting Anne guiltily admits that most of what she feels is relief. "He was just so sick, and he suffered so much, and I did too, and the house was always full of people, so it didn't even feel like my home anymore, it felt like a hospital."

Anne wants to "get through" her grief, which to her means that she wants to be able to return to the way life was before her husband got sick. What she doesn't want is to feel sad, and to avoid sad feelings she concentrates on remembering "how bad it was at the end. I don't think about the time before, because if I do I just feel sad and what's the point of that? I hate that feeling. I hate feelings. What good can they do?"

Attachment-oriented researchers interested in the differences evidenced in relational patterns throughout life point to the role of internalized mental models that develop within the first social interactions with primary caregivers (Fraley & Hudson, 2017; Simpson & Rholes, 2017; Theison et al., 2018). These experiences create representations about the self and others, which become the guiding framework for expectations and responses to future relationships (Bowlby, 1969, 1982; Ainsworth, 1979; Sroufe, 2016; Simpson & Rholes, 2017).

Similar to securely attached infants in the Strange Situation, securely attached partners are able to engage in independent activity away from the attachment figure. Security "transforms the relationship into a goal-corrected partnership, creating the conditions for a confident and autonomous exploration, including the establishment of secondary bonds" (Fávero et al., 2021, p. 3; Hazan & Selcuk, 2015).

These findings related to the establishment of secondary bonds bear on LeRoy's concept of a "loss hierarchy" (LeRoy et al., 2019). Expanding upon Sbarra and Hazan's (2008) original model, they suggest that "the degree to which an individual's physiological systems remain dysregulated depends on the state of one's attachment hierarchy – "namely, whether an individual continues to seek their lost partner for support as their main attachment figure" (p. 391). Some degree of longing and searching for the lost partner is to be expected in grief. But to recover from the loss, an individual's attachment hierarchy must be reorganized such that, over time, they can direct their attachment-related needs toward a new primary attachment figure a process that is likely to present difficulties for grievers who have not developed a network of bonds outside of their primary partner relationship.

Death of a Child

One of the most consistent findings in bereavement research is that the death of a child has a significant and sometimes very long-lasting impact on most parents – especially on mothers (Buckle & Fleming, 2011; Lundorf et al., 2017; Meisenhelder et al., 2020).

Mothers express intense feelings of pleasure and satisfaction when they are able to protect and comfort their children; they experience heightened anger, sadness, anxiety, or despair when they are separated from the children, or when their ability to protect and comfort the child is threatened or blocked.

(George & Solomon, 2008, p. 835)

The literature suggests that the death of a child (including adult children) is experienced as an event that is out of the developmental order of life and one that may engender profound feelings of helplessness and failure on the part of the parents. This is true regardless of the cause of death; however, parents who see the death as being one that they believe they could have prevented (e.g., SIDS deaths, suicide, drug overdoses) are particularly vulnerable to feelings of guilt and failure (Feigelman et al., 2012; Goldstein et al., 2018; Lichtenthal et al., 2013; Zetumer et al., 2015).

Empirical studies have demonstrated that bereaved parents can experience high levels of problematic reactions, including intense sadness, guilt, depression, and yearning for the child; increased levels of marital tension or estrangement from the other parent (although increased divorce rates have not always been found). Furthermore, these effects last longer than those arising from other forms of kinship loss (Zetumer et al., 2015; Zhao et al., 2020).

In a review of research on parental grief after the death of a young child, Morris, Fletcher & Goldstein (2018) examined findings from 42 studies focused on the identification of risk factors associated with complicated grief in this group of parents. While bereaved parents generally recover day to day functioning, many report a permanent state of yearning that does not diminish over time. The researchers report that the loss of a young child "from virtually any cause" represents a "significant burden of complicated or prolonged grief. The severity and chronicity of grief experiences following the death of a young child "is potentially a distinct subtype of grief, deserving of attention in its own right in future research and diagnostic formulations" (Morris et al., 2018, p. 321). In an investigation of the long-term effects of child loss on parental health, Zhao et al. (2020) found significant disparities in health outcomes and social integration in a sample of 1,828 bereaved parents compared to 4,739 non-bereaved parents, with the most severe and enduring adverse health effects in parents who lost their only child.

Studies of maternal grief after the sudden and unexpected death of an infant point to a high level of risk for significant grief related complications in this population (Goldstein et al., 2018). A study of over 400 mothers whose infants had died aged between two and four and were involved with support groups in the United States, South Africa, Australia, New Zealand, the United Kingdom and the Netherlands found that symptoms of prolonged grief disorder, including daily, intrusive emotional pain or yearning were "common, distressing, and persistent … with discernible symptom profiles" (p. 5). In comparison with the prevalence of 9.8% prolonged grief disorder in bereaved adult life partners one year after a loss (Lundorf et al., 2017), Goldstein et al. found that 57.1% of these young mothers had PGD at 1 year and 41.3% had PGD in their third-year post loss (Goldstein et al., 2018, p. 5). Rates of role confusion, anger, and diminished trust in others remained constant.

Attachment and Child Loss

To understand bereavement, Bowlby (and most subsequent attachment theorists) have largely focused on the model of a distressed child seeking reunion with a caregiver/attachment figure. However, Bowlby also discussed an additional and crucial behavioral system: *the caregiving system* (George & Solomon, 2008; Mikulincer & Shaver, 2007; Solomon & George, 1996). Other neurologically based researchers and theorists have likewise described the biological basis of the caregiving system and its manifestation in adult intimate relationships (Coan, 2008; Nelson & Panksepp, 1998; Panksepp & Biven, 2012). As with attachment behaviors, caregiving behaviors are biologically rooted in the vital need to protect the helpless human offspring, and as such, confer an evolutionary advantage on the infant who is the recipient of such behaviors (Archer, 1999). Also like attachment behaviors, the caregiving behavioral system can be understood as having a set-point goal: nurturance, protection, and ultimately, survival of the child (George & Solomon, 2008; Mikulincer & Shaver, 2007). As such, an extremely diverse range of behaviors can be seen as falling into the category of caregiving behaviors. Anything from a mother nursing her infant, to a parent earning an income to support the family or put a child through college, can be broadly understood as caregiving behaviors. And lastly, like attachment behaviors, the caregiving bond reflects an intense affective bond between the caregiver and the child and tends to be particularly activated by separation and threat. *In short, the caregiving behavioral system is the reciprocal of the attachment behavioral system, but it has a different goal – the protection of another person (usually a dependent child), rather than protection of the self.*

Simply put, parents serve as a secure base and a safe haven in times of distress for their offspring, but in healthy family functioning, the reverse is *not* true, at least with young children. Parents seek proximity with their distressed child, not to assure their own physical survival, but that of their children. Of course, successfully protecting and nurturing of a child can engender powerful feelings of gratification and accomplishment in a parent – key elements of the psychological identity of parents. It has also been postulated that parents are "wired" by evolutionary forces to try to ensure that survival of their genetic legacy (Simpson & Belsky, 2008). In this very broad sense, caregiving does involve a parent's attempt to survive, psychologically and genetically. It is also true that the role of caregiver and care-recipient can and often do reverse. This can be observed when adult children assume the role of caregiver and attachment figure for their aging and more dependent parents (Field & Wogrin, 2011; Nuttall et al., 2021). Additionally, it has long been noted that in dysfunctional family systems, younger children often take on the role of a psychological (or even physical) protector of their parents, a premature reversal of these roles sometimes referred to as a "parentified child".

But this is generally viewed as a pathological deviation from the normal positioning of parent and child in healthy family development (Walsh & McGoldrick, 2004).

We believe that in order to appreciate the impact of child loss on bereaved parents, it is crucial to understand this fundamental difference in the goal or set-point of caregiving behavior. Unlike the common attachment theory formulation that grief in adults is similar to separation distress in a child who has been separated from an attachment figure, when a parent loses a child, much of the emotional pain endured by a bereaved parent has to do with the perceived failure to protect and nurture the child – ultimately, to keep the child from death. In a very real sense, the feelings that bereaved parents report after the death of their child are the mirror-image of the attachment-based feelings that a child may experience upon separation from their parent(s). Perhaps most prominent of these are the intense feelings of yearning for reunion with the child, a kind of *caregiver proximity seeking* that reflects the deep feelings of purpose and pleasure that nurturing and protecting a child may provide. Likewise, there may be protest at the separation from the child through death, although most commonly this anger is directed at the self and manifests as guilt over the child's death, not anger at the child for abandoning the parent (the suicide of a child may be an exception to this). Bereaved parents can also display a tremendous amount of attachment related anxiety about the child's well-being that is accompanied by an urge to search for their child. All of this occurs despite the parent's cognitive understanding that their child is dead. In short, parents display attachment type behaviors and emotions after the death of their child, but they are the result of bonding with their child as the recipient of their caregiving efforts, not as the loss of an attachment figure. The primary aim of the behavior, rather than providing safety and security for the parent, is to provide this for the child – a persistent response, even when the child is deceased. Put differently, the caregiving behavioral system may stay activated for a considerable period of time after the death of a child, and the gradual deactivation of it is a central component of the grieving process for grieving parents.

So: are the theories of child loss sufficient to capture the experience of losing a child? Yes and no. It depends on how broadly we define "theories of child loss". If we cast a wide net, and include insights from neuroscience and attachment research, maybe we come close; if we include literature and art, maybe we come closer still. In his novel about the death of Abraham Lincoln's 11-year-old son, author George Saunders describes the depth of Lincoln's suffering, and his need to lift the boy's body from the coffin and hold his son in his arms.

> Sinking his head into the place between chin and neck, the gentleman sobbed, raggedly at first, then unreservedly, giving full vent to his emotions.
>
> (Saunders, 2017, p. 157)

In Saunder's imagining of this moment, Lincoln struggles to understand why he has come, what is this need to visit the crypt and hold his son's body. In answering his own question Lincoln expresses feelings that we have heard expressed many times by bereaved parents.

> *All over now. He is either in joy or nothingness.*
> *(So why grieve? The worst of it, for him, is over.)*
> *Because I loved him so and am in the habit of loving him and that love must take the form of fussing and worry and doing.*
>   *Lincoln in the Bardo*, George Saunders, 2017, p. 157[2]

Death of a Sibling

Attention to the impact of sibling loss has until recently been limited, as compared to other relational losses. Fanos observed in 1996 that when a child dies, we recognize the devastation of parents, but overlook the unique grief of siblings. Research has been scant in terms of the impact of sibling loss and attention to the needs of bereaved siblings (Davidson, 2018).

Much of the available research has focused on the effects of sibling loss in childhood (Marshall & Davies, 2011). although recently there has been an increase in studies of adult sibling loss (Holland & Rozalski, 2017). Clinical experience, as well as memoirs and other narrative accounts, tell us that the loss of a sibling at any age can have a significant and lasting impact on surviving siblings (Holland & Rizalski, 2017; Kaiser, 2014).

In 1989, Kenneth Doka defined disenfranchised grief as "the grief that persons experience when they incur a loss that is not or cannot be openly acknowledged, publicly mourned, or socially supported" (p. 4). Some observers have suggested that given the lack of support offered to bereaved siblings, and the relative lack of research on sibling grief, the designation of disenfranchised applies here (Davidson, 2018; Schuurman, 2022). Disenfranchisement may also help to explain the sense of isolation and alienation from others that is prevalent among surviving siblings (Funk et al., 2018). Jill Ker Conway (1989), writing of her brother's death when he was 21 and she was 15 described the lasting effects of this loss.

> After my brother Bob's death, it seemed as though I had lost the capacity for emotional responses. Daily life was in black and white, like a badly made film. He had been like the sun in my universe. I realized I would always be trying to live out his life for him.
>
> (Conway, 1989, p. 121)

The prevalence and persistence of sibling grief were the subject of a Swedish population-based study by Sveen et al. (2014). The group included

174 young adults who were between 12 and 25 years old at the time of their sibling's death from cancer. The average time since loss was 6.3 years. Respondents completed a questionnaire designed to ascertain the extent to which respondents had worked through their grief over the sibling's death (Sveen e. al., 2014). Reporting on their findings, the researchers found a high incidence of unresolved loss, with a majority (54%) of study participants stating that they had worked through their grief "not at all" or "to some extent". Lack of social support, a hallmark of disenfranchised grief, was among the factors identified as contributing to ongoing grief.

A longitudinal study by Bolton et al. (2016) examined the prevalence of mental disorders and treatment use among bereaved siblings in the general population. Results revealed that at two years after the death, 25% of bereaved siblings aged 13 and older were diagnosed with a mental disorder, vs. 17% of controls. The bereaved group also had higher rates of almost all mental disorders compared to controls, including twice the rate of suicide attempts. Herberman, Fullerton and Ursano (2013) examined the association between types of loss (i.e., sibling or close friend) and relationship quality (i.e., depth and conflict) and complicated grief, depression, somatic symptoms and world assumptions in bereaved young adults (17–29 years old), 66 of whom had lost a close friend and even a sibling withing the previous three years. Nineteen percent of the group met criteria for complicated grief. Respondents who lost a sibling reported greater depth in the relationship and were also more likely to have complicated grief (57% vs. 15%). The sibling loss group also reported significantly higher levels of depression, somatic symptoms and lower sense of meaningfulness, benevolence in the world, and self-worth as compared with those who lost a close friend or who had not experienced a loss.

Although the consequences of sibling loss in adulthood have begun to draw attention, Wright (2016) argues that "the adult sibling bond is not generally recognized as significant, which can leave the bereft sibling feeling isolated and misunderstood" (p. 43). In her review of research on adult sibling loss Wright cites evidence of a range of psychological problems in this group, including depression, complicated grief, fearfulness, a negatively changed worldview, increased depressive symptoms, and regret about not spending more time with the sibling. The sibling bond is based in genetics, in shared life experience, in mutual memories of our younger selves. Siblings grow up by our side and occupy a particular place in our relational geography. Even if the relationship was not ideal, when an adult loses a sibling, the result is an emotional space that is not easily filled.

Attachment and Sibling Loss

As with the other losses being described in this chapter, it is useful to examine the function that siblings play in each other's lives in order to understand the impact of this type of kinship loss. For many adults, the sibling relationship is the longest continuous relationship in their life, spanning childhood, adolescence, adulthood, and on into later life. They provide continuity to an individual's identity and sense of personal history in a way that is unmatched by other relationships. Siblings (usually older siblings) may also serve as role-models for how to deal with parents, other authority figures (e.g., teachers), and peers. They thus can be an important source of learning and new information about the world for younger brothers or sisters, particularly around differentiation from the family of origin.

Depending on the nature of the sibling relationship, their birth order, and the family dynamics surrounding their childhood, siblings may serve as important additional adjunct attachment figures during childhood development, providing psychological security, support, and an important intimate relationship. They may help to counteract some of the negative effects of dysfunctional attachment dynamics between children and parents in the family, mitigating the effects of neglectful or abusive parenting. Of course, sibling relationships can also be a source of significant conflict and competitiveness during childhood and can sometimes have a major impact on the development of emotional insecurity and low self-esteem, particularly when parents selectively favor one sibling over another. The reciprocal of this family dynamic for the favored child is a sense of guilt, unworthiness, and sometimes hyper-responsibility for a sibling who is openly out of favor with the parents.

For some siblings these functions may continue into adulthood and even old age. They include serving as a foundation of emotional support and identity, as well as later functions of financial support or practical help in childcare, management of aging parents, etc. This can have obvious benefits when the adult sibling relationship is close and more or less egalitarian. However, it can also have predictable disadvantages when the siblings continue to act as rivals or antagonists towards one another. The emotional gravitational pull of family of origin dynamics between siblings, even among otherwise well-functioning and autonomous adults, is a common clinical problem (Jordan et al., 1993).

With a specific interest in attachment as a factor in sibling loss, Charles and Devon (2006) investigated the association between attachment style and coping methods in young adults who experienced the death of a sibling in their lifetime. The investigators predicted that securely attached and preoccupied individuals would be more likely to use social support strategies than individuals with nonsecure attachment styles, and dismissive–avoidant and fearful–avoidant individuals would be more likely to use distancing strategies than the other attachment styles (p. 82). While their first prediction was born out results, a contrary finding was that regardless of attachment style," sibling loss seems to stimulate greater support seeking than other stressor". The researchers urge clinicians to be attuned to the effects of sibling loss, which may not be readily apparent.

> Even when the child appears to have adapted quite well to the loss, clinical data show us that failure to effectively grieve and to work through the relational fears and inhibitions that may be associated with such a loss can be quite pervasive and longstanding ... We have each worked with young adults who appear to be socially and emotionally quite resilient, and yet behind this facade there may be quite severe fears that inhibit the individual from attaching too closely to others. Being aware of this potential, given the individual's history, may help the clinician to be more attuned to what may be quite subtle signs of unresolved loss and concomitant difficulties in forming deep and lasting attachments.
>
> (p. 86)

Attention to feelings left over from childhood also need to be identified and addressed when working with an adult grieving the loss of their sibling. This may be a time when regrets about unhealed wounds and words of love not expressed weigh heavily on the griever. The following vignette portrays the depth of such feelings and illustrates how painful narratives about the past can be revised in a way that relieves some measure of the bereaved's suffering.

Max

Max, a man in his late sixties, came to speak to the first author after the sudden death of his brother from what appeared to be a heart attack. Max described his older brother, who was six years older than Max as "the smartest person I ever knew and the fairest person I ever knew." His brother "spent a lot of time" with Max when he was a child and took him to basketball games and baseball games and to the movies. Asked what his brother would say to him now, if he were able to address Max, Max replied tearfully that he would "probably say something about the Yankees or about Trump."

P. (smiles) Yeah. And what would you say to him?

M: I would say "I love you". (he begins to cry). I never said it. And he never said it to me.

It was very hard when my brother left. I was 14. I wrote him a letter and asked him to come back. That's how upset I was. I asked him to come back. He came back at Thanksgiving.

I haven't thought about this, I'm remembering it now. He came home, and a lot of family was at the house, and someone said that I had written my brother a letter asking him to come home. They said that. They made fun of me. And I didn't say anything, I just went to my room, like I was going to do homework, but no one would have believed that, because I never did homework.

P: That was so unkind, and it must have hurt you. It hurts, when we show how we feel, and somebody makes fun of us for feeling that. You were an emotional person – you still are. That's the kind of person you are.

*M: I was in my room, and my brother came in. It's so weird, I'm just thinking of this now. He came in, and he said, "Listen, you're OK. I know you love me, and I love you. Forget about them." Shaking his head, Max repeated: "That's so weird, that I'm remembering that now. **He did say it.**"*

Death of a Parent

What is lost when a parent dies?

The impact of losing a parent, like other kinship losses, is influenced by when in the lifecycle the loss occurs. For young children, the death of a parent can be the loss of a loving and comforting sanctuary, a place of refuge from everything in the world that is unfamiliar and uncaring. In this passage, author James Agee takes us inside the mind of a child to suggest an answer to the question of what parents provide, and what a child loses, when a parent dies:

> *I hear my father, I need never fear.*
> *I hear my mother, I shall never be lonely, or want for love.*
> (Agee, 2009, p. 76)

For adults, the impact of the loss is different, but the feelings may be distressingly similar. At any age, the loss of a parent can throw a person off balance and leave them with a sense that they are in some way *less than* who they were when the parent was alive. Some piece of a identify, of knowing who one is (my mother's daughter) and to whom one belongs, is lost when a parent dies.

Research on the grief of parentally bereaved children, adolescents and adults has provided a picture of the difficulties that are common to grievers at different stages of life. These findings present a general picture of grief response, the specific nature of which in any case is impacted by other moderating and mediating variables.

Children

The grief of children who have experienced the death of a parent has been extensively studied and findings illustrate the heterogeneity of their response and adaptation to this loss. Common children's grief reactions include sadness and crying, anxiety (including about their own or others' safety), guilt, anger and acting out, physical difficulties including somatic symptoms, illness and accidents, problems at school, sleeping difficulties, and vivid memories. While many grief reactions abate, others can persist or emerge later (Cockle-Heard et al., 2021).

A substantial contributor to the heterogeneity of children's responses to parental loss is their age at the time of the death (Hunter & Smith, 2008). The nature and persistence of grief are also influenced the developmental stage of the child at the time of the loss. Writing about these differences in terms of Erikson's stages of development, Sekowski (2000) argues that this model has been underutilized as a framework for understanding attitudes toward death and response to loss. Authier (2022) notes that these developmental differences not only influence a child's response to loss, but in addition, can affect the therapeutic alliance:

> At the extreme they could contribute to trust issues with their grief counselor if the loss occurred during infancy to 12 months, impair their ability to be autonomous if 1 to 3 years of age, increase guilt issues if from age 3 to 6, lessen their ability to be industrious in age 6 to 12 and negatively affect one's self concept age12 to 18 ...
>
> (Dr. J. Authier, personal communication).

The ongoing development of a child's understanding of death presents a challenge for clinicians working to establish a therapeutic alliance with a young client. Knowledge of these age-related differences is a prerequisite for work with bereaved children.

Studies of children's response to the loss of a parent have focused on school age children, with a concentration on studies of the effectiveness of grief support programs for bereaved children and their caregivers. In a systematic review of evaluations of support programs for parentally bereaved children and their caregivers, Bergman, Axberg, and Hanson (2017) reported positive effects for a variety of interventions, including groups for children, family interventions, and guidance for parents, The authors conclude that these studies, 15 of which involved randomized control groups, demonstrate that relatively brief interventions can have positive effects for both children and the remaining caregiver's health.

A question frequently posed to professionals by grievers and by people anticipating a loss concerns the relative impact of sudden traumatic death, vs. anticipated death, as in the case of a long illness. Findings concerning how the nature of the death affects children's grief suggest that losing a parent through prolonged illness can cause higher levels of maladaptive grief or posttraumatic stress for children than losing a parent through sudden death (Bylund-Grenklo et al., 2021). Prolonged illness offers an opportunity to prepare the child for their parent's death, but research suggests that this opportunity is not used to the child's benefit (Cockle-Heard et al., 2020). One of the reasons cited for this gap in care is the reluctance of some parents to upset their children by discussing the parent's illness. However, when no support was provided before the death, provision afterwards was perceived to be more challenging. Time, and the opportunity to build trusting relationships with families, was seen as prerequisite to easing parents fears and helping them find ways to prepare their children for their parent's death. Pilot programs designed to encourage communication with children in anticipation of a parent's death have proven useful for some families (Weber et al., 2022).

No one can deny the difficulty of having to tell a child that their parent is dying. Whatever findings suggest regarding the importance of communication, the final decision about end-of-life communication rests with the family. Whatever their feelings about the child's implicit understanding that something is wrong, and their belief that the child will be better served by being told some version of the truth, there will be times when a clinician will need to stand with the family in their decision not to disclose the facts of the parent's illness. The empathic clinician understands that not all decisions at the end of life conform to a hypothetical best-case scenario.

Adolescents and Young Adults

Guzzo & Gobbi (2021) reviewed research from 1987 to 2020 on parental loss in adolescence. The authors based their selection of studies on the World Health Organization (2021) definition of adolescence as ten to 19 years old. The discrepancy with other research with regard to age is a complicating factor in interpreting results. Nevertheless, the findings from this review shed light on the large range of reactions and responses observed in adolescents who have lost a parent.

The grief of adolescents and young adults has been the subject of several qualitative studies designed to provide a deeper understanding of the impact of parent loss on this age group. Porter & Claridge (2021) report that the bereaved young adults they interviewed faced "unique challenges related to their developmental stage" (p. 191). Emerging adulthood is a time when many young people are transitioning away from their families of origin and developing their own independence; yet they are often not fully certain of their ability to function without the support of the safety net provided by their parents.

Another study examined prolonged grief symptoms among 224 undergraduates who had lost a loved one within the previous two years (Klingspon et al., 2015). Participants who lost a parent reported a number of stressors in addition to the stress of the death of the parent.

The decision to leave or to. stay at home after the death was fraught with conflicting emotions. Some respondents were resentful about putting their lives on hold, while many who chose to leave felt guilty about their decision.

A study of young adults aged 16 to 28 who lost a parent to cancer found that they experienced poor psychosocial well-being over the first year and a half after the loss (Lundberg et al., 2020). Taking a longer view, Bylund-Grenklo et al. (2021) interviewed a group of 622 young adults (18 to 26) who had lost a parent to cancer from six to nine years earlier. Participants were asked about their experience of grief in the first six months after the death. Data from this part of the questionnaire was used to identify the group that, during the stage of acute grief, agreed with the statement "I had a way to grieve that felt okay." Alternative responses offered to participants included "I clenched my teeth, built a wall around me and lived on as if nothing had happened"; and "I withheld my grief to protect my other parent" (Bylund-Grenklo et al., 2012, p. 3)

More than half (57%) of the cancer-bereaved teenagers responded that they *had not* had an okay way to grieve. These experiences of acute grief were associated with difficulties in grief six to nine years' post-loss, measured with the single item question: "Have you worked through your grief?" with responses ranging from "No, not at all" to "Yes, completely." Respondents who had not worked through their grief reported being overwhelmed by grief, being discouraged from grieving, or concealing their grief to protect their other parent. Clinical recommendations based on these emphasize the importance of communication with young adolescents faced with the loss of parent. Respondents who were told about the parent's impending death, and who had had an opportunity to talk with the dying parent about matters that they perceived as important were more likely to have had an "okay way to grieve" in the acute post-loss phase (Bylund-Grenklo, 2021, p. 11).

Adulthood

The death of an elderly parent, which is the most common form of bereavement in the developed world, is typically the least disruptive of losses for adults (Balk, 2013), although many factors, including the nature of the relationship and the level of dependency influence bereavement in adults after the death of a parent. Another consideration in parentally bereaved adults is the likelihood that they have experienced previous losses of family members and friends. The accumulation of loss can lead to what Kastenbaum (1969) was the first writer to refer to as "grief overload". Even if they have not had many previous losses, parentally bereaved adults tend to feel that in losing their parents, they have been "orphaned", an uneasy feeling that is compounded by a heightened awareness of their own mortality.

Attachment and Loss of a Parent in Adulthood

Attachment theory suggests that by the time adulthood is reached, the relationship between the child and their parent has been internalized as a working model of both interpersonal connection, and emotional security. In addition, the need for attachment figures has been largely transferred to other important persons in the individual's life, including their spouse, siblings, and close friends (Jordan et al., 1993). The death of an older parent is likely to produce sadness and nostalgia over the loss of a key figure from one's past, and perhaps someone who continues to play an important role in the family as a grandparent. But it typically does not produce the intensity of attachment related feelings of insecurity, anxiety, and yearning in adults who had developed a secure attachment with their parent during childhood, and have subsequently transferred that attachment to partner and other adults (Moss et al., 2001).

All of this presumes, however, that the grieving adult is relatively secure in their attachment orientation and that they have the necessary psychological and social resources to support healthy adaptation to loss. When an anxious, avoidant attachment or disorganized orientation originating in childhood is sustained into adulthood, the death of a parent may produce a considerably more complex and problematic response. In these cases, the process of differentiation from the parents has been only partially completed, and the developmental work of transforming the relationship into one of mutual respect among equals may have important lacunae that become apparent in bereavement. For example, winning a parent's approval may continue to be a strong motivation for contact between parent and child, and the failure to win the parent's esteem a major source of concern for the anxiously attached adult child. Or, for an avoidantly attached offspring, interaction with their parent may continue to be filled with resentment and conflict that is managed by emotional and geographical distancing. Still another variation involves substantial financial and emotional dependency on the parent by the child. This is frequently accompanied by a failure to make successful connections with a life partner outside the family of origin and/or a failure to create a successful work/career trajectory without the help of the parent. In summary, when there has been a truncated process of differentiation between parent and child, and something other than a secure attachment style has evolved between them, then there is likely going to be an upsurge of attachment related emotions and complicated grief reactions upon the death of that parent(s).

Janice and Albert

A middle-aged woman named Janice and her husband, Albert, sought couples therapy for on-going marital conflict and unhappiness. It quickly became apparent to the therapist (JJ) that the husband had a very hostile and unresolved relationship with his self-absorbed, abusive, and alcoholic father, with whom Albert had developed a very avoidant attachment style. He continued this pattern with Janice, so that her angry demands that he provide more intimacy and support in the marriage were usually met with a defensive withdrawal on Albert's part. In contrast, Janice was an only child, and she was heavily involved in a mutually co-dependent relationship with her widowed mother – her father having died when Janice was five years of age. Janice and her mother had thus been mutual care-takers for one another for most of Janice's life. They had multiple daily contacts by telephone and in person. This level of contact was fueled by her mother's 20-year battle with cancer and Janice's need to protect her mother. This need to provide help to her mother was accompanied by significant anxiety about how Janice would cope without her only parent. Janice had worried for years about the well-being of her mother, essentially since the death of her father. Albert, in turn, was resentful and critical of what he perceived as his wife's over-involvement with her mother, and what he believed was his mother-in-law's manipulative use of her illness to keep Janice closely enmeshed. Perhaps predictably, as the mother finally moved closer to actually dying, Janice experienced a tremendous upsurge of anxiety about the loss of her "only friend", and an even greater amount of caregiving involvement on her part. After her mother died, Janice went into a significant depression, reacting not only with sadness about her mother, but with deep feelings of being alone in a world where she felt unable to fend for herself – reminiscent of what a five-year-old child might feel if her parent had died.

This case vignette illustrates some of the dynamics when attachment related problems are transmitted intergenerationally (Jordan et al., 1993). The loss of the father for a young mother and her five-year-old daughter set up a deep and fixed pattern of dependency and mutually anxious attachment between the pair. The normal close involvement between a five-year-old child and her parent became filled with anxiety about feared separation that warped the developmental processes of healthy separation between the two, so that Janice, although demanding more intimacy with her husband, did not feel psychologically free to engage emotionally with him. The husband, although he resented his wife's enmeshment with her mother, also was mystified about how to provide the emotional security that his wife craved, and that might have allowed her to have a more balanced and differentiated relationship with her mother. This difficulty on the part of the husband could be directly traced to the avoidant attachment style that he developed in his family of origin, where closeness to a parent was emotionally (and sometimes physically) dangerous – and distance was the only safe refuge from the risks of intimacy.

CONTINUING BONDS

Until relatively recently, mental health professionals have operated under the assumption that the normal work of grief necessarily involves confronting the reality of the physical death and relinquishing the emotional attachment to the deceased, sometimes called the griefwork hypothesis (Worden et al., 2021). Note that this was not Bowlby's assumption (Bowlby, 1980), nor is it the view represented in some long-standing models of the mourning process, among them the Two-Track Model of Bereavement (Rubin et al., 2012). However, the fullest expression of this perspective of an ongoing relationship came with the publication in 1996 of the ground-breaking book *Continuing Bonds* (Klass et al., 1996) which was later updated (Klass & Steffan, 2018).

Klass et al. propose that most bereaved people around the world and throughout recorded history have maintained some type of psychological connection with their deceased loved ones, despite their physical absence. This important shift in our understanding of the mourning process has led to a considerable amount of theoretical and research activity over the last 15 years, including by attachment theorists (Boelen et al., 2006; Kosminsky, 2018; Rubin et al., 2012; Wood et al., 2012). In the remainder of this chapter, we will explore the concept of continuing bonds (CB) with the deceased, and its implications for an attachment informed approach to grief therapy.

The concept of continuing bonds with the deceased as a positive outcome of bereavement has gained widespread clinical acceptance, and a number of techniques have been proposed that seek to enhance the CB relationship (Neimeyer, 2012f). Despite this change in practitioner views, research evidence has been mixed and complicated as to role of CB has in facilitating bereavement recovery. For example, Field suggests that not all CB are necessarily adaptive or helpful, and that the usefulness of maintaining a CB with the deceased (particularly in partner loss) is dependent on the form it takes (Field & Filanosky, 2010; Field et al,, 2003; Kosminsky, 2018) and the amount of time since the death (Klass & Steffan, 2017).

Field has also offered an empirically-based framework for understanding and distinguishing between adaptive and maladaptive CB between the mourner and the deceased (Field, 2006, 2008; Field et al., 2005). Building on the theoretical work of Bowlby, Field posits that healthy bereavement adaptation requires acknowledgement of and accommodation to the fact of the death, i.e., recognition that the deceased has physically died and cannot ever be available again in this fashion. For some mourners, this unalterable reality is unbearable. It produces what Bowlby called a mentally "segregated system" (Bowlby, 1980), which could also be described as a dissociated state of mind. In the literature of traumatology, dissociation is a primary human response to unbearable trauma of all kinds for which there is no escape (Schore, 2002b, 2002c, 2013). Thus, death results in a permanent and unfixable trauma for the bereaved. In essence, the mourner operates with two separated states of consciousness, one in which the reality of the death is acknowledged, and the other in which the death is not recognized. Note that this is not the same as believing that the loved one is in heaven – a conviction that acknowledges the physical reality of the death on earth. Instead, Field describes this as the mourner continuing to behave *as if* the deceased has not died – and in extreme cases, to consciously believe this to be the case. Signs of this process can include great distress at making changes to the deceased's belongings, active avoidance of triggers associated with the death (e.g., refusal to attend the funeral or visit the grave), and speaking of the deceased in the present, rather than past tense.

Field notes that these types of continuing bonds, which involve holding onto *external* aspects of the relationship with the deceased, are common in the early days and weeks of mourning, particularly after sudden and unexpected death. However, externalized continuing bonds gradually give way to an acknowledgement and acceptance of the fact that the loved one is dead. This in turn makes possible a transformation in the form of the connection with the deceased, what is referred to as an *internalized* continuing bond This revised bond is characterized by an acceptance of the reality of the biological death (with its attendant emotional grief responses) and a newly reorganized psychological and/or spiritual connection with the deceased (Field, 2006, 2008; Field & Wogrin, 2011; Pearlman et al., 2014; Scholtes & Browne, 2015). To cultivate this revised bond, mourners reflect on memories of the deceased and identify their own values and goals. They may continue to hold the decease as an internalized attachment figure.

To summarize, Field argues that adaptive CB can be distinguished from maladaptive CB by the extent to which the mourner has transformed the attachment to the deceased from one of an external relationship with a living person to an internal psychological connection to a deceased person – a transformation that acknowledges the reality of the physical death. Field and others have provided empirical support for this model, demonstrating that people who manifest an external connection have significantly poorer bereavement outcomes, while those with a transformed and internalized connection show better outcomes (Field & Filanosky, 2010; Field et al., 2013).

IMPLICATIONS FOR AN ATTACHMENT APPROACH

What are the implications of the continuing bonds perspective for attachment informed grief therapy? A number of authors have addressed this topic (Ho et al., 2012; Kosminsky, 2018). As originally conceptualized by Bowlby, attachment theory emphasized the important role of internalization of attachment relationships as the basis for healthy developmental separation. Thus, what allows the developing child to tolerate separation from his or her attachment caregivers is the internalization of a secure relationship with them. Analogously, CB theory and research suggest that the internalization of the relationship with the deceased allows the mourner to tolerate the permanent separation created by death. It follows from this that, psychologically speaking, *the deceased may continue to serve as an attachment figure for the mourner.* The form and function of this attachment may serve a number of different purposes that are worth enumerating. Most prominently, as the following case illustrates, the mourner may continue to use the deceased as an important source of felt security and safe haven, particularly in times of distress.

Susan

Susan was a middle-aged widow with a very anxious attachment style who sought grief therapy with the second author after the sudden death of her husband of many years. Susan's attachment history included being raised by a mother who herself was raised in foster homes after the early death of her own mother. Susan was subjected to neglect, empathic failure, and devaluing verbal abuse from her mother. Susan's relationship with her husband (also raised in an abusive family environment) included genuine aspects of affection and intimacy, coupled with considerable conflict and hostile dependency. When her husband died, Susan was deeply saddened, but also tremendously frightened about her ability to cope in the world without her partner. She expressed an intense yearning for her husband's return, and a similarly desperate need for the therapist's sustained attention and care. With the help of the clinician, Susan was gradually able to step back from and observe the dynamics of her dependency on her husband, and to begin to manage her affairs without him. But the clinician also encouraged Susan to maintain a continuing bond with her deceased husband as a supportive attachment figure. For example, the clinician suggested that Susan trust what she believed were signs of her husband's watchful presence over her (e.g., the appearance of rainbows or jet contrails at just the time when she was feeling distressed). The therapist also actively supported Susan's efforts to consult with her husband by asking for his guidance in prayer and contemplating what support and advice he would offer her if he were alive.

This vignette illustrates not only that the perceived availability of the deceased can serve as a general source of comfort and reassurance for the mourner, but that the relationship may be used in ways that are similar to the period when the deceased was alive. In the case of Susan, her fears about making decisions and taking risks (such as buying a new car) were made easier by her use of her husband as a resource for making important decisions that were difficult for her to make on her own – a function that is a direct continuation of the role that he played in the marriage before his death.

Beyond serving as a safe haven during periods of distress, the deceased may also function as a secure base for exploration. For example, in cases of spousal loss where the dying partner offered their blessing for adaptation to a changed world, including remarriage after the death, the mourner may use this symbolic support from the dead partner to counteract feelings of disloyalty to the deceased, and to make necessary changes in carrying on without them.

Saul

Saul, who was widowed after the death from an illness of his beloved wife, rather quickly became involved with a single woman who had been close friends with his wife. Shortly after this new relationship began, while shopping for clothing in the same department store that he and his deceased wife had visited many times, he ran into a doctor who had managed his wife's care at the end of her life. The two men chatted fondly about Saul's wife. Without knowing about the new relationship, the doctor concluded the conversation with a firm statement that "I know that she would want you to be happy and find someone else." Saul found this conversation to be much more than just a chance occurrence. Rather, he had a powerful sense that his deceased wife was watching over him and had sent the doctor to him as a messenger with her wishes for how he should go forward. This encounter helped to resolve Saul's conflicting feelings about whether he should be getting involved with someone else after his wife's death. In addition, one of the effects of the new relationship was that Saul began exploring new activities and developing new interests outside of his work life – activities that "my wife always encouraged me to do".

The deceased may also continue as the recipient of the mourner's caregiving behavior. This is most clearly seen in the response of bereaved parents, who may continue to engage in symbolic caregiving behaviors such as tending to their child's grave or keeping their memory alive by consolidating and sharing stories about their child with others. Klass notes that this is one crucial function for parents of bereavement support groups such as Compassionate Friends, i.e., collectively holding and keeping alive the memory of the deceased child, thus allowing the CB to develop (Klass, 1997, 1999). All of these behaviors can be viewed as a continuation of the parental role with the child, and a reinforcement of the CB between parent and child.

Allison

Allison was deeply bereaved by the death of her adolescent daughter in a motor vehicle accident. They had had a close relationship, despite the strains that adolescent development had introduced in their lives. Caregiving for her daughter had always been Allison's first priority. After the death, Allison felt lost, without no sense of purpose beyond caring for her other, younger child. At one point, when she was talking about this void and the pressure that she felt from her husband to "move on" by making changes in her daughter's bedroom, the therapist (JJ) suggested that Allison consider taking a part of the room and converting it into a "shrine" – a dedicated memorial to Allison. He noted that the creation of family shrines for deceased loved ones, particularly children, was a common cultural tradition in many societies. Allison went home and immediately went to work on developing the shrine. She found great comfort in selecting photographs of Allison and some of her jewelry and other objects for the space. She also found that the ritual of keeping fresh flowers at the shrine, which required ongoing attention from Allison, was a source of devotion to her daughter that allowed Allison her to feel closer to her child. She reported that when the yearning for her daughter was particularly intense, she could go and sit before the shrine and talk with her daughter in a way that allowed her to remember the happy moments they had together, rather than the sadness about her absence. Allison has also been able to begin changing and discarding some of the other objects in the room, so that it can be used for other purposes.

A CB with the deceased may also entail more abstract functions that may or may not have been a part of the living relationship. For example, bereaved parents and siblings will sometimes report that the death of their child/sibling has provided a new sense of purpose and inspiration for their life (Lichtenthal et al., 2013).

Maria

Maria was devastated by the suicide of her 24-year-old son. This event was profoundly transformative for Maria, whose role up until her son's death was primarily as a housewife and mother to her children. After a period of time spent healing from her loss, Maria became a dedicated activist on behalf of other people bereaved by suicide in the U.S. Maria has organized survivor bereavement support groups in her state and has become a vocal proponent of the need for suicide prevention and postvention. Maria came to see this work as a living memorial for her son, as well as a way of restoring to her own life a sense of meaning and purpose that had been shattered by the suicide of her son.

These vignettes illustrate some of the many ways that maintaining a bond can be a source of comfort and reassurance to the grieving individual. Should we then to assume that continuing bonds are always of benefit to the bereaved, and that maintaining such a bond should be a goal of grief therapy?

ARE CONTINUING BONDS "GOOD" FOR THE BEREAVED?

The answer to this question is that like the relationship with a living person, a continuing bond with a deceased person may be helpful, or unhelpful, for the griever. Continuing bonds

> cannot be unilaterally described as having either a beneficial or a detrimental effect on the course of grief ... Given the role of attachment security in CB, individuals who enjoy a secure relationship with a living person are likely to

benefit from the bond they maintain with that person after they have died. Conversely, someone whose anxious or avoidant orientation to attachment interferes with their ability to sustain healthy, growth-promoting relationships is at greater risk for having CB that are problematic.

(Kosminsky, 2017, p. 112)

Finally, it is important to understand that, as with attachment relationships with a living person, a CB with the deceased may also change and grow over time (Malkinson et al., 2006; Rubin et al., 2012). Rubin and his colleagues note that this bond may have all of the characteristics of a relationship with a living person – affection, dependency, hostility, etc., and that it is possible for the relationship to transform over time from a disturbed and disturbing one into one of affection and support within the mourner.

SUMMARY

The relationships considered in this chapter are adult versions of the attachment bond between an infant and their caregiver as described by Bowlby. The loss of an attachment figure at any point in life deprives us of the benefit conferred that person, among them the "homeostatic regulation around physiological *and* psychological set points … ."

Accordingly, this experience portends not only emotional distress, but also autonomic hyperarousal, a loss of self, sleep difficulties, and many other challenges.

(Sbarra and Manvelian, 2021, p. 278)

The infant/caregiver bond, which in Bowlby's theory is the prototypical attachment relationship, provides the infant with the help they need to survive and grow, both physically and psychologically. When that support is provided the infant will gradually develop a capacity for self-regulation. But the dyadic nature of emotion regulation persists, to one degree or another, throughout life: humans do not "grow out of" their need for other people.

In this chapter, we have considered a number of relational factors related to bereavement, with particular attention to differences in bereavement associated with the kinship relationship to the deceased. Our relationships with parents, siblings, partners, and children serve many different purposes, fill many different needs, and are subject to many different kinds of expectations. These needs and expectations have a significant impact on people's grief responses. The violation of the expectation that their children will outlive them affects the intensity of parents' grief; the same may be true for a wife who did not expect that her husband would leave her to face life alone. Another important variable considered in this chapter is the nature of the continuing bond with the deceased. With respect to both of these variables, attachment theory provides a framework for understanding differences in grief response, and sensitivity to these aspects of people's grief is integral to attachment informed grief therapy.

In the next chapter, we examine another very important element of the response to bereavement – the mode of death – and focus on the profound ways in which homicide, suicide, and other forms of traumatic death affect bereavement. Attachment theory will again serve as our organizing principle for understanding how this factor affects bereavement, and how to provide effective therapy to the bereaved.

NOTES

1 "Separation" by W.S. Merton. Copyright 1993. Used by permission of the Wylie Agency.
2 Excerpt(s) from *Lincoln in the Bardo: A Novel* by George Saunders, copyright 2017 by George Saunders. Used by permission of Random House.

6

TRAUMA AND THE MODE OF DEATH

When someone we love dies, we feel the pain of separation and yearn for their return. The severity of these responses is subject to substantial variation, and up to now we have focused on how personal and relational factors contribute to these variations in how people respond to and cope with significant loss. But some deaths engender an extra burden of suffering for the mourner over and above these factors. In these instances, the *mode* of death – the manner in which the actual dying occurred – tends in and of itself to invoke reactions of shock, horror, rage, fear, guilt, and vicarious suffering in the mourner. These reactions can come in response to what the mourner saw, heard, touched, or smelled at the death scene. Or they can emerge simply from what the bereaved *imagines* the death scene looked like, and what they believe their loved one may have suffered as they died. The response of the bereaved in these cases involves a fusion of the grief and trauma responses that has been described as *traumatic bereavement* (Barlé et al., 2017; Boelen, 2020; Heeke et al., 2019; Pearlman et al., 2014).

In this chapter, we will examine the nature of traumatic losses and the grief they engender and offer some observations on different types of traumatic deaths. We will review the neurobiology of the trauma response, and briefly survey the empirical literature on the impact of exposure to a traumatic death. We will also outline the role of attachment relationships,

DOI: 10.4324/9781003204183-9

both early and current, in ameliorating or exacerbating the effects of a traumatic mode of death.

Sarah

Sarah sought grief therapy for her self-described complicated grief, three years after the suicide of her young adult son. The son had been depressed, living at home, and in considerable conflict with his parents. Sarah found his body hanging in the young man's living quarters in the basement of their house. He had been dead for several hours, and his mother realized with utter horror that she had slept through the night with her son's lifeless body hanging in the room below her own bedroom. Sarah recalls vividly every detail of the morning when she made that terrible discovery: how her son's face looked, how his body felt, and how the police and emergency medical responders acted. In addition to intense yearning for her son and self-blame for not preventing his death, Sarah was tormented by the memories of that morning, which have barely subsided in the three years since her son's suicide.

Raquel

Raquel's husband was piloting a small plane when a sudden change in weather conditions led to a loss of visibility and a rapid, uncontrolled descent. He survived the initial crash but died shortly after he was transported to the hospital. Raquel had spoken to him the previous evening and encouraged him to wait until another pilot more familiar with the plane could accompany him, but her husband, in characteristic fashion, had "made up his mind to leave the next day." Raquel feels guilty for not having tried harder to talk him out of making a solo flight, while at the same time, she is angry at her husband for what she sees as his stubborn insistence on taking an unnecessary risk. She knows that he was barely alive after the crash and can't stop thinking about what his last moments were like.

Suicides, accidental and natural disaster related deaths, and war or terrorist related casualties are all examples of deaths that would be considered traumatic. Other sudden deaths, as in cases of stroke, cardiac arrest, or seizure, for example, can also be terrifying, and the aftereffects of fear and helplessness can be felt for a considerable length of time. Studies of the effect of admission to Intensive Care Units (ICUs) suggest that these experiences can result in lingering symptoms of trauma for patients and families (Burki, 2019).

The link between traumatic loss and problematic grief is one that makes intuitive sense: suddenly, and in many cases, violently, someone who was with us, or at least someone we imagined would be with us again, is gone from the world. There is no time to prepare, no time to make amends, no time to say goodbye. We want to know the details of the death, and at the same time we can't bear to know them. These kinds of sudden, life-threatening events are easily understood as having traumatic potential. But the caregiving experience in illnesses such as cancer can also be traumatizing and can burden the griever with intrusive and disturbing memories of the loved one's agonizing decline and death.

Jane

Jane's husband died after a prolonged illness that ended in three years of decline, a period of sustained suffering punctuated by intermittent medical crises and loss of function. Jane was his primary caregiver and knows that "I did everything I could". She also knows that her husband "needed to go – he couldn't go on the way he was, every day was torture." As tears make it difficult for her to continue, Jane says: "I understand my grief, I accept that he's gone. But what I want to know is – how am I supposed to make sense of the last three years? What am I supposed to do with those memories?"

Research and meta-analytic reviews lend substance to these expectations concerning the increased risk of problematic grief in survivors of traumatic loss. In the first meta-analysis of prolonged grief disorder (PGD) Djelantik et al. (2020) synthesized 25 studies of grief following unnatural deaths such as accidents, disasters, suicides, or homicide with the goal of computing the pooled prevalence of PGD and possible causes of varied estimates in this group Whereas previous estimates of PGD hover at around 10%, "approximately half of the bereaved individuals" in the pooled sample "might develop symptoms which meet the diagnostic criteria for PGD" (p. 156). Some sub-groups are particularly vulnerable to PGD.

Our results imply that bereaved parents who lost their only child, and bereaved individuals following violent killings such as suicide, accidents, homicide, and war-related deaths are most vulnerable for developing PGD.

(Djelantik et al., 2020, p. 156)

THE NATURE OF TRAUMATIC DEATHS

What is it about certain deaths, such as suicides, homicides, and accidental deaths, that evoke the trauma response? In their review of research concerning grief in response to traumatic loss, Barlé, Wortman and Latack (2017) offer the following description of traumatic death:

A death is considered traumatic if it occurs without warning; if it is untimely; if it involves violence; if there is damage to the loved one's body; if it was caused by a perpetrator with intent to harm; if the survivor regards the death as preventable; if the survivor believes that the loved one suffered; or if the survivor regards the death, or manner of death, as unfair and unjust. Other deaths typically regarded as traumatic include those in which the survivor witnessed the death; those in which the mourner is confronted with multiple deaths; and those in which the survivor's own life is threatened.

(p. 128)

In addition to grief, traumatic deaths elicit profound feelings of shock, confusion, and above all, helplessness in the survivors. Since they are frequently perceived by the mourner as involving human volition, and therefore human error or malevolence, traumatic deaths are also more likely to provoke rage at others (e.g., a perpetrator or God) as well as a diminished sense of self-worth and intense feelings of guilt for not having prevented the death. Compounding and underlying all of these effects is what Kaufman (2002) has described as a "loss of the assumptive world": the collapse of the griever's system of beliefs about the benevolence and justness of the world, the health and continued presence of loved ones, and other expectations that contribute to a sense of predictability and safety in one's personal world (Barlé et al., 2017; Currier et al., 2008; Kauffman, 2002; Parkes, 1975).

Traumatic deaths, then, intensify the pain of loss and produce symptoms that are often frightening and overwhelming in their severity and persistence. Research on the neurobiology of trauma helps us understand the prevalence of traumatic grief among survivors of traumatic loss.

THE NEUROBIOLOGY OF TRAUMA

The neurobiology of the trauma response has been studied extensively in the last three decades (Michaels et al., 2021; Schore, 2002, 2012, 2019). Mammals (including human beings) have evolved a complex neurobiology that allows the animal to detect and protect themselves from threats in the environment, such as predators that could pose a danger. This emergency response system involves the rapid recognition of risk and subsequent behavioral response by the animal to deal with the danger. The amygdala, a crucial part of the limbic system of the brain that is associated with emotional memory, decoding of the emotions in facial expression, and appraisal of danger, produces an extremely rapid appraisal of the threatening stimuli (see Chapter 3). This is followed by activation of a neuro-hormonal cascade that runs from the hypothalamus to the pituitary gland to the adrenal glands (termed the HPA axis), and results in the body being flooded with stress hormones (e.g., cortisol). Simultaneously, the perception of a threat produces a swift activation of the autonomic nervous system (ANS). Specifically, there is a response by the sympathetic nervous system (SNS – the metaphorical "gas pedal" of the ANS). These two reactions (activation of the HPA axis and the SNS) produce a sudden arousal in the organs and systems needed for action – an increase in heart rate and blood flow to the large muscles of the arms and legs, and a shutting down of unnecessary processes such as digestion in the GI system. Visual and auditory attention is also greatly narrowed to focus on the specific source of the threat. All of this prepares the animal to either rapidly flee or to attack the threat – the so-called "fight or flight" response. Subjectively, this hyper-arousal of the SNS is experienced as tremendous rage or fear.

In situations where overcoming or escaping a threat are not possible, there is a third response which involves the opposite of this hyper-arousal of the SNS. This is the "freeze" response, which involves hyper-activation of the parasympathetic nervous system (PNS – the metaphorical "brakes" of the ANS). This is a shutting down of the body's intense push to attack or escape, and a replacing of it with passivity and constriction – an energy conservation strategy that Porges has noted involves activation of the dorsal vagal nerve (Porges, 2011, 2017, 2021). In human beings, this response is accompanied by the subjective experience of emotional numbing and psychological dissociation – depersonalization, derealization, and amnesias for events. This dissociative response is the "escape when no escape is possible", a psychological way of fleeing from a situation that cannot be physically controlled or evaded (Schore, 2002, 2019).

To summarize, we can think of mammals as having a normal baseline range of emotional arousal – not too high or intense, and not too low or constricted. When traumatized, the animal is knocked out of this emotional comfort zone by the traumatic event, and moves into a hyper-aroused bodily state, dominated by the SNS, and sometimes followed by a hypo-aroused state, dominated by the PNS.

THE TRAUMA RESPONSE IN HUMAN BEINGS

In most mammals, this adaptive emergency response dissipates quickly once the threat is gone, and the animal's physiology returns to baseline. Learning also occurs, as the animal's brain associates the danger with the particular stimuli linked to this encounter (sights, sounds, smells, specific locations, etc.). Human beings, however, can become "stuck" in either a hyper-aroused or hypo-aroused state – or oscillate between the two. We call this condition post-traumatic stress disorder (PTSD), and what appears to happen is that the neurophysiology of the individual does not reset itself back to its normal oscillatory range (Foa et al., 2009; Herman, 1992, 1995; Porges, 2017; Teicher et al., 2019).

Another factor that makes an emergency more complicated in human beings is the fact that the trauma reaction can be evoked not only by confrontation with a physical threat to one's well-being (e.g. someone being accosted by a gun-wielding burglar), but also when a person is confronted with a situation that is massively *psychologically* threatening, even if it presents no physical danger. This is true because human beings live in a world of socially and intra-psychically constructed meanings (Neimeyer & Raskin, 2000). As noted in the beginning of this chapter, this assumptive world of the individual reflects the person's sense of self, their expectations about the fairness, safety, orderliness, and controllability of the world, and their beliefs about the value or risks of forming attachments to other people. The experience of traumatic death challenges, and can in some cases utterly obliterate, this reassuring constellation of assumptions (Currier et al., 2008, 2006; Djelantik et al., 2020).

Don and Janice

Don and Janice sought therapy with JJ after the murder of their young adult son in a convenience store robbery. The young man was working as a clerk at the store when two masked and armed men entered the store and demanded money. Their son complied with the robbers, but another clerk in the store pressed a button in the store that set off an alarm to summon the police. The couple's son was shot as the startled and panicked robbers fled the store. The son died on the way to the hospital in an ambulance.

Imagine the experience of these parents, as they try to make sense of what has just happened. While understanding that murder happens to some people, Don and Janice have heretofore found their world to be safe for themselves and their children. They may even believe that their moral actions and careful adherence to the teachings of their religion ensure that they and their loved ones will be protected by God. Don and Janice may also believe that as conscientious and cautious parents, they can protect their offspring from danger. They may operate on the conscious or unconscious assumption that as long as they anticipate and plan for the future and adhere to the "rules" of proper and moral behavior, they can prevent bad things from happening to their family. As a result of their past experiences, Don and Janice may also assume that human beings are basically good, and that if they live a moral life and stay away from bad people, they will not be harmed. All of these basic assumptions about oneself and the world are likely to be violated for Don and Janice by the apparently random murder of their son.

Understanding this key aspect of traumatic deaths helps us to understand and respond in a helpful way to the needs of a traumatically bereaved person. Consider for example what might occur after Don and Janice arrive at the Emergency Department of their local hospital. The parents are permitted to view their child's body, and insist on seeing his face, which has been damaged by a gunshot wound to his head. The death of a child does not usually present a risk to a parent's immediate physical safety, but it can be immensely threatening to their sense of identity, self-esteem, and well-being. As we described in Chapter 5, their caregiving/

protective responses are likely to be powerfully activated by the news that their son has been shot, along with profound shock and grief when they arrive at the hospital to find him already dead.

The reactions of these newly bereaved parents are very likely to include responses that are the equivalent of the fight, flight, or freeze responses of animals that are in the grip of intense threat. For instance, Don, a normally peaceful and mild-mannered person, may fly into a rage upon getting the news of his son's death and then viewing his body – wanting to find and attack the perpetrator, or perhaps even attacking the doctor who brings the unbearable news (fight response). In contrast, his wife may scream and attempt to bolt from the room – a sign of an instinctive need to flee from the enormous threat to her psychological well-being posed by this terrible news and to summon help (flight response). Perhaps Janice may then become profoundly withdrawn over the next few days and weeks, refusing to leave her bedroom or interact with anyone (freeze response). All of these reactions are rooted in the same physiological process experienced by an animal fighting with, fleeing from, or trying to hide from a predator – only in this case, they serve as a desperate protective response for the survivor's psychological self from a reality that is so radically different and painful from the world they have known that it is experienced as incomprehensible, unreal, and unbearable (Van der Hart et al., 2006).

A third important aspect of traumatic bereavement is that, unlike most other traumatic events, the "danger" to which the individual is reacting persists. In most other traumatic events (e.g., involvement in an automobile crash), the danger is real but temporary, and a continuing emergency response is no longer necessary or appropriate. Much of our understanding of trauma has emerged from the experience of soldiers facing such real, but temporary life-threatening combat situations. Veterans with PTSD are having their nervous system continue to react as if they were still in a war zone, even if they are now safe and at home (Van der Kolk, 2014). Remember, however, that the trauma response can be elicited by psychological danger, not just physical danger. *In traumatic bereavement the psychological threat includes separation, the permanent absence of the deceased through death.* In this sense, all separation-based losses through death may include some degree of trauma since the individual can never "escape" the threat of separation from their loved one. This is why an important aspect of grief therapy involves the facilitation of a psychological continuing bond with the deceased (see Chapters 5 and 10): this bond helps reduce the perceived threat involved in separation from the loved one through death. It is also why helping clients who are traumatically bereaved almost always involves helping them with affect regulation and meaning reconstruction as part of the work (see Chapters 9 and 10) (Boelen & Lenferink, 2020; Eisma & Stroebe, 2021).

Death, particularly when it is sudden, can leave survivors with a sense of unreality and a feeling that they cannot make sense of the strange new world in which they find themselves. It often initially seems impossible for them to believe that life will ever return to anything approaching the normality that existed before the death, or that they will ever be "themselves" again. But in most cases, these conclusions are not borne out, at least, not entirely. The griever eventually finds that things are not as bleak as they had anticipated they would be. They miss their loved one, sometimes terribly, but they also come to see that life without their loved one still holds possibilities for meaning, for love, for joy. Several recent accounts of grief have suggested that the reason for this has to do with the brain: how it receives, processes, and makes order out of the chaos of sudden loss (Hollinger, 2020; O'Connell, 2022; Shulman, 2018).

It is a struggle for the brain to make sense of grief, and this struggle is the subject of neurologist Lisa Schulman's account of her husband's death. Referring to the "traumatic dissociation" that acts as a defense in early grief, she writes:

> What we often experience during grief corresponds to many common neurologic deficits: the fog of confusion, the inattention, the visual neglect (holes in my visual field that block perception of his personal belongings around the house.
>
> (Schulman, 2018, p. 103)

While it can be of helpful in preventing the griever from full, excruciating awareness of the loved one's death (as well as all of the implications of a permanent separation from the loved one), traumatic dissociation can lead to a feeling of unreality:

> We vacillate from the comfort of magical thinking to the uneasy feeling that we're not making sense – that we're going crazy.
>
> (p. 103)

In Schulman's view, the emotional shock of traumatic loss results in changes in the brain that are comparable to the changes that can result from a traumatic brain injury.

> Whether physical or emotion, brain trauma is trauma. The key questions are whether these changes in brain function are reversible and how we can enhance recovery and healing.
>
> (p. 103)

In summary, we can say that traumatic deaths are ones in which the mode or circumstance of the death evokes a powerful, biologically "wired-in" emergency response in the mourner – the trauma response. This response is neurophysiological and involves the whole-body, and can add greatly to complications in the overall mourning process. It is evoked both by the threat of perpetual separation from the loved one, and in the case of unexpected, violent, and sudden deaths, the horror of the way in which the loved one died.

Drawing on cognitive behavioral theory, Boelen et al. (2015) gathered self-report data from 496 individuals who were bereaved within three years. The investigators examined the role of seven cognitive-behavioral variables in mediating the impact of violent loss, including: a sense of "unrealness" about the irreversibility of the separation; negative cognitions about the self, life, and the future; and catastrophic misinterpretations of grief reactions. Among these,

> negative cognitions about the future, catastrophic misinterpretations and depressive avoidance were all significant independent mediators of the linkages between violent loss and symptom levels of PGD and depression. Negative cognitions about the future, catastrophic misinterpretations, and depressive and anxious avoidance emerged as unique mediators of the association between violent loss and elevated PTSD severity.
>
> (Boelen et al., p. 382)

These findings underscore that role of cognitive–behavioral variables in emotional distress following violent loss and the impact of negative cognitions in problematic grief. Many adult trauma survivors struggle to incorporate information that would allow them to make more accurate assessments of threat in their current environment. These individuals "lack the ability to use disconfirmatory information within their now harmless environments" to update let go of residual danger-related expectations that have resulted from the traumatic exposure (p. 9). These findings suggest that "increasing individuals' negative to positive updating skills may help reduce PTSD symptoms and improve current PTSD treatments" (p. 9). Once again, we see the advantages of flexibility in the ability to adapt, to cope, to manage stress. We will continue our discussion of cognitive factors in adaptation to loss and address the clinical applications of CBT in griefwork in Chapter 8.

EARLY LIFE STRESS AND RESPONSE TO TRAUMA

Studies suggest that the risk of trauma related symptoms in grief may be increased due to the mourner's previous experience with traumatic losses or other traumatizing experiences. Early relational trauma in particular is a risk factor for a prolonged, problematic grief response (Barlé et al., 2017; Boelen, 2016; Haim-Nachum et al., 2022; Lobb et al., 2010). This associ- ation is consistent with the finding from traumatology that a significant risk factor for developing PTSD after adult exposure to a traumatic event is a history of traumatic abuse as a child (Van der Kolk, 2014) which can affect brain development and immune system functioning (Baumeister et al., 2016; Iob et al., 2022; Teicher et al., 2016, 2020), and also likely creates fearful and negative expectations (i.e., assumptions) about the world that, even when they have been dormant for many years, may be reactivated by the experience of a traumatic loss in adulthood.

While early life trauma has been identified as a risk factor for subsequent trauma response, it is also true that not all of those who experience early trauma demonstrate this vulnerability. Research on the role of early life trauma in response to violent loss has addressed questions about the mechanisms underlying these effects and what factors contribute to greater or lesser symptom severity. Haim-Nachum et al. (2022) report that the impact of Adverse Child Experiences (ACES) on trauma response in adulthood was only significant when it was experienced in childhood, but not in adolescence or adulthood, a finding that they relate to rapid development of the brain in the first years of life and the heightened susceptibility of the brain to be "imprinted" by early traumatic experiences while the child (and their incompletely developed neurobiology)is still relatively young. Among other effects, early exposure to trauma may impact the limbic region, resulting in a vulnerability to trauma which may only become evident if adversity occurs later in life (Haim-Nachum et al., 2022; Luby et al., 2019).

ATTACHMENT AND TRAUMATIC BEREAVEMENT IN SUICIDE LOSS SURVIVORS

Studies of the relationship between attachment orientation and grief among suicide loss survivors suggest that secure attachment is associated with lower incidence of complicated grief in these cases. In accounting for these findings, researchers point to two likely meditational aspects of secure attachment. First, securely attached individuals are more trusting of other people, making it more likely that they will seek out social support, which is itself a predictor of better adjustment to loss.

> It is plausible that secure individuals view others as symbolic safety nets because they are accustomed to depending on them and receiving attentive care from them. Thus, they allow themselves to rely on others in times of stress, a function which may serve as a resilience factor in CG.
>
> (Levi-Belz & Lev-Ari, 2019, p. 134)

Secondly, and related to this first characteristic, securely attached individuals are more inclined to disclose their feelings to others. Self-disclosure has also been found to be negatively correlated with the incidence of complicated grief in suicide survivors (Levi-Beltz, 2015). In a report on their study of protective factors against complicated grief among suicide survivors, Levi-Beltz and Lev-Ari suggest that self-disclosure "may help survivors develop a more comprehensive narrative of their loss" (Levi-Beltz and Lev-Ari, 2019, p. 134). These findings accord with those of Feigelman et al. (2018) demonstrating that high levels of disclosure concerning the death event (suicide as well as accidental deaths) were associated with lower levels of difficulty in grief response.

Interestingly, Levi-Beltz and Lev-Ari found that proficiency in self disclosure and secure attachment style could *compensate for each other* in their protective effects. That is, proficiency in self-disclosure was a protective factor in grief even among individuals identified as having an insecure attachment orientation, and people with secure attachment orientation had reduced complicated grief even if they were not inclined to self-disclosure. Accounting for this finding, they propose that in both cases, grievers are able to draw on their particular strengths to seek the support they need.

Levi-Belz and Lev-Ari (2019) conclude that the combination of lower social support and less self-disclosure among insecurely attached grievers increases vulnerability to complicated grief. Securely attached grievers not given to self-disclosure also have lower levels of CG. This finding is accounted for by the observation that people with a secure attachment orientation are generally able access the resources they need for dealing with stressful situations, whether these resources are internal or external. As a group, they tend to find ways to get the support they need. With respect to providing support for suicide survivors, their findings underscore the vulnerability to complicated grief of people with personality traits associated with insecure attachment. These traits can prevent the griever from accessing support and having the opportunity to make some sense of their loss. Clinical recommendations focus on encouraging emotional expression and modifying internal working models to encourage utilization of social support.

Thinking back to the discussion of mentalization and epistemic trust in Chapter 2, we note that these findings support what Allen, Fonagy and others have reported regarding the role of mentalization and epistemic trust in how people develop and sustain relationships. Trust in the therapist can provide a scaffolding for trust in others; and may make a person Having come to trust the therapist, an individual may be more disposed to trust others; having found value in the therapeutic relationship, the griever may be more inclined to reach out to others for support.

Individual Differences in Suicide Grief

Perhaps the most important consideration in work with suicide survivors, as with bereaved people generally, is sensitivity to the particular meaning of the loss. We emphasize this here because suicide, which is usually violent and to many people is inherently incomprehensible due to what Jordan (2020) has called the "perceived intentionality" of a suicide (i.e., suicide loss survivors usually see that death as an intentional choice made by the deceased), can take on vastly different meanings. Care must be taken to leave room for expression of the range of feelings in survivors. Even the assumption that the survivor is suffering from traumatic grief should be held in check until we have the opportunity to hear the bereaved's story. An excerpt from the first author's notes illustrates this point. All that was known prior to our first meeting was that Marie's husband of 42 years had died by suicide.

In this first meeting, Marie, an energetic 72 years old, told me that the story she wanted to tell me "doesn't start with David's death." After listening to her talk about her husband for a few minutes, I said:

> PK: Yes. Of course you were relieved. (Slowly, quietly) You must have let out a breath at that point. Just knowing that you didn't have to worry any more about something happening that was not what he wanted.

> M: Helping him end his life was an act of love, and trust. It was hard for him to trust. But he trusted me. He trusted me to do what needed to be done.

Months later, Marie said:

> For me, his death was not the biggest trauma. And people tend to see it that way. . . and at the time I was going through it was awful . . . But in retrospect I can talk about *that* with less emotional chaos than I can talk about the loss of him in my everyday life.

> For me, *the trust that he showed in me to help him die was this incredible act of love on both of our parts. . . and that's not traumatic.*

We see in Marie's story how aspects of her husband's loss were less traumatic than might be the case in other deaths by suicide. The death was anticipated; Marie had a role in helping her husband end his life; and she was able to make sense of his reasons for wanting to do so. Most of what she felt was simply his absence: mostly what she felt was the loss of him in her everyday life.

This case illustrates a point that Rubin, Malkinson and Witztum (2020) make in describing how to apply the Two Track Model of Bereavement to cases of traumatic loss, where there is sometimes an over emphasis on addressing the trauma, with insufficient attention to relational aspects of the loss. According to the Two Track Model, the effects of traumatic loss are evident both in the griever's biopsychosocial functioning (Track I) and in their relationship with the deceased (Track II). While most of these individuals do not meet formal criteria for posttraumatic stress disorder

(PTSD), persistent complex bereavement disorder (PCBD), or prolonged grief disorder (PGD, they may experience a "significant degree of distress and dysfunction" (p. 7). By paying attention to the death story and to the nature of the bereaved's past and ongoing relationship with the deceased as well as the trauma involved in the loss, the Two-Track Model provides "rebalances the approach to the class of traumatic bereavements".

> The story of the death, the psychological relationship with the deceased, and the presence of biopsychosocial difficulties each have a part to play in assessment and intervention. Ultimately, the relational bond with the deceased is a major vector in grief and mourning. Assessment and intervention with traumatic bereavements require attention to dysfunction and symptoms of trauma as well as to the death story and the state of the relationship to the deceased.
>
> (Rubin et al., 2020, p. 1).

In its emphasis on the relational factors that affect response to traumatic loss, this perspective is in alignment with an attachment-informed understanding of grief in response to trauma. Attention to both elements of the traumatic response and to relational factors is evident in this exchange with a client of the first author whose elderly father took his own life in a particularly violent and dramatic fashion. The death was unexpected, but in discussion with the clinician the bereaved daughter was able to make sense of her father's actions, while also leaving room for her profound sense of loss.

> I always knew he was in danger. There was a direction to his life that tended toward this danger and that predisposition increased with age. . .
>
> The immediate reaction to learning that he was dead was like an airplane losing altitude, like not being able to find your child. . . I know that he felt like there was something he wanted to get away from, but also, that there was something better that he was going towards. I want to say: It's OK, but I can't help but suffer so much for losing you.

As we have suggested in previous chapters, personality is shaped by relational experience, with early relationships being the most impactful. In the context of repeated interactions with our early caregivers, we learn many things. In a best case scenario, these include a foundational view of the world as safe, and of ourselves as both competent and esteemed by others. We learn how to be a separate individual with our own distinct feelings, thoughts and ideas, while also being connected to, understanding of, and being understood by others. We also learn how to manage our internal states, including our bodily experiences (sexual arousal, pain, fatigue, etc.), our distressing thoughts ("I've made a big mistake", "Nobody likes me", etc.), and perhaps most importantly, our strong emotions (fear, joy, jealousy, attraction, anger, sadness, etc.) (Siegel, 2010, 2012a). Lastly, depending on the security of our attachment style, we develop expectations about whether being close to another person is likely to bring us comfort or distress when we are threatened. These skills may or may not, however, be up to the challenges embedded in a traumatic loss.

AFFECT REGULATION

Perhaps the most crucial factor in traumatic bereavement is one that we have already identified, i.e., affect regulation. By definition, trauma pushes people outside of their emotional comfort zone, producing intense emotional dysregulation (rage, panic, and dissociation/numbing) and autonomic nervous system arousal. People who have poor foundational skills at re-regulating their emotional arousal are likely to have even greater problematic responses when faced with the traumatic death of a loved one. Alternatively, they may have developed a relatively stable set of psychological survival skills that are nonetheless self-defeating, even damaging in their consequences for dealing with this type of loss. The use of these habitual but dysfunctional tools for coping (for example, the chronic use of alcohol to help regulate one's emotions) is likely to be greatly intensified by the traumatic death of a loved one.

In addition, the level of security of an individual's attachment style may produce problems when it interacts with the nature of the loss. For example, consider a person whose avoidant attachment style means that they generally shun intimacy and rarely disclose their inner thoughts and feelings to other people. This tendency to withdraw may be become more pronounced when the individual is very distressed, and their attachment system has been activated. Recall that attachment style is reflective of how emotion was originally co-regulated interpersonally between the individual and their early caregivers. Most losses typically produce some degree of regression in an individual's defensive style. If an individual has learned that seeking emotional proximity with others results only in disappointment, frustration, or further psychological injury, they will be faced with a significant challenge when confronted with a sudden, unexpected, and violent death. Likewise, if their experience has been that being in touch with deep emotions within themselves represents a frightening loss of control, then the intensity of their grief after the traumatic loss of a loved one will be actively avoided or minimized. Rather, an avoidantly attached individual is likely to seek the "safety" of isolation when they are upset, and to try to reduce their internal arousal through techniques such as "keeping busy" or the use of psychoactive substances (alcohol, drugs, etc.). Moreover, as Sheer and Shair point out, if the deceased played a mutual co-regulation function for the mourner (e.g., they were spouses), the bereaved person may experience major dysregulation of their physical, psychological, and social functioning (Shear & Shair, 2005). Considerable empirical evidence backs the finding that social support is a key factor in both bereavement and trauma outcome, helping to buffer people from the worst effects of these difficult life experiences (Cacciatore et al., 2021; Dyregrov & Dyregrov, 2008; Levi-Belz, 2015; Vanderwerker & Prigerson, 2004).

In contrast, consider a mourner with an anxious attachment style. This individual's early experiences with caregivers have taught them that attachment figures are unreliable and unpredictable in their availability, so that desperately maintaining proximity to attachment figures is the only way to assure their accessibility. In the initial surge of support that usually accompanies a traumatic loss, this person may feel helped by their social network. However, the intense need for the continual presence of others, coupled with the typical withdrawal of social support over time, may create a spiral of ever-increasing neediness in the mourner and corresponding frustration and burnout among people supporting that individual. As the social network begins to withdraw, the anxiety of the mourner increases and becomes overwhelming for others around the individual. This can then lead to feelings of abandonment, unworthiness, and depression. In addition, recall that traumatic deaths are also frequently perceived as being preventable, meaning that someone is at fault for the death. The anxious mourner may be overcome by ruminative guilt over the circumstances of the death and painful feelings of unworthiness for failing to prevent it. This combination of a great internal need for reassurance and comfort, coupled with poor skills at self-soothing, may lead to very complicated grief reaction.

MEANING-MAKING AFTER TRAUMATIC BEREAVEMENT

The principles that we are outlining here around affect dysregulation as a result of traumatization apply equally well to other domains of functioning that may be impacted by a traumatic death. These include physiological dysregulation (e.g., sleeplessness, loss of appetite, etc.), cognitive dysregulation (e.g., difficulty with concentration; absent mindedness), and interpersonal dysregulation (e.g., becoming irritable or confrontational with a martial partner). And as we have suggested earlier in this chapter, the survivor of a traumatic death is very likely to have their assumptive world damaged by the loss as well.

Harriet

Harriet, a 49-year-old mother of two, sought grief therapy with the second author after the death of her young adult son in a hiking accident. While hiking in the southwestern region of the U.S. in exceptionally hot weather and rugged trail conditions, her son became separated from his hiking companion and lost on the trail. After an extensive search, his body was found by a rescue team three days later. He had fallen and injured his leg and had died of exposure and dehydration. Harriet had many complex reactions to the death of her oldest child and only son, including guilt, regrets about problems in their relationship, and disturbing images of what her son's final hours were like (see Chapter 10).

In addition to the traumatic nature of the death, there was another trauma related factor that complicated Harriet's mourning process, and made the task of providing assistance to her more difficult. Harriet seemed to feel an inordinate sense of guilt about her son's death, given that it was the result of an accident that no one could have foreseen, and for which no one could reasonably have been held accountable. She ruminated about her perceived failures as a mother, and at times questioned whether her son's death was a punishment from God for her inadequacies. Over the course of the treatment, the therapist began to explore these feelings of guilt and responsibility in more depth. What emerged was a revelation in one session that Harriet had been sexually abused by both her grandfather and her father from the ages of about 6 through 10. The abuse stopped when Harriet was finally able to tell her mother, who confronted Harriet's father about the abuse. However, Harriett's mother provided almost no support for her daughter or help in putting the abuse in some kind of perspective and neither of her parents ever talked with Harriett again about this issue.

What became clearer through the therapeutic dialogue was that the abuse had left Harriet with a profound sense of shame, unworthiness, and a chronic thought of self-blame ("When bad things happen, it's my fault"). Although she carried a tremendous amount of anger about her abuse and the lack of protection from her parents, for the most part Harriet was excessively concerned with avoiding conflict with other people, and maintaining their positive regard for her. She was quick to take responsibility for any problems that occurred in her relationships, but when she did so, often ended up feeling resentful toward the other person. This pattern showed up in both her marriage, and at times in the relationship with the therapist.

This vignette illustrates the dynamics that can be evoked when a traumatic death befalls someone with an earlier trauma history, particularly developmental or relational trauma resulting from abuse and neglect by early caregivers (Herman, 1992, 1995; Van der Kolk, 2014). Harriet's difficulties were complicated by the loss of a child, by the nature of her son's death (sudden, unexpected, and involving a painful dying process), and by her early life experiences with attachment figures. In such situations, the therapist needs to be aware of, and with appropriate timing and client cooperation, attend to the synergism between the vulnerabilities created by the earlier traumatic experiences and the emotional injuries created by the traumatic circumstances of the current loss. For Harriet, the probable nature of her son's death had left her with deeply disturbing feelings of anguish at the suffering of her child as he died. These were addressed by a technique of going over her fantasies about what the dying process had been like, and at one point helping her retell the death in a different and more bearable way (called "restorative retelling" – see Chapter 10). In addition, the death of her son had reactivated and greatly intensified all of the painful and debilitating feelings that Harriet originally experienced in her earlier relationships with her caregivers. These included strong feelings of self-blame, along with resentment that she had no choice but to accept this blame. These confusing feelings became an additional major focus of her grief therapy.

All of this essential therapeutic work could not have been accomplished without the establishment of a relationship of trust, openness, and sensitive attunement on the part of the grief therapist to the complicated feelings involved for this client. As a sexual abuse survivor, creating a sense of psychological safety in the therapeutic relationship was a crucial but slow and delicate process for the clinician. Emphasizing the collaborative nature of their work together, and carefully respecting Harriet's autonomy about the content and speed of the therapeutic process, was paramount in creating a venue in which she could feel understood rather than judged, and supported rather than coerced. Once the abuse was revealed, and with Harriet's permission, the therapist began a gentle exploration of the impact of the abuse on Harriet's assumptive world and feelings, and their relation to her feelings about her son's death. By "tacking" back and forth between her past experiences and her current grief, Harriet and the therapist were together able to gain perspective on the meaning of the loss of her son for her. Gradually, Harriet was able to sort out which feelings were coming from which events, and also to understand better the role that her earlier abuse had played in her current grief. By the end of treatment, she was better able to experience her son's death for what it was: a tragic accident, but one for which no one was at fault, and for which she had a right to grieve deeply. It also helped her to understand and process the feelings of shame and unworthiness generated by her early abuse.

SUMMARY

Many things influence the course of grief, and in this chapter, we have focused on one of the most important of these factors, the circumstances surrounding the death. The difficulty a griever experiences in making sense of and coming to terms with a significant loss is intensified when the death is sudden, unexpected, and violent. Further complications arise if the survivor is present at the time of death or in the immediate aftermath. But those who were not present at the time of death can also be plagued by intrusive images that linger for months or years. If the death was the result of human error – or intention – and is therefore seen as having been preventable, the griever has yet more psychological obstacles to overcome. Yearning and sorrow are weighted down by layers of guilt, blame and angry protest. The result can be a sense that life is not worth living, or that it is at any rate not sustainable, given such a burden of suffering. A mourner's early experiences with key attachment figures lays a foundation for many of the capacities that enable a person to deal with all kinds of life stress. While traumatic loss has the power to crush the strongest and most resilient of human beings, early environmental advantages, including but not limited to the provision of a secure relational base, have been found to prepare people to deal with all kinds of life stressors, including traumatic loss.

Clients who come for help in dealing with these kinds of losses are some of the most challenging for clinicians, and not only because of the depth of their pain. Traumatic deaths are a slap in the face of our most closely held and cherished beliefs about what the world has in store for us now and in the future. In facing a fellow human being who has experienced such a loss we, along with them, must confront a reality so painful and frightening that we can be forgiven for wanting to hide. We can be forgiven for feeling helpless. That helplessness is the core of trauma, the black pit in the center of the fruit of life. To help someone who has suffered a traumatic loss, we must be able to give room to our own fear, and yet rise above it, always remembering that we are here not to take away a person's grief but to help them find ways to move with and through their suffering, to gradually recover their ability to experience moments of calm and relief, and to gently encourage them to extend the time they spend in living their lives in the present, wounded but still open to life and what it still holds.

The capacity to address the complex and layered grief of a mourner who has experienced a traumatic loss, or has lived through multiple traumas in their life, requires a solid understanding of attachment dynamics and the crucial role of the therapeutic relationship in fostering change in bereaved persons. We turn our attention to these and other aspects of the therapeutic encounter in the following two chapters.

Part III

CLINICAL IMPLICATIONS: TOWARD ATTACHMENT-INFORMED GRIEF THERAPY

Bowlby hoped that his work on the role of attachment in infancy and its impact throughout a person's life would provide an impetus for changes in public policy and the development of clinical approaches incorporating his concepts. He was disappointed by the initial lack of interest in his ideas outside a narrow band of academics (Holmes, 2013). In recent years, however, Bowlby's ideas, particularly those having to do with the importance of secure attachment in infancy and childhood, have been integrated into public and privately funded health, education and welfare programs in the US and elsewhere (Hunter & Flores, 2020. Likewise, the task of translating attachment theory into practice has been taken up by an ever-increasing number of clinicians and researchers (Allen, 2021; Eisma & Stroebe, 2021; Kosminsky, 2017, 2018).

Danquah and Berry (2013), in an introduction to their collection of essays exploring the applicability of attachment theory to clinical practice with adults, expressed the hope that the material presented would provide readers with a new perspective on how to identify and treat a range of clinical problems for which people seek help (Danquah & Berry, 2013). Our purpose here is similar with respect to grief therapy. In this chapter, after briefly reviewing our assumptions about the value of bringing an attachment perspective to grief therapy, we present an overview of our

DOI: 10.4324/9781003204183-10

clinical model. We then elaborate on elements of this model in the chapters that follow. Chapter 8 addresses how the therapeutic relationship is used in attachment informed grief therapy. In Chapter 9, we focus on how to strengthen self-capacities, particularly emotion regulation, in order to allow clients to better tolerate and integrate difficult feelings. In Chapter 10, we discuss the reconstruction of meaning in adaptation to loss and illustrate the application of an attachment informed approach to facilitating this process.

7

A MODEL OF ATTACHMENT INFORMED GRIEF THERAPY

When I married Ritchie, it was the first time in my life that I didn't have to perform to have someone love me. The first time there was someone who always had my back. And the first time I didn't have to worry that all of a sudden the peace would just explode. That's what Ritchie gave me.

Anyway, I guess I lost my security blanket.

Bereaved spouse

I never know how I'm going to feel from one minute to the next. It's like there's a gremlin inside me who gives me all this pain, and then just at the moment when I can't stand it anymore, he stops, and then just when I start to feel a little better, he starts it up again. I feel like two people. One person who can have a good day and can go out and do things. And another person who doesn't want to do anything or see anyone. I just can't imagine how those two people are ever going to be one person.

Bereaved parent

At some point in life, most people will experience the death of someone they love and will struggle with a range of thoughts and feelings, beginning, in many cases, with confusion, disbelief, and a longing for the person to return. Depending on the nature of the relationship and a person's capacity for independent survival, this longing may be overlaid with the fear that

DOI: 10.4324/9781003204183-11

they will not be able to withstand the emotional and physical impact of grief. Faced with the prospect of an indeterminate future filled with painful longing, bereaved people sometimes express a desire for their own death. The recently bereaved often have little interest in going anywhere or seeing anyone. There is a sense that they are carrying something very heavy, and there is no way for them to put it down.

In Bowlby's view, these emotional and physical features of grief are the adult equivalent of the response shown by many young children when they are separated from their attachment figures, a combination of protest, despair, and collapse. In adults as in children, the distress caused by separation is a deterrent to engagement and exploration. Once the attachment behavioral system is triggered, it will remain engaged until the connection to the loved one, and with it, a sense of safety and emotional balance, is restored, or until the individual adapts to living in the world without the deceased. A part of the mind – what people often refer to as "my rational self" – knows that the person has died, but this knowledge does not dispel the desire for their return and sometimes the acute sense of disbelief that the loved one is "really, really gone". Adding to the difficulty of accepting the irreversibility of death is the bereaved's past experience of the deceased as an omnipresent figure in their lives. How can it be that the lost loved one will not return, when they always *have* returned: this parent, this partner has *always been there*, or at least, *somewhere*, and if not physically present could be expected to reappear at some point. Like many of the expectations that give predictability and meaning to our lives, the expectation that *someone who has always been available will continue to be available* is wired into the network of neural connections that constitute our individual perception of reality (O'Connor & Seeley, 2022). This difficulty in accepting, or even believing in the reality of the death seems to be particularly pronounced in situations where the death was sudden and completely unexpected.

The conflict between wanting physical reunion, and knowing that it is impossible, and the disorientation that this conflict produces, resolves for most people over time. For some, a brief course of supportive counseling will facilitate the natural healing process that is considered a "normal" grief response (Worden, 2021). However, a substantial percentage of the bereaved will continue to experience symptoms associated with acute grief for an extended period, and it is with these people that the support offered by grief therapy can be most helpful (Neimeyer & Jordan, 2013; Worden, 1991, 2018). This support can take many different forms, and can include a variety of techniques depending on the needs of the client, the skills of the clinician, and the setting in which the therapy is provided. While techniques may vary, the attuned presence of a therapist who validates, clarifies, and helps the client explore feelings and needs brought on by a significant loss is fundamental to most forms of grief therapy. In this sense, grief therapy is essentially a collaborative effort in which client and clinician work together to identify and address obstacles to integration of the loss, including fears concerning the bereaved's ability to survive without the deceased, unresolved conflicts and questions about the life and death of the deceased and the need to deal with changes in life circumstances brought about by the death (Mikulincer & Shaver, 2021; Rubin, 2012, 2017).

We propose the following as a general definition of grief therapy, one that reflects our own view regarding the importance of attachment in understanding the process of bereavement and the role of the grief therapist.

A DEFINITION OF GRIEF THERAPY

Grief therapy is a concentrated form of empathically attuned and skillfully applied social support, in which the therapist helps the bereaved person re-regulate after a significant loss by serving as a transitional attachment figure. This includes addressing deficits in affect regulation and mentalizing related to both the loss at hand, and early neglect or trauma, as needed. In an environment that encourages exploration and growth, the bereavement therapist supports the bereaved in experiencing and tolerating feelings relating to grief, integrating new information and skills, and developing a new self-narrative that incorporates the impact of the loss. The goal of grief therapy is integration of the loss on a psychological and neurological level. Successful grief therapy encourages a state of flexible attention to the loss, and to the relationships, roles and experiences that are still available to the bereaved individual, in order that they may re-engage in life, without relinquishing their attachment to the deceased.

This definition directs attention to attachment as a factor in adaptation to bereavement and as a factor in the design and delivery of grief interventions. It does not change the goal of grief therapy (Worden, 1991, 2009, 2018) but it does reflect our understanding of the therapeutic process by which that goal is reached. This understanding is consistent with the emergent shift in the paradigm of psychotherapeutic change described by many clinician/researchers (Cozolino, 2017; Schore, 2019). These writers argue that what transpires in psychotherapy happens not only through cognitive, language-based interventions, but through the emotion rich, right brain to right brain communication between therapist and client, a connection that serves an affect regulating function not unlike that served by the secure connection between parent and child (Siegel et al., 2021). The regulatory function of the therapeutic relationship is particularly important in grief therapy, where the painful feelings that bring clients into treatment are often a consequence of the loss of a significant attachment figure.

ASSUMPTIONS GUIDING ATTACHMENT INFORMED GRIEF THERAPY

In line with the many researchers and clinicians whose work has been cited in earlier chapters, we regard variations in attachment experience and orientation as critical factors in understanding how people form relationships with others, how they respond to the death of a loved one, and how they utilize the resources they bring to the tasks of adapting to significant loss. This analysis, along with contributing to our understanding of the roots and trajectory of normal and problematic bereavement, has implications for the practice of grief therapy, and it is to these that we now turn.

The assumptions on which our approach is based are summarized below.

Assumptions Related to Attachment Informed Grief Therapy

Concerning attachment:

- Early attachment experience impacts neural development and lays down a template for relationships with other people.
- Early attachment experience has a formative and lasting impact on the development of an individual's attachment orientation, their set of expectations about subsequent close interpersonal relationships.
- Early attachment experience has a formative and lasting impact on core self-capacities and self-identity, in particular capacities related to mentalizing and self-regulation.
- Attachment orientation is a factor in how people cope with adverse life events in general and with the death of a significant attachment or caregiving recipient figure in particular.

Concerning grief:

- Loss of an attachment relationship is dysregulating and destabilizing; separation distress in childhood is mirrored in the distress that accompanies the death of an attachment figure or a caregiving recipient in adulthood.
- Reregulation in the aftermath of loss, like the recovery of emotional balance in infancy, is a dyadic and transactional process that is facilitated by, if not dependent on, the engaged, attuned presence of one or more other people.

Concerning problematic grief:

- Attachment related problems that persist into adulthood are often present in complicated grief.

- Difficulties related to affect management and self-regulation are present in many survivors of early abuse or neglect, and often interfere with their adaptation to later losses. Self-regulation involves capacities for both the tolerance of strong affect that may be associated with loss, and maintenance of the coherence of the mourner's self and world narratives.
- Traumatic loss is a risk factor for problematic grief independent of attachment orientation. However, previous trauma, including early relational trauma, amplify the effect of adult traumatic loss and compound the likelihood of protracted dysregulation.

In what follows, we will expand on the definition of grief therapy and illustrate how the therapeutic relationship functions to support the bereaved individual in becoming better equipped to tolerate distressing affect and acquire new information and skills. Just as all of these are functions that attachment figures serve for a growing child, they are all important components of grief therapy. Our discussion of each of these highlighted functions will then be expanded in the remaining chapters.

THE THERAPEUTIC RELATIONSHIP

Because it involves the loss of attachment, Bowlby regarded bereavement as a period in which attachment related needs are likely to be intense, making the quality of the therapeutic relationship particularly important. In counseling the bereaved, Bowlby emphasized, "the patient's experience of the therapist's behavior and tone of voice and how he approaches a topic are at least as important as anything he says" (Bowlby, 2005, p. 180). Based on our own experience and on our reading of the robust body of empirical research, we believe that the foundation of all successful grief therapy (indeed all psychotherapy) is the development of a trusting, emotionally safe, and psychologically nurturing therapeutic relationship (Okamoto et al., 2019; Norcross & Lambert, 2019). Emphasis on the primacy of the therapeutic relationship is a distinguishing feature of attachment informed approaches to therapy (Berry & Danquah, 2015; Holmes & Slade, 2018). While the effectiveness of therapy for bereaved individuals has been studied for decades (Allumbaugh & Hoyt, 1999; Aoun et al., 2018; Jordan, & Neimeyer, 2003) relatively little attention has been paid to this fundamental element of interventions for the bereaved.

As illustrated in Chapter 4 and further elaborated in Chapter 8, the development of a strong therapeutic bond depends on an array of strengths and aptitudes, some teachable, some innate, and some that are refined over years of clinical practice. These are not simple, one-dimensional traits but composites of the clinician's emotional, cognitive and behavioral repertoire.

As clear as the problem at hand and the goals of therapy may be, what happens between a grieving client and the therapist happens in the moment. Empathic attunement, a prerequisite for effective grief therapy, depends on the clinician's ability to maintain a stance of flexible accommodation to client attachment needs, which vary from person to person and from session to session over the course of the mourning process (Norcross & Lambert, 2019; Sekowski & Prigerson, 2022). The warm and nurturing approach that is comforting to some clients, particularly those with an anxious attachment orientation, will be off-putting to those who prefer more psychological distance. Some clients will be hungry for soothing words and will want to be assured of the therapist's continuing availability; others will be looking for a time limited intervention and will insist that what they need are tools to help them work through their grief and get on with their lives.

With every client, the ability to build a trusting therapeutic relationship will be subject to that individual's prior relationship experiences – good, bad, or indifferent. Early relational trauma, such as is often reported by clients with a disorganized attachment style, raises the stakes and the difficulty of establishing a strong therapeutic bond. British psychiatrist and Bowlby biographer Jeremy Holmes has urged clinicians to recognize that "disorganized clients are going to find it massively difficult to trust us" and advises a slow, indirect approach that lets the client's narrative emerge in their own time.

> So if you ask someone how their childhood was and they say, "Just normal childhood", this is an individual who can't bring to mind their actual experience and the feelings associated with that experience. Move in the direction of helping them regulate emotion, bring emotion into the room at a pace that they can tolerate.
>
> (Holmes, 2022)

As this comment, and the preceding discussion suggests, difficulty in managing emotion is often observed, and readily identified, in clients with a history of early abuse or neglect. Hill (2016) makes the case that a person doesn't have to have suffered abuse to have problems with regulating emotion. Hill explains that these clients are prone to a "moderate degree of dysfunctionality" which, being less evident, may be overlooked. In these clients there is "some modulation of the degree of intensity of affect but not enough to stay regulated ... This 'subclinical' dissociation is debilitating but not necessarily disabling, and often passes unobserved" (Hill, 2016, p. 160).

STRENGTHENING THE CAPACITY TO TOLERATE EMOTION

Attachment theory draws many parallels between the role of attachment security in childhood and in adulthood. In childhood, relational security is associated with flexibility in emotional expression and behavior. In other words, securely attached children are able to experience a range of emotions, and to express them in a spontaneous and unconflicted manner. In contrast, the emotional awareness and expression of insecurely attached children is subject to what they have learned are the preferences of unreliable or rejecting caregivers (Holmes, 2010; Wallin, 2007). In adulthood, relational security confers comparable benefits with regard to social and emotional functioning. The ability to experience, acknowledge, and manage emotion is a singularly important indicator of mental health (Kraiss et al., 2020). Difficulties in emotion regulation are a defining feature of many psychiatric diagnoses (Ein-Dor & Doron, 2015) and remediation of these difficulties has become a major focus of treatment of these disorders (Sekowski & Prigerson, 2021). In the context of bereavement therapy, it can reasonably be assumed that addressing deficits in emotion regulation can positively affect the course of bereavement in clients who are struggling to cope with sadness, yearning, and other grief related feelings.

In keeping with what we have learned about the impact of insecure attachment on the development of emotional tolerance and self-regulation, we must expect that many clients with problematic grief will need help building these skills, either because they come to the therapeutic encounter with a basic deficit in these skills from early relational experiences, or because the loss itself has been sufficiently traumatizing that even a securely attached person may be significantly dysregulated by the death (see Chapter 6). Compounding the difficulties caused by a lack of internal resources, these mourners may also be lacking in social support and other external resources (Logan et al., 2018). As discussed in Chapter 4, depending on their characteristic manner of response to painful emotion, these mourners will tend to over-use one of two secondary regulatory strategies: either becoming immersed in the loss (hyperactivating) or suppressing awareness and behaviors related to the loss (deactivating) (Mikulincer & Shaver, 2021).

Whether in childhood or adulthood, we grow through experiences that challenge, but do not overwhelm us. As Ogden (2009) and Ogden and Fisher (2015) explain, the ideal therapeutic environment provides a level of arousal that is comfortable but not *too* comfortable. An attuned grief therapist works with clients to create a balance between too much, and too little engagement with their emotional reactions to the death. Through moment-to-moment awareness of a client's physical and emotional state, the therapist continually seeks to expand the client's emotional awareness and affective flexibility.

In a similar vein, Holmes describes the ideal therapeutic balance between nurturing and confronting the client. Successful therapy requires that the therapist initially accommodate to the role "allocated by the patient's unconscious expectations" (Holmes, 2013, p. 18.). With avoidant, deactivating clients, this might mean that the therapist starts with an analytical approach, engaging the client intellectually before making the move to engage them emotionally. With anxious, hyperactivating clients, it might involve a degree of "boundary flexibility," such as an exchange of messages between sessions. Over time, the therapist modifies their approach in order to move the client in the direction of an enlarged pattern of interaction, one that expands the client's relational repertoire.

Beth

A highly anxious client sought treatment following the death of her mother. The day after their initial session, the therapist received a request from the client for an appointment over the weekend. The therapist responded by reminding the client that she did not offer weekend appointments. The therapist received, and responded to, several additional communications from the client. Feeling increasingly agitated by the client's intrusions, she decided that she would have to have a conversation about boundaries with the client, a prospect she dreaded. But on further reflection, she decided on a different approach. At their scheduled appointment the following week, the therapist commented: "Well, I want you to know that you were very successful in communicating to me **just how anxious** *you are. In fact, when I was thinking about seeing you today I became a bit anxious myself, and I thought* **this is how she feels all the time.***"*

This exchange was important for several reasons. It established, once again, that there were limits to the clinician's availability, but at the same time conveyed that she was very conscious of the level of the client's distress. Client and therapist were able to share a moment of levity, which diffused any lingering resentment that might have remained on either side, and from that point forward a strong therapeutic bond developed. Secure in the knowledge that this relationship was in place and that she could fall back on it if needed, the client was able to begin to allow some distance from the clinician. The clinician also taught her a number of self-soothing techniques, and as she became more confident about her internal resources for self-regulation, the client was able to address ongoing conflicts with members of her family that were compounding the distress related to her mother's death.

Of course, some clients will resist any move on the clinician's part to promote the client's independence, including suggestions about how they might learn to manage their emotions more effectively. They may regard such efforts as yet another example of someone telling them that they should get a hold of themselves and get back to the business of living. In counseling the bereaved, it is important for clinicians to be careful to not make premature attempts to get clients to move toward a resolution of their grief.

A clinician's ability to sense when and how to give clients a gentle nudge in order to broaden their emotional and behavioral range is one of the pillars of clinical wisdom in grief therapy described more fully in Chapter 8. In the following exchange, the clinician suggested to Robert, 44, whose father had died eight months prior, that he begin thinking about looking for work:

> R: *I don't want to hear this. All I really wanted today was to be soothed. I feel like you're sticking pins in me.*
>
> PK: *I'm sorry you feel that way. My instinct, you know, is to soothe you. My impulse is to soothe you. But if all I do is soothe you, nothing will ever change.*

This exchange was followed by a nod from the client, who jokingly concluded the session by announcing that he was never coming back (he did).

The ability to gradually accommodate to a loss occurs through repeated interactions of this sort, always within the context of a secure bond. To maintain that sense of security the clinician must be sensitive to the client's state of mind and their tolerance for emotion and closeness within the therapeutic relationship (Muller, 2010).

RESTORING MENTALIZING

> Mentalizing is the key to self-regulation and self-direction ... By integrating *a sense of self and a sense of connections with others*, mentalizing enables us to manage losses and trauma, as well as distressing feelings such as frustration, anger, sadness, anxiety, shame and guilt. (emphasis added). Mentalizing, we manage these feelings *without* resorting to automatic fight or flight responses or efforts to cope that are ultimately self-destructive or maladaptive.
>
> (Allen, 2003, p. 93)

Described in Chapter 2 as the ability to understand what is happening in one's own mind, as well as in the minds of others, the capacity to mentalize develops in infancy within the security of an attuned, nurturing relationship, and as Allen explains, is an essential component of healthy self-regulation of emotion (Allen, 2013). In the context of grief therapy, impaired mentalizing and emotion regulation become targets of treatment when these impairments complicate grief and amplify the difficulties associated with integrating loss. Problems in mentalizing are most often apparent in people with a history of early attachment trauma, many of whom exhibit characteristics of disorganized attachment (Hesse, 2008; Main & Hesse, 1990). Learning to mentalize can help a person make sense of their past, including the past relationship with an abusive parent. Being able to look back on a confusing and frightening time from a place of safety, the adult who survived can take their place next to the child who could not escape.

INTEGRATING NEW INFORMATION AND DEVELOPING NEW SKILLS

We believe that working with people who are grieving involves not only helping them come to terms with their loss, but helping them build, or rebuild, connected, productive lives. For many people, this will require learning new skills. Broadly speaking, we can identify three categories of skills that mourners acquire as they heal from their losses. The first are the skills involved in emotional and cognitive self-regulation.

Sam

Sam was disturbed by his bouts of weeping at work after the death of his beloved daughter in a boating accident. He worked in a mostly male work setting, where his periodic weepiness was viewed as being at best a socially awkward lapse in self-control, and at worst as a dangerous distraction from his responsibilities on the job, which required vigilant attention. Over time, Sam settled on a strategy of allowing himself to cry on his way to and from work while driving in his car, but actively suppressing his tears while he was at work. With appropriate cautions about the risks of "driving while crying," the therapist supported Sam's acquisition of this adaptive skill in self-regulation, given the realities of his work environment.

The second category of skills includes self-care skills that may have deteriorated since the death or may never have been well developed by the individual. These skills include care of the physical, emotional, and spiritual self. For example, recent evidence suggests that exercise can be a potent antidote for depression, including the depressive symptoms that accompany bereavement (Stanton & Reaburn, 2014). It is common for us to inquire about the exercise history of the bereaved clients with whom we work, and after taking into account the health and age of the individual, to encourage them to begin some kind of regular physical activity, ranging from simply going for regular walks to starting exercise programs at a gym or health club. In similar fashion, we may encourage an individual whose religious practice has lapsed to resume their involvement with their faith community, as well as their solitary practice of prayer.

The third group of skills often needed by mourners includes the ability to manage their relationships with other people, particularly the changes in relationships that have come about as a result of the death:

Patricia

Patricia found that many people treated her differently after the death of her daughter to suicide. Some people who related to her were intrusive, often asking questions about the details of the death and demanding an explanation for something that Patricia could barely understand herself. By contrast, other friends and work colleagues avoided any mention of the death when they were with Patricia, or simply avoided having contact with Patricia at all (for example, crossing to another aisle when they saw her in the grocery store). The death of her daughter had placed Patricia in the very unfamiliar social position of having to actively manage her boundaries and protect herself in relationships with other people in ways that she had never needed to do before. This became a focus of her work with her grief therapist,, as she decided how she wanted to handle the complex reactions of other people to her new status as the "Mom of a child who killed herself." She also considered suggestions offered by her therapist about ways that other suicide survivors have learned to deal with people's insensitive intrusions or hurtful avoidance.

These examples illustrate the new repertoire of skills and knowledge that bereaved persons will need help with developing. Also evident in these examples are the social nature of grief and the role of a bereaved person's environment in either facilitating or complicating their integration of loss. Part of a grief therapist's role is to encourage clients to identify and connect with people in their lives who are supportive, and as much as possible, to limit contact with people who make them feel worse than they already do (Jordan, 2020).

MEANING-MAKING AFTER LOSS: THE DEVELOPMENT OF A REVISED SELF-NARRATIVE

The relationship with an attuned support person helps the bereaved client to stay present with painful emotions and to gain perspective about the changed self and world created by the death. Some of this information may become the nucleus of a new life narrative, one that replaces a storyline built on negative beliefs about the self, an exaggerated sense of responsibility for problems in a relationship, or a general expectation that relationships with others will be hurtful or disappointing. In the case of traumatic bereavement, the mourner's beliefs about their ability to control what happens **to** them and to the people they care about may be shattered by the death (Cacciatore, 2017). In such cases, meaning making will involve the reconstruction of these beliefs to consider existential realities that can no longer be denied.

Kanesha

Kanesha, a married woman in her late twenties sought grief therapy after the sudden death of her younger brother to a cerebral hemorrhage. Exploration of her history revealed an extremely abusive history with both of her parents, with her father being unpredictably and terrifyingly violent towards his children, and her mother being extremely manipulative in keeping her daughter attached to her as a support person. This latter behavior included feigning heart attacks and blaming her daughter for them when, as an adolescent, Kanesha wanted to begin dating. Kanesha and her brother formed an alliance of mutual protection in order to survive the abuse from both parents, with Kanesha taking a lead role in trying to shield her younger brother from harm. When her brother died as a young adult, Kanesha became depressed and suicidal, developing a kind of magical thinking about her responsibility for keeping her brother alive, and her unworthiness for having failed to do so. Therapy with JJ focused on helping Kanesha examine the roots in her abusive childhood of the narrative that she had constructed about her brother's death and her role in it. With the therapist's support Kanesha was also able to confront the reality that random but terrible things can happen to anyone without being a judgment about that person's worth.

In their review of variations in grief response related to early attachment experience, Sekowski & Prigerson (2022) propose that adults who report early abuse or neglect may exhibit "exaggerated and contradictory states of mind" in attachment relationships owing to a combination of fear and distrust, on the one hand and the need for closeness and safety on the other. Describing the particular attachment related needs of these bereaved clients, whose adverse early experience is associated with disorganized attachment, the authors conclude that for these bereaved persons, "the most important task may be to construct a coherent narrative of the relationship and the death" (Sekowski & Prigerson, 2022, p. 1820).

The development of an expanded self-narrative is also an important element of recovery for people who are seriously in doubt about their ability to survive without the person who has died. The loss of a spouse is painful for many people, but it can be disabling for a woman whose core self-narrative, learned in the context of her early relationships with care-givers (as well as societal expectations about the gender roles of women), is that she does not have the strength or skill to manage on her own. Similarly, a widower who believes that he is inept at dealing with emotion may feel overwhelmed by the prospect of caring for his bereaved children. In these situations, the therapist can often help a bereaved person find evidence of aptitudes they claim not to have and skills that may have been underutilized or even devalued in the past. Helping bereaved people realize that they are stronger, kinder, more resourceful, and more resilient than they believe themselves to be can provide a powerful infusion of hope for people who doubt their ability to function in the world without the deceased.

REVISING THE NARRATIVE OF THE RELATIONSHIP WITH THE DECEASED

According to the Two Track Model (see Chapter 4), the factors that influence how a person adapts to relational loss can be grouped into two domains: their day to day functioning, and the emotional valence and intensity of their ongoing relationship with the deceased (Rubin et al., 2012). Like many parents who lose a child, Sylvia struggled with the feeling that she should have done more to save her daughter, who died after an extended illness. In Sylvia's case, however, this feeling was amplified by Sylvia's lingering sense that her daughter had not loved her.

Sylvia

Sylvia, a woman in her eighties, was referred to PK by her physician and friend, who reported that she seemed "very down, maybe depressed." Sylvia confirmed that she was not feeling herself and noted that since her 23-year-old daughter's death she had not been able to forgive herself for failing to be more available to her during her illness. Based on information collected in the first and second sessions, it became clear that Sylvia had endeavored to be more of a presence in her daughter's life, but that her daughter had in fact resisted Sylvia's intervention. Subsequent sessions focused on identifying Sylvia's interpretation of her daughter's response, and what became clear was that to Sylvia, her daughter's refusal to accept her help "proves that she didn't love me."

This discussion helped pave the way to Sylvia's understanding that her pain was a composite, not only of grief and guilt, but of resentment and a feeling of rejection. She mourned the lost opportunity to build a better relationship with her daughter, one that would have allowed her to be closer to her daughter during the final stages of her illness. Sylvia was invited to "introduce" her daughter, and in the course of doing so, she talked about her daughter's fierce independence and her refusal to be "pitied or babied" by friends and family. As she talked about her daughter, Sylvia came to realize that her daughter's behavior was not a personal rejection, but a reflection of a life-long pattern of wanting to take responsibility for herself and not depend on others. Sylvia was able to see that in backing off in response to requests from her daughter, she was honoring her daughter's wishes.

Following this work, Sylvia was able to imagine having a conversation with her daughter, articulating her own concerns, and expressing what she thought would be her daughter's explanation for her steadfast refusal to accept help. During this conversation Sylvia found that she was able, for the first time since her daughter's death to recall many instances in which her daughter had clearly communicated her love and gratitude for Sylvia's support and care. After two months Sylvia reported feeling "much more at peace" about her daughter, having realized that "a lot of what was hurting so much was the feeling that my daughter didn't love me, and now I realize that that just isn't true."

THE RECONSTRUCTION OF MEANING AND
PURPOSE IN LIFE

The central role of meaning making in recovery from loss has been elaborated by Neimeyer and his colleagues, both in terms of theory and empirically supported clinical practice. In this view, bereavement is fundamentally a process of meaning reconstruction, through which the mourner must find a way to accommodate not only the loss of the person who has died, but aspects of personal identity that were linked to that person (Gillies & Neimeyer, 2006; Neimeyer & Sands, 2011). Someone whose role as caregiver provided a sense of purpose, or whose relationship with a spouse or child was central to his or her identity, will have to reconfigure their sense of self, and will benefit from guidance in establishing a new basis for their identity. In such cases the first task of therapy is often to help the bereaved client understand their sense of dislocation.

Janet

Janet, 56, moved in with her father after her mother's death and took care of him until he died several years later. Although she had often felt resentful about having to spend most of her free time taking him to doctors and cooking him special meals, she now felt letdown, lethargic, and unsure about what she will do with the rest of her life.

The therapist engaged Janet in a discussion of what had been most fulfilling to her about caring for her father, and of what the loss of her identity as a caregiver meant to her. Jennifer came to understand that her lethargy was mostly caused by the sudden vacuum of purpose and meaning in her life. This was a powerful realization for her because, unlike the loss of her father, it was something over which she had control. Janet now saw her emotional state as a problem that she could attack as she had attacked her father's medical problems.

In the months that followed, Janet began to expand her base of social support and to pursue interests that had been sidelined during the period of her father's illness. Through a process that has been described as "mapping the terrain of loss" (Kosminsky, 2012). Janet was able to differentiate her yearning for her father from the secondary effects of losing her identity as a caregiver. The shift from hopelessness to purposefulness and from isolation to engagement that Janet was able to make was the end result of changes in her thinking, her emotions, and her behavior. This kind of reorganization of the self is what we hope to see in our bereaved clients.

The following clinical vignette illustrates the use of several techniques used in AIGT.

These include:

• Psychoeducation about grief as a form of attachment loss

- Discussion of the client's attachment history
- Introducing strategies to strengthen emotion regulation
- Identifying and addressing fears about the future

Jane, who was introduced in Chapter 4, is a woman in her early seventies whose husband died three months before her first meeting with the therapist. His death came at the end of a three-year period of progressive decline, during which time Jane was his primary caregiver. In response to my questions about her childhood, Jane described being "constantly on high alert" because of her mother's mental instability and erratic behavior. With no support from her father, Jane adapted to her situation by becoming extremely self-sufficient and "needless." Psychoeducation focused on explaining how our experience of being cared for in childhood influences our feeling of safety in the world, our feelings about other people, and how we handle emotion.

What became clear was that for Jane, her marriage to Richie was little short of miraculous in healing her early deprivation and filling her heart with love, understanding and a solid sense of belonging. Seeing her marriage, and her loss, in this way, was both unsettling and revelatory, bringing her in touch with the magnitude of what she had lost.

J: As bad as 2020 was, I don't want it to be the new year because it's a year when he's not going to be there. And there's nothing I can do about it.

PK: When you say "there's nothing I can do about it" ...

I just want to say - you're an extremely practical person. And I get a small sense sometimes that if you think there's nothing you can do about something, your next thought is that you should just push it off to the side, forget about it, dismiss it.

I'm not suggesting that you dwell on things that you can't do anything about. On the other hand – that doesn't mean that you have to dismiss it, it doesn't mean that you have to dismiss the deep painful feelings it brings up, just because the source of those feelings is something you can't do something about.

J: With my mother there was no point having feelings. Since Richie died, with a lot of people I know, I feel the same way I did then. People don't want to know how I feel.

PK: Yes. When people don't respond to your needs ...

J: I do basically what I did then. I perform. Then, I performed academically or on the playing field. That was my life. Now, I perform for people. I read something that said that people like me are more likely to have headaches and irritable bowel syndrome. That's me.

PK: You somaticize your emotions.

J: Exactly. I somaticize my emotions.

PK: It really speaks to what you didn't get from her. You didn't get the kind of love and nurturing that a child needs and that connects them to their mother. When people grieve the loss of their mother, that's what they're grieving - the feeling of being seen, and valued, and loved. That unconditional love: what they're grieving is the loss of all of that. The feeling that no one else is going to love them the way their mother loved them.

J: That's where Richie comes in. He was my secure attachment.

PK: I know. And when people lose their secure attachment - a lot of times it's their mother. But this loss for you - has overtones of the kind of terror that a child feels when their mother is unavailable. You're absolutely right. Richie gave you what you never had, what you maybe thought you never could have. Richie was like a miracle for you.

J: He was.

PK: When you talk about the way you operated as a kid - there was never any room for you. Everything that you did, everything that you were, was a defense against your mother's explosions. It's like you were constantly operating behind enemy lines, in enemy territory, trying to stay low, feel out what was going on.

J: Absolutely.

P: What happens then is that everything you knew, everything you feel gets suppressed. So that you don't even know at a certain point what your feelings are, because your feelings don't matter. You just shut them down ... And with Richie, there was such a depth of love, and understanding and compassion that he drew you out of yourself.

J: To lose that . . it impacts you for life. Even though you may go on, and live your life ...

PK: Yes, I understand. I get all of that.

I just want to say – and take as much of this is as you can and ignore the rest - I just want to say that what you just said about how that kind of experience stays with you - that's true, of course. All of our experiences are layered on top of one another, from the earliest to the latest, and when there's a disturbance on top, in the present, that disturbance can be felt all the way down to our core.

*That's the part of you I want to speak to now. And what I want to say to the part of you that's all the way down in the core is: "You don't have to go back to your bunker. It's OK to have your feelings. I'm here. I'm listening. **You're** here, **the you that you are now is here,** and you can listen.*

SUMMARY

A good therapist, like a good parent, does any number of things, and usually multiple things at the same time. A therapist provides a secure base from which clients can explore thoughts, feelings, and environments that they would otherwise avoid, and also helps them to reflect on the behavior and feelings of others (i.e., to mentalize). A therapist encourages a hopeful, realistic view of the client's potential for healing and growth, and this positive regard promotes a more positive sense of self in the client. Grief therapists do many of these same things in the course of helping clients cope, adapt, and come to terms with loss.

Advocates for the use of attachment theory in psychotherapy have generally argued that it is best viewed not as a particular "brand" of psychotherapy, but rather as a framework that supports all forms of psychotherapy. Insights from attachment theory, which have been supported by neuroscience research, have direct application to the development of treatment strategies for the bereaved, particularly in cases where bereavement is complicated by problems related to early trauma.

The loss of a significant person is a uniquely stressful event, one that is qualitatively different from other types of stressful events, including other types of losses. Attachment informed approaches to psychotherapy put particular emphasis on aspects of therapy that contribute to the creation of a strong therapeutic bond. The reassurance and sense of safety that a strong therapeutic bond provides are particularly important for someone who has recently suffered a significant loss. The case examples included throughout this book convey our belief that the therapeutic relationship is central to work with the bereaved and a sense of what this commitment to the primacy of the relationship looks like in practice. In the following chapter we offer a more systematic discussion of what we regard as the core capacities that support the development of a strong therapeutic alliance in attachment informed grief therapy.

8

THE THERAPEUTIC RELATIONSHIP: CORE CAPACITIES OF THE ATTACHMENT INFORMED GRIEF THERAPIST

What is it about the experience of being listened to and feeling understood that is so valuable to someone who is bereaved? How is it that one human being can provide comfort and facilitate healing for another, even in the worst of times? And what does this most basic of human needs teach us about our role in providing grief therapy?

J: Why do I still need therapy? I don't need to talk to you every week, but there are times when I still do.

PK: Maybe it's because all of your adult life you had someone you could talk to about anything. And maybe now, a year after losing Richie., sometimes there are things you need to talk about that are hard to talk about with other people, even people who love you.

J: (Nodding). Yes.

Carol

Carol entered grief therapy shortly after the suicide of her son. The first session was extremely sad for client and therapist alike, as Carol recounted the details of her son's

DOI: 10.4324/9781003204183-12

death, and her shock, confusion, and profound sorrow at his loss. Her despair was palpable, and she wept for much of the session. At the end of the meeting as they were about to part, the therapist (JJ) followed a human impulse to somehow offer comfort in the face of this wrenching sorrow. He said "Do you need a hug?" Carol said "Yes" and they embraced for a moment as the therapist simply said "I'm so sorry"

Unaccustomed to hugging new female clients at the end of first sessions, the therapist later wondered "What's going on here? Why did I do that?" Early in their next session, he said to Carol, "I don't usually end first sessions that way – what was your experience of that?" Without a moment's hesitation Carol replied "It was fine. I felt like you understood."

In this chapter we examine the relational aspects of grief therapy and elaborate on what we consider the pivotal role of the therapeutic relationship in fostering recovery from loss. Decades of research have established that the therapeutic alliance is a critical variable in the effectiveness of all psychotherapy (Allen, 2013; Norcross & Wampold, 2018; Norcross & Lambert, 2018). Although some notice has been taken of the importance of the therapeutic relationship in the field of thanatology (Iglewicz et al., 2020; Neimeyer, 2012; Larson, 2020; Pearlman et al., 2014) historically very little attention has been paid to this central aspect of grief therapy. Our purpose here is to address this gap.

We begin with a brief review of the theory and robust body of research on the therapeutic relationship as it impacts general psychotherapy outcomes. We will then look at the linkage between this literature and the insights from attachment theory and neurobiology presented in earlier chapters. From there we will move toward a formulation that recognizes the grief therapist as a *transitional attachment figure* for the bereaved individual, one who provides a safe haven and a secure base from which re-regulation of the self and exploration of the changed world without the deceased becomes possible. Lastly, we will expand on what we see as the core relational capacities that are intrinsic to the practice of effective grief therapy. Like all of our recommendations regarding treatment, what we have to say reflects our attachment informed understanding of how people recover from and integrate major losses into their on-going life experience.

HISTORICAL VIEWS OF THE THERAPEUTIC RELATIONSHIP

With the development of psychoanalysis, Sigmund Freud revolutionized the practice of psychiatry and laid the foundation for modern psychotherapy. Central to this new method was a focus on the emotional reactions of the patient to the therapist. This unconscious transference of feelings about the client's parent(s) and other caretakers to the relationship with the therapist became the cornerstone of psychoanalytic treatment. The idea of the therapist as a "blank slate" grew out of this approach to psychotherapy, with the clinician remaining, in effect, a non-specific human presence, onto which the patient's feelings could be projected and then "analyzed". This way of thinking also proscribed personal disclosure on the part of the therapist, who, it was understood, should reveal as little as possible about themselves or their personal history.

In contemporary models of psychodynamic treatment, exploration of the client's reactions to their therapist remains a cornerstone of the process. What has changed is the idea that the therapist should strive to be a non-reactive and generic human presence. In the view of modern psycho-analytic theory, the therapeutic encounter takes place in an "intersubjective field" – a place where the unique minds of the therapist and the client come together (Ammaniti & Gallese, 2014). In this view, therapy is a relational process, and the therapist makes explicit use of his or her own experience as a therapeutic tool. Thus, in modern psychodynamic psychotherapy, the therapist is much more likely to share their own personal experience of what is going on for them in the relationship as a way of clarifying the relational dynamics and of modeling the value of self-disclosure in intimate relationships (Epstein, 2022; Kealy & Ogrodniczuk, 2019; Wallin, 2007).

The other major psychotherapeutic approach that has influenced grief therapy is the client-centered tradition, founded by Carl Rogers (Rogers, 1951, 1957). As with contemporary psychoanalytic methods, client-centered therapy emphasizes the importance of the therapeutic relationship as a curative factor but directs the therapist to maintain a specific type of thera-peutic stance towards the client: one of unconditional positive regard, emotional empathy and warmth, and congruence. In client centered approaches, the therapist has always been seen as an authentic, thinking, feeling human being – not a neutral presence. This clinical posture approximates the approach that has been adopted by contemporary psychodynamic clinicians. Both of these approaches embody a shift in emphasis from content to process. What the practitioner says is not more important than how they say it and how they engage with the client (Allen, 2013; Epstein, 2022).

Research on the factors that correlate with therapeutic effectiveness has consistently validated the importance of the therapeutic bond (Allen, 2022; Norcross & Wampold, 2018).

Over the past 20 years the American Psychological Association Presidential Task Force on Evidence Based Practice has amassed evidence demonstrating the importance of the original Rogerian relational variables, as well as the skill of the clinician at customizing the therapy to the particular personality and defensive style of the client. This includes the clinician's ability to arrive at and maintain consensus goals for treatment with the client, their willingness to gather ongoing feedback about the progress of treatment (particularly negative feedback), their ability to repair "ruptures" that develop in the treatment alliance (Eubanks et al., 2018) and their skillfulness at managing their own "counter-transference" reactions to the client (Norcross & Wampold, 2006, 2011, 2018). The "corpus of psychotherapy research" has consistently demonstrated that the "largest chunk of outcome variance" involves individual therapist differences and the emergent therapeutic relationship between patient and therapist, regardless of technique or school of therapy ... What is missing in treatment guidelines, now across five decades of research, are the person of the therapist and the therapeutic relationship. As a consequence of this omission, "the vast majority of current attempts to develop treatment guidelines" are "seriously incomplete and misleading, both on clinical and empirical grounds" (Norcross & Wampold, 2018).

In the remainder of this chapter, our goal is to operationalize many of these empirically supported variables in the form of what we call the *Core Capacities* of the attachment informed grief therapist. These are the capacities that enable the clinician to use the therapeutic relationship as a means to enhance the bereaved client's sense of trust, safety, and feeling understood, and hence the effectiveness of grief therapy.

CORE CAPACITIES OF THE ATTACHMENT INFORMED GRIEF THERAPIST

We make a distinction between the Core Capacities of the attachment informed grief therapist, which we see as foundational skills, and some of the specific techniques that are described in Chapters 9 and 10. Techniques are explicit procedures used by the therapist at particular times to achieve a particular goal(s). For example, the grief therapist might have a client do some letter writing to the deceased in the service of resolving some "unfinished business" or strengthening the continuing bond with the deceased. When applied with wisdom, skill, and an empathically derived knowledge of the client, such techniques can be invaluable tools in grief therapy.

In contrast to techniques, the Core Capacities presented here are applied throughout the course of therapy, primarily in the service of building, maintaining, and repairing the therapeutic alliance between client and clinician. From the perspective of our model, as outlined in Chapter 7, these capacities help the clinician become a trusted attachment figure for the bereaved client, one who uses the relationship itself to underpin the healing process.

Core Capacity One: Fostering Emotional Safety and Trust

Emotional and physical safety is the cornerstone of all secure attachment relationships, including the therapeutic relationship. Mammalian species are hardwired to pay attention to potential threats in their environment;

for human beings, the threat can be psychological as well as physical. Early experiences of threat, particularly when experienced at the hands of caregivers, are laid down in memory and continue to influence how the individual sees the world. Someone whose early experience with caregivers compromised their attachment security will approach a potentially threatening interpersonal experience (such as therapy) with a learned attachment style meant to protect themselves from interpersonal threats. By definition, threat activates the attachment system, whether secure or insecure. For clients with a secure attachment orientation, the likelihood of being able to use the clinician as a transitional attachment figure is usually high. Difficulties in establishing a secure bond are more likely to arise when the client is avoidant anxious or disorganized in their attachment orientation (Wiseman & Egozi, 2021; Talia & Holmes, 2021).

The loss of a significant person in someone's life often results in a state of heightened psychological vulnerability, which can contribute to the individual's sense of talk therapy as emotionally threatening (Thomson, 2010). It is no wonder, then, that building trust is the first order of business for grief therapists. *The literature on grief therapy and attachment suggests that the clinician must be able to modify and customize their approach to a given client's attachment orientation if the therapy is to be successful* (Mikulincer et al., 2013; Sekowski & Prigerson, 2022; Talia & Holmes, 2021).

How does the clinician build trust with a bereaved client? Our answer is "One step at a time." Recall that a parent engenders secure attachment in their offspring by being reliable in their availability, predictable in their responses, affectively attuned to their child, and skillful in alleviating distress and increasing positive affect in the child. These same principles apply when a grief therapist works to build trust with a bereaved client, particularly one who comes to the encounter with an insecure attachment style – one whose early attachment experiences have left them with expectations that close relationships will lead to emotional disappointment, injury, or abandonment. Just as with the relationship between parent and child, the sense of "felt security" is not created in a single interaction between therapist and bereaved client. Rather, it is the result of repeated interactions in which the therapist proves to be available, trustworthy, benevolent, and skillful in their actions.

Therapeutic Distance

Mallinckrodt, Daly, and Wang offer a useful model of the evolution of therapeutic distance over the course of treatment (Mallinckrodt et al., 2009). While originally formulated to describe treatment for attachment-based problems in the client's interpersonal life, it also has direct applicability to work with bereaved clients with insecure attachment histories. The authors recommend that the practitioner, particularly at the beginning of therapy, adjust their own style to reflect the client's attachment-based requirements for feeling safe. Over the course of treatment, the clinician may gradually move toward a style of engagement that then challenges the client to explore different ways of being in a close relationship. We propose that in attachment informed grief therapy, the therapist monitor and adjust the therapeutic distance with regard to three relevant domains presented by the client: their relationship with the deceased, with their own grief reactions to the loss, and with the therapist as a helping attachment figure.

Building Trust with the Avoidantly Attached Bereaved Client

In Chapter 4, we discussed some of the factors to consider when working with a client whose attachment style is generally avoidant. As we noted, in the beginning of therapy, the clinician will need to go slowly in asking the client to focus on and tolerate exploration of all three of these domains. They will need to adapt to the client's style and pace, without pathologizing it or communicating impatience (Zech & Arnold, 2011). Over time, as the therapeutic alliance grows, however, the clinician will gradually encourage the client to relate to these three domains in a different way – one that helps them to decrease their psychological distance from their continuing bond with the deceased, from their own grief reactions, and by extension, from the therapist. This evolution over the course of therapy helps to increase the client's repertoire of coping tools as they learn that allowing themselves to approach their loss is a tolerable experience – one that actually leaves them feeling better than simply avoiding it.

Mark

Mark entered grief therapy with the second author only in response to his wife's urging after the death of his older brother in combat in the Middle East. Mark acknowledged that he missed his brother, but also told the therapist that he was "not one to cry in my beer about things like this." Mark felt that he had done as well as could be expected with the loss and believed that because he had been able to continue working and supporting his family, he was okay. However, his wife revealed a different, more complex story. In a joint session with Mark and the therapist, she indicated that her husband was becoming more and more withdrawn from her and their two children. He was drinking more heavily, sleeping poorly at night, and had recently had three episodes when he uncharacteristically exploded verbally at her or one of their children. She also reported that Mark was reluctant to talk about his brother, despite her attempts to encourage him to do so.

Understanding that Mark was having trouble integrating this painful loss, the therapist decided that he needed to go slowly with him in the beginning. He decided to concentrate on building a relationship with his client. While offering Mark a rationale early on for why he thought grief therapy might be helpful and stating that he believed that Mark's symptoms were related to his grief, he also told his client that his goal was not to get Mark to "spill his guts" each week. In fact, he explained that his wish would be for Mark to be able to "visit" his grief from time to time at a moment of his choosing, and even symbolically to "visit his brother" through memories of their life together during the sessions, so that he would be free to address the other important things that needed his attention in life now, such as his wife and children.

Following this pathway, the therapist began by asking Mark to tell him more about his life now, what he enjoyed and was interested in, and what his goals and ambitions were for his future. They sometimes chatted amiably about sports teams that they mutually admired, or about the work that Mark did and the achievements of his children. As this progressed, the therapist began to inquire about Mark's brother in relation to these particular topics - did he and Mark share an interest in sports (yes); did they talk about how their work and family life was going (yes); were there particularly happy memories or stories about Mark and his brother from childhood (yes). Over the course of the sessions, the therapist would casually point out how important Mark's brother had been in his life, and what a "hole" had been created by his death.

As the trust between them grew, and Mark began to open up and become invested in the therapy, the therapist started to focus more on the details of his brother's death, and how life had been for him since his brother's demise. Eventually, he was able to ask Mark to share what he thought and felt when he first got the news of his brother's death, what the funeral had been like for him, and more about how he managed his "visits" with his grief now. Mark wept for the first time in that session but reported in the following session that it had helped – he had been able to sleep better after that and seemed less possessed by the thoughts about the horror of his brother's death and his yearning to have him back. Further work in the therapy involved the use of some directed techniques, such as having Mark write a letter to his brother, and also visit his brother's grave to read the letter, accompanied by his wife and children. All of these efforts helped Mark to both confront his grief and to be able to "put it away" when he needed to do so.

Building Trust with the Anxiously Attached Bereaved Client

In keeping with our definition of grief therapy, the goal of the attachment informed grief therapist is to help the client develop flexible attention to the loss (see Chapter 7). In the language of the Dual Process Model of grief, this means being able to move towards a "loss orientation" at times and places of their own choosing. For example, in the previous example, the therapist was able to help Mark move towards his brother, towards his own grief about the loss of his brother, and towards a closer and more self-disclosing relationship with his therapist. In contrast, for the client who has an anxious attachment style, the clinical approach might be quite different with regard to these three domains. Here, the most difficult therapeutic work often involves gradually helping the client to flexibly move *away* from their grief – that is, to be able to move towards a "restoration orientation." Work with these clients also typically involves transforming the nature of the continuing bond with the deceased in a way that continues the relationship but recognizes the reality of the physical death and separation. It may also require helping the client to scale back the emotional dependency that the anxiously attached client often forms with their grief therapist.

Carmella

Carmella felt bewildered and frightened after the death of her husband of 25 years after a difficult struggle with cancer. Carmella described their relationship as "perfect" and reported feeling more overwhelmed than she had ever been in her life. She portrayed her husband as "a rock," someone who she could always rely on to help her when she felt unsure or afraid. Carmella had great difficulty handing many of the family tasks without her husband, she yearned intensely to be with him, and although not actively suicidal, she frequently expressed indifference as to whether she lived or died.

Not surprisingly, Carmella frequently looked to the therapist (JJ) for reassurance and support. Her feelings spilled out more or less continuously in their sessions, as she wept frequently and expressed a great deal of hopelessness about ever feeling better. She talked mostly about her husband's illness and dying experience, and also had trouble ending the sessions, frequently wanting to tell the clinician "just one more thing." Based on Carmella's way of relating to him, the therapist knew that he would initially need to provide some extra support for his client. He told Carmella that he knew she was in tremendous pain, and was also frightened about coping without her husband. He suggested that strengthening Carmella's ability to take care of herself might be one of the major goals for their work together. He also indicated that there might be ways that Carmella could "not let go, but instead find a different way to hold on" to her husband – a goal which Carmella liked. The therapist also allowed Carmella plenty of time to tell her story in her own way and pace, took seriously her suicidal ideation, and offered extra contact time between sessions via e-mail "check-ins."

Over time, the therapist pointed out to Carmella the competencies she had but did not recognize. He also noted when Carmella had a little easier session ("you didn't cry quite as much this week"), praising her slow but steady progress. He began to ask Carmella about the things that she was learning that gave her some relief and encouraged her to do them more deliberately when she found herself upset (e.g., gardening). The therapist encouraged Carmella to join a widow/widowers bereavement group, not only for the support, but for the chance of making new friends, something that Carmella tried and liked. He also began suggesting that Carmella resume some of the activities that she had enjoyed doing earlier in her life. They discussed engaging in some of these activities with her adult children (going to new restaurants), but also joining a book club where she could begin reading and discussing the literature that she loved.

Lastly, another major component of the therapy consisted of helping Carmella transform the psychological attachment with her husband. The therapist introduced a new idea to Carmella: that although she could not have her husband physically back in her life, she could continue to have a relationship with him, and even count on him as an important source of support. He encouraged Carmella to begin writing to her husband, and also writing back what she felt he might say to her after reading her letters. Over time, Carmella described a growing sense that her husband was now watching over her. She enjoyed talking with him every evening before she went to bed. After about a year, Carmella and the therapist agreed to gradually reduce the frequency of their meetings.

Building Trust with the Disorganized/Unresolved Client

As discussed in Chapter 4, clients with a Disorganized/Unresolved attachment style are often the most emotionally wounded of our clients (Beeney et al., 2017). Typically, they present for grief therapy not only with issues of a current loss, but with a great many characterological issues that result from early experiences with caregivers who were abusive, neglectful, or abandoning (Sekowski & Prigerson, 2022). People with this classification often have a defensive or guarded edge to their style of relating to people (including the therapist), while also craving contact and support. They also typically suffer from one or more psychiatric and/or substance abuse disorders. Establishing a trusting and productive working alliance with them in treatment can be no small task, and the therapist's understanding of attachment dynamics and the role of early relational history is often crucial to helping the client.

Allan

Allan, a 37-year-old single man, presented for grief therapy with the second author after the cancer death of his girlfriend, Sandi. Their relationship had been a stormy one, filled with considerable conflict and numerous separations, followed by reconciliation. Their last reconnection happened when Sandi was diagnosed with ovarian cancer, and Allan returned to be with her. Both Allan and Sandi were heavy drinkers, and suffered from bouts of depression, although Allan's depression was expressed more often as explosive outbursts directed at Sandi. Allan's drinking had increased since Sandi's death, as had some occasional suicidal ideation. Allan had also recently been fired from a job for excessive absenteeism.

Allan's early history included several losses and disrupted attachment relationships. His father abandoned the family when Allan was four years old. His mother began to drink heavily. The family moved frequently as she struggled with financial problems and depression. Three and a half years later, his mother remarried a man who was a stable provider, but who was physically and verbally abusive to Allan and his mother. Conflict between Allan and his stepfather increased in his adolescence, and he moved out of the house at age 17 and joined the Army. Over the years, he maintained periodic contact with his mother, but continued to avoid and despise his stepfather.

Clinical work with Allan occurred over the course of several years, during which Allan would do a piece of work with the therapist, and then drop out of treatment – only to return when new problems (or resurgence of old ones) surfaced in his life. In the first episode of treatment, Allan's narrative about the loss of Sandi, and even more so about his childhood, was very fragmented. He was clearly uncomfortable discussing his thoughts and feelings, and had difficulty putting them into a coherent narrative. Allan mainly wanted help with his disrupted sleep and the problems that his drinking was creating in his work life. Allan stayed in therapy for only a short time but returned about two years later after he had remarried and found himself having intense arguments with his new partner. A year and a half later, when he became a father at the age of 41, Allan found himself flooded with a range of emotions that he thought he had "put behind him," and he returned for a third round of therapy. This third episode resulted in the most productive work that he and his therapist had been able to do. Allan was able to talk for the first time in depth about the impact of his early family life on his development. In their work together, the therapist and Allan were able to identify and mourn the many losses he had experienced in his life, ranging from the initial loss of his biological father, the loss of security as his family life was shattered by the stress of single parenting and his mother's increased drinking and erratic behavior, and then the further loss of his mother as a safe haven in the face of an abusive stepfather. Allan also began to talk in more depth about the impact of his relationship with and subsequent loss of Sandi. Over the course of the next two years, Allan came to better understand his use of alcohol and avoidance to cope with his painful feelings of unworthiness, loneliness, and fears of abandonment in close re-lationships. He developed a new clarity about what he wanted for himself in his life. Over time, Allan's ability to be nurturing towards and take pleasure in his new wife and son increased significantly. Likewise, his depression and need to use alcohol to deal with it subsided.

This vignette about Allan illustrates the long-term impact of early attachment insecurity that results from unreliable and abusive caregivers, including the resulting disorganized/unresolved attachment style that combines both avoidant and anxious elements. Allan's problems, while catalyzed by the loss through death of a conflictual but important adult attachment relationship, had deeper roots in the emotional damage he absorbed in his early relationships. The willingness of the therapist to meet Allan where he was in the therapeutic encounters allowed progressively deeper layers of his emotional injury and grief to be brought to light, shared, validated, and mourned during each episode of therapy. The stable availability of the therapist over a period of several years, as well as the clinician's subtle tuning of the therapy to Allan's needs and readiness to be more vulnerable, greatly facilitated Allan's growing maturation and capacity to become permanently committed to a partner and child of his own.

Additional Ways to Build Trust with Clients

We believe that the therapist also builds trust by being transparent, that is, making their intentions and perspectives clear to the client, so that the bereaved person understands how the therapist views their problems and the goals and methods of the therapy. For example, a therapist who believes that successful griefwork involves confrontation with the death would make this belief clear to the client, along with timely explanations about why they held this belief. Even if the client has some doubts about what the practitioner is saying, transparency allows the client to begin to trust that "my therapist will be direct with me – I can trust his motives and agenda, because he makes them clear to me."

As much as we strive to create a safe and non-judgmental space for our clients, there may be times when our observations or suggestions are taken as criticism, as in this interaction with Audrey, who was introduced in Chapter 4.

Audrey

A: My brother was yelling at me about my mother's estate and my sister just stood there! She didn't stand up for me! Then the next day she said "What was all that about yesterday! As if she didn't know!"

PK: How does your sister do with conflict?

A: She hates it.

PK: Ah. So could it be that she was afraid to confront him? And that she asked you that the next day because she felt bad about not standing up for you?. Maybe she wanted to give you two a chance to talk about it.

A: Okay, I see what you're doing. But do you think I'm wrong to be angry at her?

PK: Here's the thing. This isn't about my thinking that you're wrong to be angry. My only purpose here is **to help you suffer less**. When you get angry at your sister, when you feel like she's not on your side, that hurts, yes?

A: A lot. I hate feeling that way. So OK, I get it, and you're trying to tell me in a gentle way that there's another way for me to think about it and if I do that I won't hurt as much.

Note that this way of framing a suggestion that has been, or could be, taken by the client as criticism helps to preserve the therapeutic bond, but *only* if the statement ("my only purpose here is to help you suffer less"), is believable to the client. That is, momentary ruptures can be healed, but only if there is a foundation of trust and mutual good will, and the clinician is able and willing to be transparent with the client.

Additional ways of building trust include giving the client a maximum amount of control over the process of treatment, while recognizing the degree of direction or therapeutic leadership the client may need from the clinician. Many bereaved people, particularly those with an avoidant attachment style, fear that therapy will involve an involuntary surrender of control over their emotions and the privacy of their thoughts, as though therapists have the ability to read a person's mind and force them to "open up." To ease this concern the clinician needs to not only explain, but to demonstrate in their actions, that therapy is a collaborative process, with the client retaining final control over their own internal process and their disclosure of that process to the therapist. The vignette with Allan illustrates this principle, as the therapist allowed Allan to regulate the psychological distance in their relationship, including the frequency and duration of their contacts.

Finally, therapists build emotional safety and security by demonstrating warmth and genuine respect for the client as an individual. These are the core components of successful therapy identified by Carl Rogers many years ago, and they apply equally well to grief therapy today (Rogers, 1957; Harris, 2021).

The empathically attuned grief therapist will have as their goal understanding and then responding appropriately to their client's particular attachment style. They will adjust their own pacing, style, and interventions to the tolerance levels of the client. When the inevitable empathic failures occur in this process, the therapist recognizes the error, and works to repair the relationship so that it is more in synchrony with the needs of the client.

Core Capacity Two: Empathy

Empathic attunement is a vital component in a number of contemporary models of psychotherapy, including grief therapy (Allen, 2013, 2021; Epstein, 2022; Geller, 2018; Harris, 2021; Wallin, 2007). Empathy has both emotional and cognitive components. Emotional empathy involves the ability to resonate with the emotional state of another: to observe the emotional state of another person and then to experience the same emotion in ourselves. The happiness we feel when watching a delighted child play with a pet dog, or the sadness we feel when we see a bereaved mother well up in tears, are responses that often occur without any higher order cognitive modulation. In the same way that we may find ourselves unconsciously walking in step with a friend, we can find ourselves feeling in step with another person's emotions.

The resonance that connects people is not without emotional risk, however. Immersion in the feelings of a distressed person can result in emotional flooding on the part of the helper and can interfere with their ability to take appropriate action. For this reason, it is important for the empathic observer to exert what has been called "effortful control," or higher cortical modulation of resonant emotions. (Hodges & Wegner, 1997; Rothschild, 2006). This ability to maintain a "self-other" distinction ("they are in pain, but their pain is not my pain – instead, I feel bad about their distress") is crucial if the observer is to respond in an engaged and compassionate way, rather than defending themselves from pain by maintaining emotional distance. This capacity to feel the pain of a client without becoming immobilized by it is a critical empathic skill in a grief therapy (Harris, 2021).

The cognitive component of empathy involves what is generally thought of as perspective taking – that is, understanding not just what a person feels, but why they feel that way. To have perspective on another person's responses, we need to have in mind not just what is happening to the person now, but also to consider the impact that previous life experiences may be having on a person's emotions and behaviors.

An example of emotional empathy might be: "I can see from your face and body posture that you are sad." In contrast, cognitive empathy involves the recognition that "I understand that you are sad *because* your mother has just died. You had a very close relationship with her, and that makes it especially hard to lose her."

The capacity to combine both emotional and cognitive empathy in the context of a therapeutic relationship, while also holding on to the ability to differentiate between self and other, entails a subtle balancing act, and an acquired skill. On the one hand the grief therapist needs to be open to the pain of their client, and on the other hand not so open that the therapist becomes emotionally overwhelmed and triggers their own defensive processes. This "sweet spot" of empathic attunement appears to offer the most helpful stance for any caregiver of the bereaved individual, whether they are friend, family member, or grief therapist (Larson, 2020).

In addition, it is crucial that the clinician not only be able to emotionally resonate with and understand their client, *but that they are also able to successfully communicate this understanding to the client.* Empathic attunement that is not felt by the client is not really empathic attunement. The client must "feel felt" by their therapist; they must know, in a way that goes beyond words, that they have been understood, and that they are not alone (Allen, 2022; Cozolino, 2017; Siegel, 2012). The "I felt like you understood" interaction with Carol, mentioned in the opening vignette of this chapter, would seem to include all of these elements of empathy. The therapist himself felt Carol's emotional distress over the loss of her son, he reflected on the source of the distress and based on his emotional response and cognitive appraisal responded in a way that communicated his empathy and desire to comfort her. We believe that this complex integration of empathic skills is essential to an attachment informed approach to grief therapy and is a capacity that requires active monitoring throughout the therapeutic process.

This is empathy: to feel what someone else feels. Overlapping and often confused with empathy is *compassion* (Vachon & Harris, 2016) where the felt sense of another person's suffering is accompanied by a desire to alleviate it. The emphasis in definitions of compassion is on *action*. Joan Halifax, American Zen Buddhist teacher, anthropologist and activist tells us that while the "capacity to see clearly into the nature of suffering" is the first requirement of compassion, "that is not enough ... because compassion means that we aspire, we actually aspire to transform suffering" (Halifax, 2012).

Based on their many years of clinical experience and research Vachon and Harris (2016) have described compassion as a" liberating capacity" for the client and therapist.

> In the presence of a compassionate listener the client is able to fully explore and express their feelings ... Even coming from a place of limited trust in others, clients gradually come to anticipate that the clinician will listen to them without an excess of emotion, without judgement and without feeling the need to preemptively "fix" the client's grief.
>
> (Vachon & Harris, 2016, p. 267)

Harris (2021) has proposed that compassion is of "specific interest in situations of loss and grief, due to the intensity of the work and the need to provide clients with a secure base from which to they can begin the process of rebuilding their lives after a significant loss" (p.780). Harris advocates training in compassion and stresses the need to disconnect compassion from its association with "prosocial behaviors such as kindness or sympathy." Compassion is something that calls for stronger stuff: at its heart compassion is most closely associated with courage.

> It is with courage that we are able to turn toward pain and suffering rather than away from it. The ability to stay fully present requires practice, that when cultivated, enhances a sense of sustainable well-being, even in situations where significant distress and suffering occur.
>
> (Harris, 2021, p. 781)

Much of what Harris proposes as training) in compassion relates to strengthening the capacity for emotion regulation, a subject to which we will return in the Chapter 9.

Core Capacity Three: Non-Defensiveness and Attending to Relational Repair

A strain or rupture in the therapeutic alliance has been shown to dramatically increase the chances of treatment failure, including premature termination of therapy. Conversely, the ability of a therapist to successfully repair these ruptures is one of the best predictors of the ultimate success of treatment (Norcross, 2011b; Norcross & Wampold, 2011a, 2011b). Norcross identifies three common types of alliance rupture in psychotherapy (Norcross, 2011b). The first is disagreement about the goals of therapy: what does the client want from therapy, and how well does it match what the therapist is trying to achieve? The second is about the tasks of therapy, meaning the methods and processes by which therapy can achieve the agreed upon goals. And the third is the emergence of direct interpersonal strain or tension in the relationship between therapist and client. To provide an example of a rupture of the therapeutic alliance in grief therapy, consider the following hypothetical case:

Jose

Jose, a middle-aged male whose wife had recently died, entered therapy wanting help to feel less depressed and to improve his disrupted sleep cycle. The therapist, however, believed that Jose needed to be less avoidant and to confront the reality of his wife's passing, with its attendant emotions and thoughts. The therapist spent the initial sessions trying to get Jose to talk about his feelings about his wife and her death, sometimes pointing out his avoidance of the topic. Instead, Jose tried to discuss the problems created in his life by his wife's death – for example, how to handle discipline issues with his children by himself, and what he could do to get a good night's sleep. He wanted the therapist to give him some "tricks" about how to cope, while the therapist tended to avoid making direct recommendations to Jose, instead trying to help him find his own solutions to his problems. Rather quickly, Jose began to feel frustrated with the process, deciding that it was a waste of time and money. The therapist, meanwhile, was aware of becoming annoyed with Jose, deciding that he was resistant and unwilling to deal with the impact of his wife's death. This culminated in Jose not showing up for his next appointment and deciding not to return to therapy again.

In this vignette, we can see all three types of relational rupture in the therapeutic alliance. The therapist has different goals for therapy than the client (confronting the death rather than avoiding it), and different expectations about how to go about achieving those goals (getting the client to "open up" and talk about his feelings rather than offering specific suggestions about solving specific problems). As a result, tensions have arisen in their relationship.

What might the clinician have done differently in an empathically attuned therapeutic relationship?

Sensing that Jose was growing frustrated, the clinician made several adjustments, starting with the acknowledgement that they were out of synch: "Sometimes I feel like we're going in different directions here – that I'm trying to get you to do something that to you doesn't seem right. Is that how you see it? If so, that must be frustrating for you, and sometimes it is for me as well. Let's talk about how we can get more on the same page." Listening carefully to the client's explanation that he felt that he was wasting time, the clinician inquired about what would make Jose feel like they were making more progress. This led to a fruitful discussion in which Jose communicated that he needed to be able to get a good night's sleep, without thinking constantly about his deceased wife. The therapist gently remarked on how difficult that must be for him, and assured him that that they could work on some "tricks" (the client's own words) to manage his evenings more easily. The therapist suggested that Jose might be able to use their sessions as the best time to "face the tough facts," but then give himself a "break from the grief" when away from their sessions. Jose could relate to this idea, and agreed to try talk more about how he feels in the meetings, and to try the suggested sleep technique at home. By the end of the conversation, both Jose and his therapist felt that they understood each other better, and that they were now functioning more as a team.

What capacities are required of the therapist to be able to handle a rupture in the therapeutic relationship with success? Actually, all of the Core Capacities identified here come into play. Specifically, to respond well to the strain in the alliance, the therapist must maintain a genuine openness and non-defensiveness that allows the issue to be worked through. The ability to mentalize about the experience of the client, about the therapist's own experience in working with the client, and most importantly, about the differences in how they each experience the problems in their relationship, were crucial to resolving the impasse.

Human beings are continually evaluating and passing judgment on their own behavior, feelings, and thoughts, as well as those of other people; this is what our brains are wired to do in order to help us correctly read other people and situations. Although therapists strive to be aware of their own motivations and feelings, we believe that all people can think, feel, and act for reasons of which they are unaware. The defensiveness that can be unconsciously provoked in the therapeutic relationship can be invisible to both the client and the clinician, yet destructive to their alliance. As much as possible, maintaining an open and non-defensive stance and suspending one's own judgments about a given interaction or a given client, is vital to doing the work well. What differentiates a well-functioning therapeutic relationship from a less than helpful one is the capacity of the therapist (and to a lesser extent, the client) to recognize when an empathic failure is happening, and to take steps to repair the alliance.

Capacity Four: Distress Tolerance

By now, we hope that we have helped the reader to understand that grief, even when it is not debilitating, is dysregulating. This state of disequilibrium, which varies greatly in intensity and persistence, can be eased by the presence of a supportive person or persons. No matter how independent and skilled at taking care of ourselves we may become, there are times that life challenges us with more than we can manage without help from others. As adults, the need for others is generally not as constant, or as desperate, as it is when we are young. But it is a need, nonetheless, and one that tends to be particularly intense in response to loss (Vachon & Harris, 2016).

As we have noted, the relationship with an empathic grief therapist serves a reregulating function that is in many respects similar to the re-regulation that an attuned caregiver provides to a distressed child. But to serve in this stabilizing and soothing capacity for another person requires that the therapist have a high capacity for distress tolerance – for remaining "present" in the face of the emotional, cognitive, and behavioral storms that bereaved clients may bring to therapy.

This chapter began with a case example (Carol) in which, arguably, the clinician was overwhelmed by his own reactions. In hindsight, it led him to make what was probably the right response, based on Carol's feedback in the following session, but it also might have led to an unhelpful experience for the client. For example, imagine that the clinician had broken down in sobs as he listened to Carol's wrenching story. The client then might have become concerned about the well-being of the therapist and felt compelled to comfort him. Carol might also have found herself wondering "Can this person handle this? This is just like the people at my church – they don't know what to say or do with me. Maybe no one can deal with this." *One of the most difficult aspects of being a grief therapist is learning to tolerate one's own feelings of helplessness in the face of their client's profound suffering, and their presentation of a problem that is existentially "unfixable" – the irrevocable loss of a loved one to death.* Such helplessness has the potential to undermine the clinician's feelings of professional competency and efficacy. It can also bring the clinician face to face with his or her own feelings about loss and mortality.

Sarah

As mentioned in previous chapters, Sarah lost her son to suicide. In addition, she had a number of subsequent losses in her life. These losses included the break-up of her marriage, the loss of financial security, and rejection by a new man with whom she had begun to have a romantic relationship. These additional losses, on top of the grief, guilt, and feelings of failure about her son's death, had a significant effect on Sarah's sense of self-worth. They culminated in an acute period of despondency marked by significant suicidal ideation and hopelessness. The therapist (JJ) monitored this state of mind, and directly encouraged Sarah to contact him if she was having a very difficult time. She did this, and in an emergency session with the clinician, poured out her feelings of despair, shame, and thoughts of ending her life. The therapist listened carefully, with empathy and compassion, as well as some anxiety about the extent to which his client was at risk for making a suicide attempt. For the first part of the session, the therapist's goal was simply to have the client feel that they were not alone with their distress – that he "got it" about how badly she was feeling. As the session unfolded, and the therapist was convinced that Sarah felt the recognition of her emotional pain, he worked to help Sarah reflect on why she was feeling so very bad at this particular point in time. He enumerated the many losses she had experienced (not the least of which was the suicide) and normalized the feelings of unworthiness they had understandably engendered. He also noted the significant progress they had made in their work together, and gently reminded her of the resilience that she had been able to muster in the face of these devastating losses. He also offered a metaphor about what had happened to Sarah, with her "psychological immune system" having been compromised by the losses, so that her ability to ward off assaults on her sense of well-being and self-esteem were not functioning at full capacity. By the end of the session, the combination of being able to freely express her distress, having those expressions accurately heard by the therapist, and then helped to view her suffering from a different and more normative perspective, seemed to help Sarah feel better – in other words, to reregulate her emotional arousal back to a range that she could tolerate and manage by herself.

Distress tolerance refers to the capacity of the therapist to remain present for, yet not overwhelmed by, the emotional storms that grief may elicit in the client. Like a parent who listens to the fears, rage, and unhappiness of their child with calmness and compassion, and thereby helps the child to find their emotional equilibrium, the grief therapist serves a similar purpose for their client. In a very real sense, the professional caregiver functions as a kind of emotional shock absorber, softening the impact of the emotional injuries embedded in the loss (and sometimes the subsequent losses that flow from it). In this way, the clinician remains able to protect both themself, and the client, from emotional pain that could otherwise overwhelm them both.

The Liminal Space

Grief therapists are often asked "how do you listen to so many sad stories without being sad yourself?" When clients ask me (PK) this question, I explain that there is a space between us, and I am aware, as they speak to me, that they are in that space, and I join them there. And we hold their story together. We're sharing the weight of it. And because it is not my story, I can hold it in a different way, in a quieter way, and because they are with me in that space, they may be able to feel some of that quiet. I'm not afraid of their pain, and because they are in that space with me, maybe they can feel a bit less afraid. In creating this shared experience my hope is to offer what can be thought of us a *liminal state,* a state of relaxed attention that is conducive to new learning, to a different way of seeing and a different way of feeling.

Distressing Thoughts and Behavior

Along with strong feelings, bereaved clients may confront the clinician with a range of thoughts and behaviors that are distressing to the client (and often to the clinician). Hearing that a client is isolating herself from other people, abusing substances to numb her pain, or considering suicide, it is natural to feel concern and to find a course of action that will protect the client but not provoke defensiveness or a withdrawal from treatment. Clients may also behave in a guarded, sullen, or sarcastic manner, rolling their eyes every time the clinician makes a comment or ridiculing the clinician's observations. In most cases these ways of coping have their roots in the client's earliest attachment experiences with caregivers, and these defensive responses are a reflection of internal working models that developed at a time when the client was not able to develop healthier forms of self-protection. The challenge for the grief therapist is to address the problematic behavior while also keeping in mind the inner psychic pain and defensive processes that drive the dysfunctional coping patterns.

Finally, we would be remiss if we failed to mention one other form of helplessness that grief therapists must confront: their own existential vulnerability as a mortal human being. Therapists, of course, will have their own history of losses to absorb over the course of their lifetime, many of which will have shaped their own attachment style and frame of mind. And sooner or later, they must also confront their own approaching death. *In a very broad sense, all grief therapy is about the encounter by the client, and the therapist, with the uncertainty and impermanence of life itself.* While primarily focusing on the experience of our clients as they navigate what life has delivered to them, we believe that grief therapists must also work to make their peace with the transience of their own lives and emotional attachments. The recognition of their shared human experience – the need to come to terms with the reality of impermanence - can deepen the experience of mutuality between the grief therapist and client, an experience that is vital to doing the work well. This leads directly to our last Core Capacity of the attachment informed grief therapist.

Core Capacity Five: Openness, Mindfulness and Self-Knowledge

In order for the grief therapist to be of assistance to a client who is being buffeted by the disruption of loss, they must be aware of, have reflected on, and to a reasonable degree, come to terms with their own experiences of loss, separation, and psychological trauma. Of particular relevance to the ideas we are offering in this book, we would suggest that grief therapists should be attuned to their own experiences with attachment relationships, beginning with their early developmental experiences and on up through their current close relationships with partners, parents, children, colleagues, and friends. The goal is for the secure grief therapist to be knowledgeable about and accepting of their own feelings, thoughts, and bodily sensations, such that they are neither dissociated from them, nor controlled by them. This wisdom about one's own inner experience is what allows the attachment informed grief therapist to foster these capacities in their bereaved clients.

Openness

Openness has been described in Buddhist literature as a "beginner's mind" (Suzuki, 1973) – a receptivity to experience that is, as much as possible, free of assumptions, preconceptions, and prejudices. In the context of grief therapy, openness involves maintaining a non-judgmental stance regarding the experience that the client brings to therapy. It also means retaining an uncluttered curiosity about the client's unique way of construing their loss, as well as their relationship with the deceased and their attempts to live in the world without their loved one. Openness also denotes the therapist's willingness to refrain from prematurely coming to conclusions about who the person in front of them is, what they are capable of, and what they need from therapy. This approach is in marked contrast to a medical model of mental health intervention, in which therapy is deemed to be a mostly technical process in which rapid diagnosis of the patient's problem(s), followed by a straightforward application of the appropriate treatment, is regarded as the therapeutic ideal (similar to diagnosing a brain tumor, and then performing brain surgery to remove the tumor according to a standardized protocol). Lastly, openness implies what Wallin describes as the "flexibility and freedom" of the secure therapist (Wallin, 2014) – the capacity to change, adjust, and even stretch themselves beyond their usual professional comfort zone to meet the client where they need to be met.

The capacity to stretch, to improvise, and to meet the client where they are aspects of psychotherapy that feature in the work of the renowned hypnotherapist Milton Erikson. Erikson is best known for his use of "teaching tales," essentially extended metaphors designed to invite a patient to look at their problem in a different way. Erikson also made generous use of puns and playful humor. The psychologist Stephen Gilligan has adapted and built upon the work of Erikson, who was his teacher and mentor. We find it helpful to utilize what Gilligan has described as "three energies" of psychotherapy: tenderness, fierceness, and playfulness (Gilligan & Dilts, 2022). Consider as an example the way in which the tone of the following question alters its meaning. Let's say that the client has just said something along the lines of "I am just a mess. I can't do anything right." Circumstances can trigger such feelings, but if they are there to be triggered, it's because somewhere along the line the client learned to think about themselves this way. The therapist is interested in knowing where these beliefs come from, and so might say: "Where did you get that idea?"

In a tender voice, this is a gentle invitation to consider where (and from whom) they learned to see themselves this way, and beyond that, to consider whether this is a fair and true assessment of the sum total of who they are as a person.

Now consider the same statement expressed as a challenge: "Where did you get *that* idea?" Here the message is more direct: someone taught you that. Who do you think that was? Was it fair, then? Is it fair, now?

And finally, humor. Humor, in the midst of grief, can have the same effect as taking a breath, or having a sip of cool water when the throat is parched. Shared laughter a is a bonding agent in relationships, and in the right moment with the right person, can strengthen the bond we have with a bereaved client. A smile, offered to the client, often elicits a smile in return, with the result that both client and therapist experience a stress-reducing release of neuropeptides (Sonnby-Borgstrom, 2002) and neurotransmitters such as dopamine (Palmieri et al., 2021). Imagine responding to a client who states that "I must have the craziest family you've ever heard of!" A surprising number of clients claim this dubious distinction. The response here might be *"Wherever did you get that idea?"* in a tone of warmth and humor. Or one of us (JJ) when a client would apologize for using too many tissues, may respond with a gently teasing remark, something like "Oh, no problem. I buy them by the caseload at Costco …".

Like self-disclosure, humor is something we use sparingly and with therapeutic intent. A simple example is this exchange with a client who tends to disparage her own emotions. She has been talking for several minutes about how much she misses her husband.

Anne

A: Sorry, I don't mean to whine.

PK: Yeah, really, I can't stand it when people talk about sad things (said with a smile, which is returned). Of course, you're sad, He loved you. And the memory of his love is bittersweet.

A: See I don't want to talk about those things. I want to talk about cleaning out the freezer, I want to talk about replacing the carpets. I don't want to feel those feelings.

PK: Well, good luck with that because you know what, **you are feeling those feelings.**

While it is by no means universal, the inclination to mirror another's sorrow and to offer sympathy is a fundamental feature of human nature; we are wired to recognize and to resonate with other people's emotional states. But tenderness is just one element of authentic human relationships, and with therapeutic intent, we vary the tone of our communication with bereaved clients.

Mindfulness

Mindfulness can be understood as an extension of this stance of openness – essentially the clinician applying this same attitude of openness toward his or her own experience on a moment-to-moment basis. A number of theorists have noted that while mentalizing denotes the clinician's ability to reflect with *depth* on their own mind and the mind of their client, mindfulness points to the therapist's ability to reflect on the great *breadth* of the mind and of human experience (D. J. Siegel, 2010; R. D. Siegel, 2009; Wallin, 2010). Emerging from hundreds of years old Buddhist and Hindu meditation traditions, mindfulness practices have entered into western approaches to therapy as both a valuable generic skill of self-aware clinicians, as well as a specific therapeutic technique in various clinical situations (Epstein, 2022; Vachon & Harris, 2016). For the clinician, the practice of mindfulness entails awareness of the continuous changes in their own subjective experience while conducting therapy: thoughts, emotional reactions, and bodily sensations that arise during their time with a client. In line with modern psychodynamic therapy, this "data" about the therapist's own experience becomes part of the inter-subjective field to be examined, understood, and where helpful, shared with the client (Orange, 2010). As an example of this aspirational goal of remaining open and mindful, consider the following case example:

Wilma

Wilma entered therapy with JJ seeking help for her grief after multiple losses: of an important romantic relationship, of a beloved pet, and of her own physical functioning after it was compromised by a medical error that led to a permanent disability and chronic pain. She had previously been a relatively optimistic and resilient individual, but this series of losses, in close temporal proximity, had left her distressed and bitter. During one session, the therapist needed to end a few minutes early, due to another commitment. Wilma accurately felt the therapist's anxiety about ending the session, and felt cut-off and betrayed by it. At some point Wilma became unable to contain her anger at the therapist's manner, and she let loose with a verbal barrage, telling him that she felt abandoned by everyone in her social network, all of whom were "getting sick of me feeling sorry for myself – now even you." The therapist was aware of the bodily reactions (tightening in the stomach) and strong feelings of anger and shame that Wilma was evoking in him. He had to work hard to sit with these reactions, neither suppressing them, nor acting to defend himself against her attack. Instead, he struggled to reflect on what Wilma must have been feeling in response to what she experienced as the avoidance and dismissiveness of everyone in her social network, which now included her therapist. But he also worked to honor his own experience of feeling unfairly criticized. He expressed empathy to Wilma about how painful it must be for her to feel "unseen" by those around her and apologized if he had provoked this feeling in her. And he also clarified what he thought had been going on within himself in terms of his own need to end slightly early. He shared that he often felt at a loss as to how to talk with Wilma in a way that did not leave her feeling angry and hurt. His response led to a productive discussion with Wilma about her feelings of abandonment by many people in her life, as well as an empathic apology on her part for becoming so angry. Both Wilma and the therapist agreed that some life situations create dilemma's that are just unsolvable, leaving everyone feeling helpless and upset, despite everyone's best efforts.

Self-knowledge

Self-knowledge is the work done by the therapist to develop insight about their own sources of emotional pain and injury. It includes reflection on their own motivations for doing what they do with clients, and their own characteristic ways of psychologically protecting themselves when they feel threatened. It incorporates both the cultivation of mindfulness about one's interior experience – thoughts, feelings, bodily sensations – and deliberate effort at mentalizing or reflecting on that experience with a minimum of distortion or avoidance. Attachment theory, offers one useful way to think about the therapist's mode of reacting to their clients (Mikulincer & Shaver, 2007). And as Wallin points out, it is useful to understand that in addition to having an overall attachment style, each of therapist can fluctuate between different states of mind with regard to attachment at different points in time – sometimes on a moment to moment basis within the ebb and flow of a therapy session (Wallin, 2010, 2014).

When the therapist is in a secure state of mind with regard to attachment, or towards a particular client, they are in a balanced position towards their own experience and towards the communicated experience of their client. They can empathize with their client's feelings and thoughts yet differentiate between the client's experience and their own. Moreover, they can keep perspective about why their client feels, thinks, and acts the way they do. As Wallin notes, there is room for "two minds" – that of the clinician *and* that of the client (Wallin, 2007). Secure clinicians are also balanced in their need to seek certainty, order, and security for themselves and their client, and to explore the ambiguous and sometimes anxiety provoking possibilities for new meanings and behaviors with the client. In other words, clinicians with a secure attachment style are able to balance their own need for attachment security with their need for exploration. Clinicians in a secure frame of mind can be flexible in their stance with the client, sometimes taking the lead and acting as the "expert," while at other times being guided by and even corrected by the client. Mistakes in the therapeutic relationship are experienced mostly as opportunities to learn, rather than painful examples of failure. And throughout the therapy, the clinician is free to stay focused on the crucial process-oriented question that is central to good therapy: "what does my client need from me right now that will be of help?"

When clinicians are in an anxious (or preoccupied) state of mind with regard to attachment or a specific client, they are likely to be focused on the client's feelings and thoughts, to the exclusion of their own (Wallin, 2014). They may be worried about how the client will react to them, or whether they will approve of what the clinician is saying or doing. They may feel angry or wounded by what the client is communicating yet feel immobilized in their freedom to react to it. They are likely to over-identify with the client's experience of grief and find themselves triggered into remembering their own experiences of loss or trauma. They may devalue clients who intellectualize their grief or who express it with words, rather than with tears and other explicit signals of emotional distress. They may at times be overly serious with a client, and fail to appreciate the humor or absurdity that is part of their mourning, even as these things are a part of life as a whole. In Dual Process Model language, they may focus on a Loss Orientation to the exclusion of a Restoration Orientation with clients. They may find that their ability to use their left-brain capacities to analyze and reflect on what is happening has been subsumed by a right brain flood of emotion. They may be preoccupied with concern about the client's well-being (e.g., their ability to ever integrate their loss and rebuild their life, or their suicidality), but uncertain about how to be of help. They may experience themselves as incompetent or inconsequential and be filled with doubt about whether they can challenge the patient or risk strain or conflict in the relationship. In its more extreme form, the therapist in an anxious state of mind with regard to attachment may fear that the client will fire them – either by leaving them for someone else (e.g., another therapist), or by dying (e.g., suicide). Conversely, they may be suspicious of clients who seem to recover too quickly and have trouble letting the client end treatment with them.

By contrast, when the clinician is in an avoidant (or dismissing) frame of mind with regard to attachment or a particular client, they may limit themselves to detached, left-brain analysis of the client and their grief, with little or no resonance with the client's emotional experience. They may find themselves being contemptuous or disapproving of the client and their style of mourning. This may be particularly true of clients who are experienced as overly emotional, dependent, or needy. They may be certain that they understand the client and what needs to be done to help them, and may be prone to blaming the client for their resistance to accepting their help, or in being slow to recover. They may be overly focused on their own thoughts and feelings, rather than the thoughts and feelings of the client. They may find displays of strong grief emotion from the client to be awkward and uncomfortable and may steer the therapeutic conversation back to ideas and words, or even to humor. They may find themselves reacting with defensive anger when challenged by a client. They may be reluctant to share anything of a personal nature with the client, even when it might be of help.

Lastly, when a clinician is in a disorganized (or unresolved) state of mind with regard to attachment, or a given client, they are likely to respond to the client with the exaggerated emotionality or significantly distorted thinking associated with countertransference to a particular client. Perhaps the hallmark of this state of mind is a feeling of psychological paralysis or immobilization, along with significant bodily cues of hyperarousal. The client may evoke strong feelings of shame, rage, fear, or helplessness in the clinician. The vignette of Wilma is an example of this kind of intense response on the part of a clinician. Therapists may also find themselves responding with a hostile use of professional skills - for example, a hostile diagnosis ("This person is just a borderline") or attacks on the client via interpretations ("Clearly, you are out to get me, and are attempting to ruin me"). Particularly relevant to grief therapy is the experience of being overwhelmed by the client's bereavement situation (e.g., death of a child when the therapist is also a parent), or their grieving style (e.g., a client whose sadness feels unbearable to the clinician). Extreme feelings of helplessness, often accompanied by global feelings of professional incompetence and inadequacy, are also markers of this state of mind. Clinician's may find themselves wishing to avoid or be rid of the client because of the painful affect they trigger. Most of these states of mind will have been triggered by a specific client, but upon reflection, the therapist might discover they are rooted in areas of the clinician's own psychological vulnerability and dissociation that have their origins in wounding early experiences with attachment figures.

The repeated experience of these types of reactions, with many different clients, suggests a possible mismatch between the therapist's personality and skill set, and their choice of profession. Nonetheless, it is also true that at one time or another, all clinicians experience reactions like these with a given client who is very triggering for them. And the appropriate response, not surprisingly, is for the professional to make use of a relationship with someone in their professional setting, such as a trusted supervisor, colleague, or therapist they respect and with whom they feel a sense of safety. Together, they can reflect on and work through the clinician's reactions to the client. In other words, the clinician must make use of a secure attachment figure – someone who can serve as a safe haven and secure base for them - to help them reregulate themselves and mentalize about their experience with the client. This use of a safe and supportive relationship, in turn, allows the clinician to better serve as a helpful attachment figure for their client – restoring their ability to be empathically attuned to their client, without being overwhelmed by them.

SUMMARY

This chapter has focused on what we believe to be the heart of attachment informed grief therapy: the therapeutic relationship between therapist and client. We began with a brief discussion of the substantial body of the theory and research on the importance of the therapeutic alliance in all forms of psychotherapy, while noting that this topic has received comparatively little discussion in the grief counseling literature. We then introduced five Core Capacities that we believe the grief therapist must cultivate within themselves in order to foster a strong, collaborative, and effective relationship with their clients. These capacities include: fostering emotional safety and trust; empathy; non-defensiveness and attention to relational repair; distress tolerance; and openness, mindfulness, and self-knowledge.

Grief support, like all psychotherapy, is about more than technique. This perspective animates and organizes the two volumes that comprise the third edition of *Therapy Relationships that Work* (Norcross & Wampold, 2018). Rather than assembling research that supports the use of specific treatment for particular diagnoses, what the editors present are studies designed to identify the contribution of *therapy adaptations and therapy relationships* to treatment effectiveness. Norcross and Wampold acknowledge that their singular attention in this edition to responsiveness as a factor in therapeutic effectiveness may unfortunately be taken to imply that, in their view "this is the only important area of inquiry" (p. 4). In fact, their actual position is much more nuanced; they do not dispute the contribution of treatment methods to patient success, but insist that attention be paid to the decades of careful research indicating that the "relational ambience of psychotherapy and responsiveness to patients prove typically more powerful than the particular therapeutic method or strategy" (Norcross & Wampold, p. 4). In line with this evidence, they (and we) endorse the argument made by Jerome Frank (1991):

> My position is not that technique is irrelevant to outcome. Rather, I maintain that ... the success of all techniques depends on the patient's sense of alliance with an actual or symbolic healer. This position implies that ideally therapists should select for each patient the therapy that accords, or can be brought to accord, with the patient's personal characteristics and view of the problem.
>
> (Frank & Frank, 1991, p. xv)

Unlike the capacities presented in this chapter, which are used throughout the course of therapy, the specific therapeutic techniques presented in the following chapters are used for targeted purposes and for selected clients. Techniques are tools, and their value is always tied to their suitability to the task at hand. While that task may be similar in its broad outlines, the awareness that we are caring for a unique human being facing a unique life event must be present in our minds and guide our work in every therapeutic encounter.

9

STRENGTHENING
SELF-CAPACITIES

In the preceding chapters we have looked at early attachment experience and adult attachment orientation as factors that impact adaptation to significant loss. As we have seen, a substantial body of research from developmental psychology, social psychology and neuroscience supports the role of attachment security in adaptation to loss, and more broadly, in people's capacity to cope with stressful life events. Coming from different traditions and posing different questions, these streams of research have converged on the importance of emotion regulation in sustaining a healthy relationship with oneself and others (Eisma & Stroebe, 2021; Cesur-Soysal & Durak-Batigun, 2022; Mikulincer & Shaver, 2019; Naragon-Gainey et al., 2018).

In this chapter, we focus on strengthening emotional self-regulation as a goal of attachment informed grief therapy, with examples drawn from our work with a number of clients introduced earlier. Helping clients learn how to manage emotion is by no means the *only* task of a grief therapist, but it is a *necessary foundation* for treatment with many bereaved individuals, as suggested by Allen:

> Thinking about our feelings while we are feeling them is essential to regulating and controlling our emotional states effectively, rather than doing something

DOI: 10.4324/9781003204183-13

impulsively to shut off the emotions. . . This is a tall order, and these are skills we develop and refine over a lifetime – not without help.

(Allen, 2003, p. 94)

The cases in which the work of such work is particularly important have been identified in previous chapters, and include people with early attachment trauma, and people who have suffered particular kinds of traumatic and kinship loss. These clients include people who, like Vince, have come to see a connection between their difficulties in dealing with grief, and their lifelong habit of suppressing or rejecting their emotions.

Vince

I'm realizing more and more that I don't know what to do with my feelings. And some of that is because in my family it didn't pay to tell someone what you were feeling. If you said something was wrong you'd just get screamed at. There was no point, and it was easier just to shut down. So now that's what I always do, I just shut down. Or I run away. I don't want to deal with anyone because I feel like I have no way to ... I don't know how to. . . what my feelings are, or how to talk about them.

For Vince, who described his mother as a "really scary person" (see Chapter 3) emotions are uncomfortable reminders of a time in his life when no one saw or heard him, a time when he was left to figure out for himself how to manage all the feelings that occupy the mind and heart of a little boy. When a child's feelings are disregarded or disparaged, he learns to keep them to himself, and eventually, to keep them *from* himself, outside of awareness. Avoidance can be a useful strategy for keeping emotions in check, but in life there are bound to be times when feelings overwhelm this approach. For many people, bereavement is such a time, a time when their way of coping with emotional distress collapses and they have no other strategy on which to fall back.

In Vince's case, the collapse of an avoidant coping strategy after the loss of a close friend precipitated an escalation of anxiety, and the appearance of troublesome physical symptoms, the combination of which led him to seek help. In therapy, Vince was able to make connections between his experience as a child, and his difficulty acknowledging and managing emotion. He learned alternative ways of relating to his feelings and practiced noticing and allowing them to surface. Soon, Vince's physical symptoms began to abate. He became more aware of feeling sad and realized that he was also angry. But as he allowed himself to feel his feelings, Vince's anxiety decreased, and he was no longer afraid that he was going to "go crazy" and "lose control."

The weeks and months following the loss of someone important in a person's life are generally a period in which they explore thoughts, feelings and memories related to the deceased. While most people manage this process without professional help, others decide, after a period of struggle, to talk to someone about their loss. Whatever other support a grief therapist or other professional provides in these circumstances, an important part of their role is to serve as a transitional attachment figure who helps the bereaved individual to achieve a degree of self-regulation sufficient for them to think and talk about their loved one without collapsing into their emotions or steadfastly avoiding them.

In this chapter, we will continue our discussion of attachment orientation as a factor in how people respond to loss, with particular attention to problems in emotion regulation that complicate bereavement in insecurely attached individuals.[1] The treatment recommendations we offer in this chapter reflect what we have described as an important goal of grief therapy, which is to support flexible attention to the loss, particularly in those individuals whose grief has been complicated by their tendency either to become immersed in their feelings or to dismiss them.

Both the Dual Process Model, and Mikulincer and Shaver's work on the role of insecure attachment in problematic grief, emphasize the need to help bereaved clients who lack core emotional regulatory capacities develop them (Eisma & Stroebe, 2021; Mikulincer & Shaver, 2019; Stroebe & Schut, 1999a). Building these capacities is also a principal component of therapy for securely attached individuals who have experienced traumatic loss. While all clients may be helped by learning how to soothe themselves and manage painful feelings, there is now substantial evidence that this work is particularly important for individuals who have experienced a traumatic loss or who are survivors of unresolved early relational trauma or loss (Eisma & Stroebe, 2021; Pearlman et al., 2014; Sekowski & Prigerson, 2022).

Given all that we have learned about the diversity of people's response to significant loss, it stands to reason that bereavement interventions must be correspondingly diverse. When we apply this principle to the use of emotion regulation strategies, the initial questions that arise are: "what is the purpose of introducing these strategies to a particular bereaved individual?" and "which emotions are we trying to help the bereaved person regulate?"

EMOTION REGULATION STRATEGIES

In the second edition of the *Handbook of Emotion Regulation*, Gross (2014) explains that regulatory processes do one of two things: they either down regulate negative emotions, or up regulate positive emotions (p. 8). He describes five "families" of regulatory processes which are explained with examples below.

Situation selection: The "most forward-thinking approach to emotion regulation" (p. 9) situation selection involves taking actions that are likely to relieve negative feelings or give rise to positive ones in anticipated difficult situations.

For example, a grieving individual may be encouraged to arrange for a low-key social activity, such as dinner with a friend, on the anniversary of a spouse's death. Visualization is another approach to helping clients plan for what are expected to be emotionally difficult situations. Visualization entails directing the client to think about the upcoming event, bring up the thoughts and feelings he or she imagines will arise at that time, and with the clinician's help, imagine what they will do to help themselves manage those feelings (Taylor et al., 1998).

Situation modification: "Directly modifying a situation so as to alter its emotional impact" (p. 9).

For example, a grieving widower might avoid driving past the cemetery where his deceased spouse was buried. At a family gathering, he might choose to avoid interacting with a family member who routinely makes hurtful other insensitive remarks about his spouse.

Attentional deployment: "Directing attention within a given situation in order to influence one's emotions" (p. 10).

Attentional deployment is often used when situation modification is not possible, for example, a widow might recall pleasant memories of her husband, or look at pictures of him taken when he was healthy and active. Techniques for redirecting attention can also be used to promote oscillation between a Loss Orientation and a Restoration Orientation (Mikulincer & Shaver, 2013). A simple way to do this is to encourage a person to let themselves think about something sad, and then redirect their attention so that they are thinking about something happy. More concretely, a widow could be coached to plan to clean out her husband's desk in the morning, and then to have lunch with a friend. The idea is to encourage an awareness of the possibility of *choosing* where one's attention is directed, rather than having one's state of mind determined randomly by external or internal events.

Cognitive change: Modifying "how one appraises a situation so as to alter its emotional significance" (p. 10).

Techniques to help clients reframe dysfunctional thoughts can be an important component of therapy with anxiously or avoidantly attached clients. Reframing can take a number of forms, from reconsidering the importance of a past mistake, to reevaluating one's ability to manage in the face of external stressors (Kosminsky, 2017; Malkinson, 2006, 2012; Neimeyer, 2012f). An anxiously attached and insecure widow, for example, might work with her therapist to recall instances in which she successfully faced adversity, in order to develop a different perspective on her ability to take care of herself and her children. She might be taught the use of the ABC model of Rational Emotive Behavioral Therapy (REBT) to minimize self-defeating thoughts (Malkinson, 2012). This activity of reframing how one looks at the self or a situation is closely linked with the meaning-making process, which will be discussed in more depth in Chapter 10.

Response modulation: Response modulation refers to "directly influen-cing experiential, behavioral, or physiological components of the emo-tional response" (p. 10).

For example, a therapist could provide instruction in deep breathing or muscle relaxation techniques or suggest that a bereaved person engage in some form of regular physical exercise.

This final category of regulatory strategies summarized by Gross includes many of the techniques that clinicians use to help people who are in distress, whether or not their distress is related to an ongoing problem or a traumatic event. We will give some examples of how we use these tech-niques, many more of which are detailed in a number of excellent clinical manuals (Greenspan, 2004; Linehan, 2015; Pearlman et al., 2014).

Addressing Emotion-Regulation Deficits: Fitting the Treatment to the Client

Bereavement is a process that involves reconstruction of meaning and identity, a rebuilding of the self that will continue for the rest of a person's life. Before that process can begin, however, someone who is grieving must find a way to manage the pain of separation. In the immediate aftermath of significant loss, that pain, and the fear, guilt and other emotions associated with it, can be disabling. The persistence of this level of emotionality is associated with anxious attachment and is what brings many anxiously attached bereaved people into treatment (Boelen & Lenferink, 2020; Mikulincer & Shaver, 2016, 2019).

As discussed in Chapter 4, anxiously attached individuals have learned to sustain or even exaggerate negative emotions in order to attract the attention and care of attachment figures (Reisz et al., 2018). This coping strategy is apparent in a tendency to ruminate on painful memories and to exaggerate one's inability to cope with current life stressors. Understanding this dynamic as it relates to bereavement is an important consideration in treatment planning. If these tendencies are not addressed, they are likely to interfere with the effectiveness of grief therapy.

In contrast, the grief response of avoidantly attached people is char-acterized by a tendency to deny or suppress the possibility that they might be having difficulty in coping with the loss, thus avoiding activation of their attachment system. A list of the emotions that avoidant individuals are most intent on downplaying could also serve as a list of the feelings that most often accompany significant loss: fear, anger, sadness, guilt, distress, anger – in other words, feelings that they associate with vulnerability. In a reversal of the regulatory strategy used by anxiously attached people, avoidant individuals direct attention away from emotion related thoughts and memories and "suppress emotion related action tendencies" (Shaver & Mikulincer, 2014) such as crying or vocalizing their feelings. Also in contrast to anxiously attached individuals, avoidant individuals operate on the principle that negative emotions are something to be managed without the help of others, who are viewed as unable, or not inclined, to provide support. Like anxiously attached people, individuals who are avoidantly attached can benefit from emotion focused interventions but given the differences in their way of managing their feelings, the type of interventions will differ.

Attachment orientation influences the individual's style of defensive strategies and the problems that arise from overuse of these strategies. It is reasonable to conclude that interventions to support emotion regulation (and grief interventions on the whole) must address the specific difficulties of each bereaved client. While these observations will be true in all cases, they hold particularly for the insecurely attached, where interventions that strengthen people's capacity to experience, understand, express, and manage their emotions can help restore the dynamic oscillation described in the Dual Process Model. As we have proposed in the preceding chapters, the specific difficulties that people with different kinds of insecure attachment orientation encounter require different treatment approaches. Table 9.1 provides a summary of some of these projected difficulties and Table 9.2 summarizes the kinds of interventions that we tend to use with clients who have these different types of insecure attachment orientations.

Table 9.1 Attachment Related Complications in Grief

Attachment Style	Complications
Anxious	Dependency in relationship; intensity of loss related emotions interferes with oscillation and integration of the loss
Avoidant	Dismissive of attachment; ambivalence about the person and avoidance of feelings about them interferes with oscillation and integration of the loss
Disorganized	Difficulty in tolerating and managing emotion and lack of mentalizing capacity interfere with processing intense and conflicting feelings relating to the deceased and interferes with integration of the loss

Table 9.2 Emotion Regulation Techniques by Attachment Style (Based on Expected Problems in Integration of Loss)

Attachment Style	Treatment Recommendations
Anxious	Emotion regulation: address cognitions that sustain negative emotions
Avoidant	Affect awareness: address negative cognitions regarding the experience of emotion
Disorganized	Establish safety: develop and/or restore mentalizing; support dosed experiencing and expression of emotion

In the next section, we present examples of techniques for emotion regulation that address the problems associated with different types of insecure attachment. Note, however, that like all therapeutic interventions, *approaches to strengthening emotion regulation should be chosen based on the needs of the individual client*; what is offered here is not prescriptive. The references cited are all excellent sources for learning more about the wide range of approaches to strengthening these capacities.

ATTACHMENT ORIENTATION AND EMOTION REGULATION

Anxious Attachment

Modifying catastrophic thoughts that contribute to negative emotions; modulating response:

Jane

I just don't know how I can live with so much pain.

When her husband was dying, Jane and her therapist (PK) had talked about many things that upset and frightened her. Caring for a loved one at end of life entails both the trauma of witnessing their slow and painful departure, and a depth of fear about their own solitary future barely captured by terms such as "anticipatory loss". The torture of this experience is magnified by an internal divide in the caregiver, who cannot bear to see the loved one suffer any further, and yet cannot bear to imagine life without them. Jane and the therapist had discussed all of this in session, with an emphasis on helping Jane express her feelings and find ways, cognitive and practical, to address her fears.

During one session, as Jane quietly wept, the clinician turned to the topic of fear, suggesting that along with the agony of missing her husband, Jane seemed also to be feeling a lot of fear. The clinician asked Jane if she remembered any other time in her life when she had felt so afraid. Slowly, gently, she encouraged Jane to let her mind drift. After a minute or so Jane said that as a child, she had been constantly worried about her parents dying, particularly her mother, who Jane now believes suffered from undiagnosed mental illness as well prescription drug abuse. As a school principal for many years, Jane was familiar with the variety of adverse effects that being raised by a parent with these difficulties can have on a young child. She understood that children need a secure home base to be able to learn, to form healthy relationships with others, to grow. Jane had not had a secure base growing up, but she had found it in her husband and had relied on it for 50 years. The clinician observed that now, faced with the loss of this security, it stood to reason that Jane was deeply afraid. But what sustained Jane's terror, the clinician suggested, was the depth of her pain. Pain, physical or emotional, can drive a person crazy; it can make a person believe that they are going to die.

> PK: I understand that you're afraid. And I know you're in pain. Sometimes it's good to be able to recognize that what's frightening us more than anything is the idea that we are not going to be able to survive the pain. Sometimes it's good to pay attention to what we're saying to ourselves about our pain. And to respond to the part of our minds that is telling us that the pain will kill us.

> Jane listened, and still crying asked, How do I do that?

> PK: First, you want to let your body and mind know that you are safe and alive, and that you're not going to die. One way to do that is to become conscious of your breath.

Jane was guided in focusing on her breath, and asked to breathe in deeply and exhale deeply, to do this a few times. The clinician explained that slowing and deepening our breathing is a way of engaging the para-sympathetic nervous system (Harris & Winokuer, 2021). In effect, we are letting our body know *that nothing bad is happening right now*. There is nothing to fight, nothing from which we need to flee.

The next suggestion was that Jane recognize when she was having the thought "I'm going to die" and to consider what she might want to tell herself instead. Nothing came to mind, so the clinician made some suggestions:

> P: "This is just pain. This is hard and painful, but I can get through it."

Jane was shown how to use tapping techniques (Parnell, 2008) that can help with affect regulation and stress reduction and introduced to the "butterfly hug", an EMDR technique that helps produce a feeling a calm. With arms crossed and a hand on each shoulder, Jane was instructed to tap on one, side, then the other, while she repeated in her mind, out loud, a positive or hopeful belief about her ability to cope. Another tapping technique is Therapeutic Tapping, which combines somatic stimulation of acupressure points with elements from Cognitive Behavioral Therapy (CBT) to address negative cognitions and deepen alternative, positive thoughts (Konig et al., 2019).

Trudy

> I wake up, I remember that he's gone, and I'm not just sad, I'm terrified.

> My parents always said I needed someone to take care of me and they were right. Now they're gone, and my husband is gone, and I can't get over this terrible feeling that I'm not going to make it.

The meaning we make of our experiences, past and present, is like the moral of a story we tell ourselves. In Trudy's case that narrative went something like: "This is what happened to me, this is how I felt, and what I learned is that I am weak and cannot take care of myself." This narrative becomes the individual's go-to interpretation of whatever painful experiences we have later in life ("I was hurt because I could not take care of myself") and the calculus on which we base our expectations about the future ("I will suffer because I cannot take care of myself)".

Trudy, who was described in Chapter 4 as having an anxious attachment style, remained tearful and hopeless five years after her husband's death, when she consulted with the first author. Notwithstanding Trudy's insistence that she was incapable of caring for herself and her two almost adult children, she had done exactly that, and arguably, had done it more consistently than her husband. Like many bereaved individuals, Trudy wanted to feel better – more energetic, less worn out, more able to manage several life challenges that were on the horizon such as selling her house, finding a new job, and finding a suitable placement for her 17-year-old son, whose behavioral and emotional problems were an ongoing source of stress for Trudy and her teenage daughter. While talking about these issues Trudy's speech and breathing became rapid Gently pointing this out, I asked Trudy to slow down and take a few deep breaths, after which she was able to proceed at a more regulated pace. I commented on how sometimes "our feelings take so much energy that we don't have much left over to do the things we want to do." I went on to suggest that one of the things we could work on together was helping Trudy manage her emotions a bit, so that she didn't always feel so tired and stressed (see *Modulating Feelings*, below). Before she left, I taught Trudy some breathing exercises she could practice at home during the week. I ended the session by assuring Trudy that she was not alone – that I would be there to help – and that together, we would help her find a way to feel better and move on with her life.

Although a clinician may be tempted to reassure a client like Trudy that she is an adult and can surely take of herself, making this observation before a strong bond has been established is likely to result in a rupture in the relationship, and even the withdrawal of the client. Following the well-established principle that we begin where the client is, not where we want them to be, we begin by offering empathy for the distress the client is feeling ("that must be pretty distressing for you. I'm sorry that you are feeling so badly'). We offer sympathy and reassurance ("Let's work together to help you feel calmer, less upset, etc.) rather than encouragement. As discussed previously, anxiously attached clients will at times sustain an agitated emotional state in order to ensure the attention and care of the therapist. Of course, we want people to know that they are not helpless. But someone like Trudy, who genuinely feels unable to care for herself, has to be helped to come to her own conclusion about her competence and strength. Faith, as we know, has to come from within, and that includes faith in oneself.

After a few weekly sessions with the clinician, Trudy was able to talk about her husband's death without dissolving into tears, and the narrative she had constructed of her own helplessness and her husband's strength began to change. With her attention gradually directed to evidence of her accomplishments and what these accomplishments said about her ability to survive independently, Trudy became increasingly self-confidant. She was able to understand the roots of her tendency toward excessive dependence, and this too helped her let go of it. Strength built upon strength, and over the next year Trudy put her house on the market and found a new job. She found a placement for her son, and after a difficult period of adjustment, concluded that it was the best thing she could have done for him. Along the way, Trudy decided to take dance classes and try online dating. In short, Trudy made the kind of progress we hope to see in people who come to us for help, especially those have been through years of unrelieved suffering. After five years of being on her own, Trudy was ready to shed the identity of "fragile china doll", an identity that no longer fit, and that no longer served her.

Modulating Feelings

To modulate feelings is to exercise control over their intensity, rather than letting the feeling overtake you. One of the many approaches to modulating feelings involves focusing on the physical sensations that accompany emotions – discomfort, tightness, rapid breathing – and "reporting" to oneself on these sensations without attaching meaning to them. Often simply shifting attention from thoughts that sustain and intensify emotions to physical sensations is enough to bring down the level of emotional arousal.

An alternative approach involves examining the emotion with the intention of identifying what information it contains ("What is this emotion trying to tell me?"). Like the approach described above, focusing on the meaning of an emotion – shifting from the physiological to the cognitive, and regarding the emotion as a source of information rather than an overwhelming force - can help a person feel more in control. Also important is the realization that emotions vary in intensity, and that there are things we can do to moderate them.

Calming Breath

The way a person is breathing is one of the most readily available measures of their emotional state, and also one of the most direct paths to changing it. People are quick to pick up on the connection between how they are breathing (rapidly, shallowly, or hardly at all) and their level of emotional and physiological discomfort. With practice, in session and at home, taking a breath becomes a habituated response to feeling stressed, and taking "breathing breaks" to regulate their internal state becomes part of clients' daily self-care. To get them started, it helps to offer some simple and easy to remember instructions, for example:

> *Sit in a comfortable position, your body softening into your chair. Soften your gaze at your surroundings, or close your eyes. Now take a slow breath in, for a count of four; hold it for a count of four; and slowly breathe out for a count of four. Do this a total of four times.*

The neediness of anxiously attached clients can produce a variety of reactions in therapists, from sincere sympathy to active resentment. The response elicited depends on a number of factors, including the therapist's own attachment orientation, what kind of day he or she is having, and the cumulative level of stress in their personal and professional life. That being said, as a general rule the desperate unhappiness of anxiously attached bereaved clients cannot help but provoke in the helping professional a desire to provide comfort and to offer someone deep in grief the hope that their pain will ease. In short, grief therapists do not need to be told to provide the comfort that anxiously attached bereaved people want. They may, however, be reluctant to employ methods that are more directive or even confrontational. Yet there will be times when this approach is what is needed to restore functioning and heal the spirit.

In Chapter 4 we met Gloria, another client of the first author whose grief was complicated by the anxious nature of her attachment. Gloria was described as someone who was "tormented by her persistent feelings of failure as a daughter; she weeps continually in session. . . only stopping brief when the therapist draws her into discussion and encourages her to breathe." Here's a bit more of Gloria's story.

Gloria

She was my everything. I just don't know how I can go on without her.

Two months into treatment, Gloria continued to weep, and the clinician often found herself drawing her chair closer to Gloria's in an effort to convey more fully her attention and care. When the clinician did this, Gloria would calm down. The resulting interaction resembled a kind of dance: Gloria would weep, the clinician would bring her chair in closer, and Gloria would stop weeping. Although she recognized this pattern, the clinician was not sure what to say or do about it. One day, when she had drawn closer and Gloria had stopped weeping, the clinician moved her chair back to its original position. Within moments, Gloria was gasping for breath, and her tears resumed. The clinician's response was likewise immediate and intense. Looking Gloria in the eyes, she said in a firm voice: "Stop! You were fine just a moment ago! Nothing has changed! You can be fine now!" And with that, Gloria stopped crying.

Many years later, this experience is a reminder of how a clinician can be drawn into the drama of a client's efforts to get her attachment needs met. Once this behavior became an explicit focus of treatment, Gloria was able to trace the history of her intense and anxious attachment to her mother and to understand how it had been reenacted in therapy. In response to the therapist's gentle inquiries, Gloria confirmed that her mother did not pay much attention to her, except when she was hurt or sick. She had learned that the surest way to ensure her mother's attentive care was to through the signaling of extreme distress.

After this discussion, Gloria gradually became less prone to prolonged crying jags, and more able to talk about changing her day-to-day routines in ways that would help her feel better and more in control. She was encouraged to find ways to soothe herself and to occupy the many hours she had previously devoted to her mother's care. She eventually returned to school and began a new career that restored some sense of meaning and purpose to her life. While Gloria learned to better moderate her emotions and create more meaning in her life, her feelings about her mother and her longing for her remained intense throughout treatment and in the several years following, when she was in periodic contact with the therapist.

The past exerts a powerful influence on how we experience what is happening in the present. While it is helpful to know this, knowing it is often not enough to keep us from reacting in a manner that is beyond our capacity to understand and modulate, nor that of those around us. Someone who, like Gloria, grew up with a mother who was inattentive except when she was sick or crying may find herself weeping in response to a therapist's moving her chair back a foot. Someone whose father died when he was young may feel panic at the thought of his teenage son going on a school trip. Jon Allen describes these as "90/10" moments, where 90% of a response is related to what is happening in the moment, and 10% is connected to past events. The idea that their response to a given situation is not unreasonable in light of their history, is reassuring to many people. As Allen writes, they are not "making a mountain out of a molehill"; in truth, there is "a real mountain in their past, and their sensitized nervous system inclines them to react to molehills as mountains" (Allen, 2013, p. 60).

In Gloria's case, what turned out to be an effective intervention (firmly instructing the client to stop crying and resume the conversation) was born of the therapist's frustration with the client's collapse into an old behavior pattern. The literature on mindfulness-based psychotherapy practices offers a good many more considered techniques for helping clients stay in the moment (see discussion of Mindfulness, below).

Finally, we turn to Trish, another anxiously attached client who benefitted from recognizing the impact of her past on her present reactions and functioning.

Trish

I never feel like I can trust that my feelings are really mine. My feelings are always so tied up with my mother, my sisters, my husband. I'm always trying to figure out what someone else wants, what would be good for someone else.

In contrast to Gloria, Trish was able to talk about her emotions without crying; she was analytical and dispassionate in describing a childhood in which she often felt alone, helpless and afraid. When she first came to therapy Trish described her mother's death as a relief. But within a short time, she began to feel frighteningly unsure of herself, and was unable to bring herself to make the decisions that were necessary to settle her mother's estate.

Trish's mother was always unwell, and as a child Trish worried about her constantly, often getting up in the middle of the night to make sure that she was breathing. Only as an adult and with input from others had she come to understand that the illness of alcoholism made her mother unsteady on her feet, drove her to bed in the middle of the day, and was the reason for her periodic, sudden hospitalizations. Trish remembered her mother as being "fine one minute and falling down the next", and she recalled her Mother insisting that it was Trish and her sisters who were making her sick, and who would be the death of her.

Early in therapy, Trish explained that there was "no point in getting angry or upset" when she was growing up because "mom would get more angry or more upset, and then she would leave the room and you would feel guilty and be afraid that she was going to die." With a slight nod of understanding, the clinician gently asked Trish what she was feeling now as she talked about her childhood then. After a few moments' hesitation she said, "Like a mess." The clinician(PK) smiled and said, "That's good to know, but that's not a feeling." Trish was shown a list of feelings and asked to choose one or two that were closest to the feelings she had when she talked about her childhood. "Fear" was Trish's response. "Because thinking about that time is hard, and I don't know if I can do it and not fall apart." The clinician noted that fear was a reasonable way to feel when you're starting to think about revisiting painful memories. "But feeling afraid is a lot different than feeling like a mess, don't you think? A mess is something you **are**; fear is something you feel." Trish nodded, and the clinician added: "And it's good to know that fear is what you're feeling, because now that you know that, and now that you've told me, I can say something that may help you feel less afraid. I can tell you that you don't have to do this alone, and you don't have to do it all at once."

Returning the following week, Trish said more about the stress of being the executrix of her mother's estate. "How can I talk to lawyers and accountants? How can I talk to anyone, when I'm afraid I'm going to say the wrong thing, make the wrong move?" Her mother had always told her what to do, and as much as she had resented her for it, Trish now realized that she had no idea of how to think for herself. She was terrified that without her mother she would have no one to go to for help when problems came up; her sisters were as useless as she was. The clinician suggested that Trish try asking herself what she should do when a decision had to be made; she might know more than she suspected. Trish replied: "I know what you're saying, but when you say it, I get very afraid and every part of my body says no." Acknowledging the fear Trish felt and why it made sense, the clinician immediately withdrew her suggestion, saying, "Well, I certainly don't want to recommend you're doing anything that your whole body tells you not to do. But I wonder, could I have a word with your pinkie?" This seemingly nonsensical inquiry was in fact an invitation for Trish to close her eyes and relax into a trance state, something she had previously found allowed her to explore ideas that were otherwise too frightening or uncomfortable to consider. In a gentle voice, the clinician began to speak of Trish's pinkie as a place where a lot of undiscovered self-knowledge could be found. Her pinkie indicated agreement (with a little nod) and the clinician continued, emphasizing that Trish had it in herself to find her way. She could always ask for help, but before asking others she could ask herself. When she opened her eyes Trish smiled and said "I like that. Because my pinkie is always with me." When she returned the following week, Trish reported that she had taken to asking herself "WWPD?" (what would Pinkie do) rather than always turning to others for answers.

The utilization of trance, as illustrated here, owes much to the teachings of Milton Erikson (Erickson & Rossi, 1979; Wigren, 2014) and to the interpretation and expansion of Erikson's work by his student Stephen Gilligan (Gilligan, 2012, 2013, 2019).

Avoidant Attachment: Becoming Aware of Feelings; Suspending Judgment

Margaret

Why am I even talking about my anger? It's stupid for me to be angry, because there's nothing I can do about it. Really, I don't see the point of this.

If the neediness of the anxious client challenges the clinician's capacity for compassion, the dismissiveness of the avoidant client can cause them to question their competence. It is important, in the face of such a person's lack of confidence in the value of therapy and frequent assertions that she doesn't need anyone's help, to remember that her presence in the clinician's office provides countervailing evidence to these claims. When allowed to take their time and draw their own conclusions, avoidant clients will often get to a point where they can let down the defenses they have erected against their feeling their own emotions, and receiving the help offered by others.

Margaret

I don't know how you listen to this stuff all day. It must be so boring for you.

Margaret's declaration in this instance was both a hedge against her fear that the therapist would openly declare her desire for Margaret to simply stop talking and leave so that she could go home, and a hint as to her attitude toward the importance of emotion, her own in particular. Margaret, a client of PK who was introduced in Chapter 4, was aware of her emotions, but she did not trust them. If she was angry or disappointed, it was only because she had unrealistic expectations of others and of life in general. If she was anxious or worried, it was only because she was irrational and unable to think clearly about whatever was causing her distress.

Contrary to Margaret's assumption, we believe that most mental health professionals and grief therapists do not usually find it boring to listen to people talk about their feelings. What can cause a certain amount of frustration is listening to someone relentlessly judge and criticize their feelings. It is important to remember, and when the time is right, to convey to the client, that the antagonistic relationship they have with their emotions may have originated as an adaptation to an early environment that was unresponsive to their feelings and needs. Antagonism toward one's emotions can also be amplified by the messages that people may be getting from their current relationships, and by the social pressure to "get over" their loss or suppress grief related feelings.

As discussed in Chapter 4, avoidance is by no means an ineffective strategy for managing emotion, but there is some evidence that it can collapse under conditions of extreme stress (Mikulincer & Shaver, 2019). At worst, the collapse of an avoidant strategy can manifest itself in impaired physical or emotional functioning. But impaired functioning is not the only potential downside of trying to overcome or ignore emotions rather than learning to live with them, particularly when the emotion is grief. Given our assumption about the importance of flexible attention in bereavement and the role of emotion in healing, we spend a fair amount of time talking with avoidant clients about how they can develop a kinder and more accepting attitude toward their feelings and themselves.

Anne

From their first meeting, Anne made it clear to the therapist (PK) that the predominant feeling that she'd had since her husband's death six months earlier was relief. Anne fortified her resolve to not feel bad about her husband's death by scrolling through online message boards for people caring for a loved one with ALS. "When I see what other people are going through, it reinforces my relief."

She avoids going into the room that was his bedroom. "When I do go in there I see him lying there on the bed." She is even more reluctant to enter the room that was his study. "All of his books, his papers, all his work is there. That room is so much who he was, I just can't go in there, it will be too painful."

She has cleared out the remnants of her husband's illness - the pills, the hospital bed – but finds herself unable to face the task of cleaning out his closet. Here, she realizes, there is a problem:

"There are also clothes of his in winter storage. Mine are there too, and I have to get them out. I'm afraid of doing that. I don't want to have to see his clothes. What do I do with all of this? I don't see how I'm ever going to be ready to do any of these things."

The suggestion made to Anne at this point was a simple one: think about what it will be like to see his clothes. Prepare yourself for what you might feel. Know that it is going to be uncomfortable but that you can do it. Feelings, whether we want them or not, tend to stick around when we try to ignore or push them away.

PK: I understand that you don't want to feel your feelings. But it seems like you're running into problems with that coping strategy. How about trying a different one?

*I think the best thing that you can do here is to start small. Don't try to clean out his study or even his closet – just get out the clothes from storage. You may not feel like doing any of these things, But here's my suggestion: think about something that you don't feel that you're ready to do and **do it anyway.***

Anne's next appointment was several weeks later. She began as she often did, by recounting her follow-up to the previous discussion.

A: The last time we spoke we talked about how every time I went into his bedroom I saw him, lying on the bed. So I talked to him, like you said.

I loved your comment last time: 'Start doing things that you don't feel like you're ready to do'. I got the clothes out of storage and it was okay, seeing his clothes.

I'm going to think about what to do about his bedroom. I feel like reality is setting in.

PK: That's part of the reason I suggested that you do these things – so that it will feel real.

A: And I put up some pictures. I had all of his pictures put away. Now I have them up. But I don't look at them.

KP: Okay, well, that's a start.

A: My daughter made a picture board for the funeral, this big thing, it's just sitting upstairs. What do I do with it?

PK: Do you like it?

A.: I've never looked at it. I've moved it around, but I've never looked at it.

PK: You're nothing if not determined, Anne. If you're not going to see something you're not going to see it.

A: The pictures bring up memories. I don't want those memories. I'm not ready for the picture board.

PK: So put the picture board in the attic. A year from now, you can ask yourself, do I feel like looking at the picture board? Knowing you, you'll probably say no (Anne. laughs).

A: I do have some pictures of him up now, there are pictures of him in every room. I don't look at them. But they are up.

PK: I really like the way that you approach this. It's like you've created your own exposure hierarchy. First you have two pictures, then you have more picture, but you don't look at them. (Anne laughs). You have a way of doing things that enables you to gradually face things that scare you.

And who knows. Maybe sometime – I think it's likely that sometime in the future, you'll say to me "I looked at some of the pictures."

Note the trust that has developed in this relationship. The clinician suggests a direction, but at every step it is Anne who sets the pace.. She remains steadfast in her reluctance to look at the picture board. She also lets it be known that as much as she is willing to do things that awaken her feelings, what she's feeling is pain, and she'd prefer not to feel it.

A: It bothers me that I'm losing that feeling of relief. I loved that relief.

PK: I know you did. It's like some kind of ice shell on your heart is melting.

A: I don't want it to melt anymore. I'm really trying hard not to let it melt anymore.

At the end, I would go into his room and he would call me sweetie, and he would say, 'oh hi sweetie'. And when he would say that it would break my heart. And I hate thinking about that. I hate feeling that feeling.

PK: What is that feeling, Anne?

A: Love. Like nobody is ever going to love me as much as he loved me. They just aren't. That just makes me so sad. Even at the end it was like the softness and kindness of his soul came through. I wish he had been horrible. That would be easier. That would be easier than "hi sweetie".

PK: *Because that was so tender. It broke your heart.*

A: *It breaks my heart to think about it even now.*

PK: *Yes, I know. You don't want to feel it. I believe that in the long run, though, feeling whatever we're feeling about someone who died is the only way for us to continue to have a connection to them. When we push away all of our memories of someone we love who has died we're disallowing any connection that we could continue to have with them.*

We are at the end of the hour, and I ask Anne to just close her eyes and think about her husband. To say whatever she wants to say to him. To listen for anything he wants to say to her.

A: *He's saying to me that we're free – both of us – and that he's at peace. He's saying that he's here and he's holding me.*

A few weeks later I received an email from Anne: "I am working on his study. My kids are helping me. I wanted to let you know that I cried. I knew you'd want to know that. And I am trying to feel my feelings."

At our next meeting Anne begins by telling me:

A: *I feel . . . I think I'm getting accustomed to the fact that he died. I just feel like I'm feeling better with the grief. But I feel . . . I don't know. . . more than right after he passed away . . . I'm feeling flat. Like I'm feeling like my life is flat a lot.*

PK: *Like there's something that **took the color out of it.***

A: *You just said it in a nutshell. Before I felt relief. I read that stupid website all the time and I just thought I was doing great. Like I was handling all of this perfectly.*

PK: *(Laughs) That's kind of funny, because people rarely say that! They'll say 'other people tell me I'm doing so great, but they don't know. . .'.*

A: *No, I really thought that I was! (Laughs). Until I spoke with you and you took all the air out of my balloon and told me I wasn't doing great and that I wasn't feeling anything.*

PK: *I don't know what that says about me as a professional, but okay!*

A: *It's the truth! And then I started to come to terms with the fact that maybe I had to start feeling a few things. . .*

*So now I think I'm feeling . . (long hesitation) a little **lonely** maybe?*

PK: *That's the word that came into my head too,*

A: *I think that might be it.*

PK: *I think so too.*

A: I'm not sure what to do with it, really.

PK: It's not a simple thing. That's why you don't know what to do with it.

A: I've been working on the bedroom. I don't see him dead anymore. And also – lately I feel his presence more. I mean, I really do believe that he's with me.

This intervention appeared to strengthen the continuing bond between Anne and her husband, enabling her to have the sense that an experience of "while his physical body is gone, his presence is still with me". For many people, this experience of the continuing presence of the loved one is central to reducing separation distress.

As the reader will appreciate, this is rewarding work, for the client and the therapist. Greater awareness of, and tolerance for emotion are goals of compassion-based psychotherapy (Gilbert, 2009; Harris, 2021; Vachon & Harris, 2016) which emphasizes the cultivation of an attitude of acceptance toward oneself and one's feelings. Rather than treating their feelings as enemy intruders, clients are encouraged to regard their emotions as the deepest and truest source of insight about the self and others. Emotions draw our attention to what lies beneath the surface of our day to day lives. They are a kind of coded message waiting for our open-minded, open-hearted attention.

Clients who have cultivated an avoidant strategy for dealing with emotion can be expected to challenge the therapist's suggestion that they might benefit from adopting a more accepting attitude toward their feelings. Such a suggestion conflicts with what they believe is a constructive approach to limiting the impact of emotions that they should not have.

- It's crazy for me to be angry at him for being dead.
- It's stupid for me to think that I should have been able to save her.
- It's been six months since she died. There must be something wrong with me if I'm still so upset.

These thoughts/statements, which we have all heard, sustain a of negative self-evaluation and drain an individual of energy and hope. Rather than helping a bereaved person to keep their chin up and carry on, this kind of thinking usually only serves to reinforce the bereaved person's sense of futility and despair.

For people who have become accustomed to managing their emotions in this way, the shift to a more emotion friendly attitude does not happen overnight. It helps to explain that like any habit, the habit of attacking one's emotions is mentally sticky, but that given time and practice, the mind can learn to let it go. Mindfulness, and the cultivation of self-compassion, practice, the mind can learn to let it go.

Soften, soothe, and allow

Sit comfortably and either close your eyes or soften your gaze. Slowly let your attention come to your breath, and as you do, become aware of any tightness in your body. Take another breath, and as you do, pay attention to what you are thinking and feeling. Notice the connection between what you are thinking and feeling, and the tightness in your body. Now, think about softening that part of your body. If your stomach is feeling tight or your heart is hurting, you can rest your hand there, and just let yourself be comforted by your own gentle touch. You can speak to yourself in a soothing way, or you can simply repeat the word soft, saying it quietly to yourself as you continue to breathe, slowly and deeply. Whatever discomfort is there, notice it, and let it be what it is. You can repeat the word "allow" on each breath. Continue to repeat the words "soften, soothe, allow".

Adapted from Germer et al. (2013)

Disorganized Attachment: Establishing Safety and Cultivating Mentalization

Children classified as disorganized by Main and her colleagues in the Strange Situation were those who, upon reunion with their caregivers, exhibited behavior that alternated in a confused and sometimes bizarre manner between approach and avoidance, and included episodic displays of "freezing" or collapse. In contrast to anxious or avoidantly attached infants, these children seemed to have no coherent internal working model directing their behavior and little ability to soothe themselves when stressed. The mothers of these children were described as "frightened and frightening," a reference to the difficulty they appeared to experience in managing their response to a needy infant, and to the behavior exhibited toward the infant.

Allen describes early trauma as a failure of mentalizing: the parent is not attuned to the child's internal state, cannot understand what the child may be feeling, and responds to expressions of need with anger, or not at all (Allen, 2013). The child feels unseen, invisible, and alone. Among the developmental deficits that result from the parent's lack of mentalizing is a lack of mentalizing capacity in the child, a breakdown in the ability to understand what other people are feeling, and to recognize internal emotional cues. Therapy, above all, is an opportunity to explore the world of emotion in the company of a reassuring guide. The therapist's attunement to the client provides a model of mentalizing, and the safety of the therapeutic environment provides a space in which the client's own mentalizing capacity can develop.

Mentalizing

The idea that understanding another person's point of view can sometimes, though not always, reduce our antipathy toward that person is not new. We have found, however, that describing something in a new way can help people *think* about it in a new way. In our experience, clients (particularly those who are more easily engaged by talking about ideas than about feelings) are interested in hearing about mentalizing, how it develops and why it is important. The idea that mentalizing is *a skill that they can learn* as opposed to an innate capacity they are lacking, is encouraging to many people. They can appreciate how learning this skill will help reduce conflict in their current relationships, and how it can also help lighten the emotional burden of anger that they have been carrying toward other people, living and dead. Clinicians can themselves sometimes view clients as irreparably deficient in certain capacities (such as mentalizing) and correspondingly assume that they are essentially, beyond help.

The clinician in the following exchange had previously explained mentalizing as a skill that Audrey (who was introduced in Chapter 4) might find helpful. This suggestion was part of a broader discussion of the toxic effect of Audrey's lingering anger toward her father on her current relationships with family, friends and co-workers. Audrey regularly got into arguments with people over what she took to be hostile or critical remarks. In the following exchange, the clinician models the skill of mentalizing, while also affirming Audrey's empathic response to her mother.

Audrey

A: So I've been living with my mother, and then my friend asked me to stay at her place for a week and take care of her cat, and my mother is asking me all these questions, like how much is she paying me, and do I really think I should be taking this on. She's still treating me like a child! She thinks I can't make my own decisions! And when I was ready to leave to go over there, she comes at me with these files and wants me to look at them, and why is she doing that right then?

PK: What do you think?

A: I don't know. . . . But it makes me so angry! Like here it is again, no one in my family knows me, no one knows who I am or what I'm capable of!

PK: I know, and that's a bad feeling, an old, bad feeling.

A: It's my whole life, that feeling.

PK: Yes. . .You felt that way so much growing up, mostly because of your father, all the criticism, the accusations, the yelling. . . . This reminds you of him, when what you're trying to do is to not think about him all the time.

A: When my mother talks to me that way it's like I never left, like he never died.

PK I know you and your mother don't always get along, and you figure that anything that comes out of her mouth is a judgment, a criticism. I'm wondering, though, what do you think she was expecting it would be like when you moved in? I get the sense from things you've said that she was looking forward to it, she was kind of happy about it. And now, even though you don't always get along, I think maybe she likes having you around.

A: That could be.

PK: Uh huh. So, is it possible that she said those things about you going to cat sit because she didn't want you to be away for a week? Maybe she's going to miss you.

A: Well, I don't know about that. But maybe. It has been kind of nice, just not being alone. We usually sit together and eat dinner. And now that you mention it, right after she handed me the files, she went into the kitchen and got her supper and brought it out to where I was standing and looking at the files, and I said, you know, these files are interesting. I want to look at them for a minute. Why don't we sit down and I'll look at them while you eat your dinner.

PK: That was kind of you.

As this conversation proceeded, Audrey's body began to relax, and she began to breathe more deeply. I noted this apparent "softening" and suggested that Audrey think about how "softening" might become a goal for her, in her relationship with her mother, and also in her relationship with herself.

A: I guess I'm carrying a lot of anger around all the time. Maybe if I could be softer with other people, and with myself, I could let some of that go. I did one of those visualizations this week, I listened to one, and it helped me go to sleep. I could do more of that.

PK: I'm glad that worked for you, and that sounds like a good idea. Just remember that you don't have to push yourself. Think about softening.

A: I want to do that. I want to be softer, especially with myself.

Feeling "softer", as Audrey imagined, is a more comfortable way to feel. When she feels softer, Audrey feels like a more mature and nicer person. She is less self-critical, and less inclined to think that others are judging her. Physiologically, she is more relaxed; her breathing is deeper, and body is less tense. All of these responses have the effect of giving her back some of the energy that her father's death, and her preoccupation with it, have taken from her.

The cultivation of what is described here as "softness" is one small example of practices that have been used for thousands of years to reduce human suffering and enhance human happiness. In the next section we discuss some of these ideas.

MINDFULNESS, FORGIVENESS, COMPASSION: DEVELOPING ATTITUDES THAT PROMOTE THE INTEGRATION OF LOSS AND OTHER PAINFUL EXPERIENCES

Mindfulness

Everything we have written in this chapter relates in one way or another to the question of how to help people manage the disruption of mental peace that is the wellspring of suffering. Drawing on the Buddhist view of suffering, Hanson differentiates between the suffering that is inevitable and that which we amplify through our response:

> Inescapable physical or mental discomfort is the "first dart" of existence. As long as you live and love, some of those darts will come your way. First darts are unpleasant . . . But then we add our *reactions* to them. These reactions are "second darts" – the ones we throw ourselves. Most of our suffering comes from the second darts.
>
> (Hanson, 2009, p. 50)

The emotional suffering we call grief is caused by the deprivation of someone or something we cherish. Deepening the wellspring of suffering is the reminder of how unpredictable and chaotic the world is, and how little control we have over much that happens to us. These are, as Hanson tells us, the first, and unavoidable darts of existence. The second darts, the ones we throw ourselves, originate in our minds, and include the negative judgements we make about our own emotional responses to loss ("What's wrong with me? Why can't I get over this?"). A further source of secondary pain is the inability, or unwillingness, to accept reality when what is real is not what we want (Bodhi, 2005). Mindfulness practices (see Chapter 8, as well), and the cultivation of an attitude that *what is, is*, can help ease people away from their struggle against reality, a struggle they are bound to lose (Jordan, 2016). In this sense, mindfulness is not simply a set of practices but a way of being that involves staying present with and accepting reality, including the reality of our own limitations and the emotional injuries that life may inevitably include.

> Originating in Eastern spiritual practices, mindfulness training has been integrated into a variety of clinical models, including CBT and psychodynamic

psychotherapy, Acceptance and Commitment therapy (ACT), sensorimotor psychotherapy, mindfulness-based stress reduction (MBSR) and internal family systems (IFS) therapy. These practices, including moment-to-moment awareness and acceptance of emerging thoughts, feelings, and sensory experiences helps create a "reflective vantage point" in which client and therapist can hold and regulate painful and traumatic experience.

(Ringel, 2019, p. 144).

Pat Ogden describes a process in which mindfulness is an integral part of the interaction between therapist and client (Ogden, 2009; Ogden & Fisher, 2015). She suggests asking questions that bring the client's attention to what is happening in the moment. "Directed mindfulness," Ogden writes, is an "application of mindfulness that directs the patient's awareness toward particular elements of experience considered important to therapeutic goals (Ogden, 2009, p. 222). In the following exchange, the clinician used this approach with Audrey, who was beginning to grimace and clench her jaw at the conclusion of her session:

A: I know I have to be more understanding with my mother. I know she's old and sick and I have to try to be nicer to her.

PK: Okay, so as you say that I notice your body is tightening again, and your jaw is clenched, and you have a scary kind of smile on your face. How does it feel?

A: (Laughing) Not very good. Like I can hardly breathe, I'm so tight.

PK: Okay, great, so how about you take a breath. And now relax your jaw. Maybe, let yourself smile, just a little. And try saying it again.

This time Audrey's voice was quieter, her tone softer, her body more relaxed. It felt better, and since feeling better is what Audrey wants, she is motivated to be mindful of the messages she sends to her body through her expressions, her tone of voice, and her breath.

PK: Remember how we talked about the messages you send to your body, about whether you're safe or not – and how if you breathe, and smile a little, your body gets the message that you're not in danger, and that helps you feel calmer and more in control.

In work with bereaved clients, mindfulness can be introduced as a way for someone who is grieving to have an interlude of peace even as they are continuing to grieve, by focusing attention on the present moment. A simple exercise that we have used with clients is to have them focus on something beautiful in the therapist's office and to simply gaze at it for a few minutes, while breathing slowly in and out (Shapiro, 2005). This exercise can be particularly helpful for clients who tend to ruminate about their loss (Zech et al., 2010).

As a final example, an invitation to focus on the present moment can be extended by bringing attention to the connection between the therapist and client. When a clients (or anyone, for that matter) is caught in worries about the past and/or fears about the future, the following can be used to ground them in the present moment.

> *Right now in this moment*, I can see that you are suffering, because you miss her so much. . . And *right now in this moment* you're here with me, we're here together. Outside, there are trees, and the breeze is blowing the branches, and right now we're just here, looking at each other, and it feels good, just sitting here together and not having to do anything but be here, now. No place to go, nothing to do. We're just here, together. Right now in this moment we can feel good about just being together.

Forgiveness

People have different views concerning the importance of forgiveness. We have had many conversations with bereaved people about forgiveness, and what we have come to believe is that while it may be a relief to forgive someone, it is not always possible. Making forgiveness a goal can sometimes interfere with whatever degree of emotional healing *is* possible, rather than facilitating healing. For example, the second author has worked a great deal with survivors of suicide loss (Jordan & McIntosh, 2011). In addition to a sorrowful separation from the deceased, suicide can frequently be experienced by the survivor as an abandonment, a rejection, or even a deliberate attempt to psychologically wound the mourner. Forgiveness of the deceased after suicide is therefore often a complex and difficult task.

For many people, to forgive either past psychological injuries, or current wounds from a recent loss can feel too much like a denial that any injury occurred at all. If someone was hurt as a child, that person may need to hold onto anger *on behalf of the child* she was, because not to do so is tantamount to failing to have the child be protected yet again. A person may be reluctant to forgive because of the perceived equivalence between "forgiving" and "forgetting." They may feel that if they forgive, the memory or what happened will recede, and with it, a piece of their past or present experience that is a key to understanding who they are and what the death means to them. People may also be reluctant to forgive because of the perceived equivalence between "forgiving" and "forgetting." They may feel that if they forgive, the memory of what happened will recede, and with it, a piece of their past or present experience that is a key to understanding who they are and what the death has meant to them. They may feel that they have a right to be angry, and that to let go of that anger would be a betrayal of some part of who they are, or of their deceased loved one. The question then becomes one of how they can retain the memory of what happened to them, and yet not remain attached in an unhealthy and self-destructive way to the person who hurt them.

One way to help clients get past feelings about old hurts in situations in which forgiveness is not possible, or not yet possible, is to guide them toward identifying some of the negative thoughts about themselves – feelings of self-blame, failure, vulnerability – that may keep those old wounds from healing (Shapiro, 2012). For example, if someone lied to them, they may blame themselves for their gullibility. If someone hurt them physically, they may hate themselves for not having fought back. These kinds of thoughts are another example of the "second dart" of suffering.

Angry thoughts associated with old hurts are "sticky" thoughts and letting go of them takes practice. Clients can be advised that what they are letting go of is not the memory of what happened, but some of the discomfort generated by the memory. It may be helpful for a person to remember that they do not have to see, or interact with, the person who hurt them. Some people like to imagine having a force field that protects them from the influence of another person. Some people like to imagine that the person who hurt them is very small, or very far away (Hayes et al., 2011). This approach can be suggested with a statement such as: "When someone is taking up too much space in your mind it can be helpful to imagine that they are too little or too distant to be concerned about." Any of the practices above for working with painful feelings can be suggested to clients who want to be able to moderate their feelings of anger. What should be emphasized in recommending these practices is that the goal is not to "forgive and forget" but to loosen the hold of negative thoughts and feelings that interfere with peace of mind and detract from the individual's ability to focus on what is important and meaningful to them.

Self-Compassion

Self-compassion is another kind of forgiveness, and another kind of letting go. What we need to let go of is the idea that we can be as perfect in reality as the ideal self of our imagination. To be compassionate is to embrace human imperfection, our own, and others. For many people, nothing is more difficult than befriending the self (Harris, 2021; Vachon & Harris, 2016).

Vince

V: This week I've been very frustrated with myself, I feel like I'm not able to say what I want to say clearly, I can't articulate . . . and I felt that in a meeting with my supervisor and I got very angry at myself last night, like, what is wrong with me? Why can't I express myself? And it's weird because my supervisor actually commented that I was well prepared for the supervision, that I presented my cases well. But I couldn't take it in, what he said. And actually it made me a little uncomfortable.

PK: Any idea what that might be about?

V: Well, you know, we've talked about how I'm not comfortable sometimes being seen. I'd rather not be seen.

PK: If someone sees you . . .

V: They're going to see that I'm not a good person. I feel like part of me is not a good person. And that's also why it's hard for me to take it in when someone says something good about me, because I don't feel like I deserve it.

And some of that is because in my family it didn't pay to tell someone what you were feeling. I couldn't do it with my mom and my dad wasn't much better. It didn't matter what I felt. When you have to pretend everything is OK when it's not, that's a burden for you.

So now that's what I always do, I just shut down. Or I run away. I don't want to deal with anyone because I feel like I have no way to ... I don't know how to. . . what my feelings are, or how to talk about them.

PK: It's hard to have a relationship with another person if you think they're going to judge you or get angry at you. And that's true for your relationship with yourself too. That's why it's important to be able to be with yourself, to accept your feelings, to accept how you are, even if it's not exactly how you think you should be or want to be. To start from the position that you're OK, that there's nothing wrong with you.

V: Like that book you gave me, that's a good book and I'm going to read it again (Huber, 2001). There's one passage in that book that I like a lot, where she talks about self-improvement. The problem with thinking about how you're going to improve yourself is that it brings you back to the feeling that you're not good enough the way you are. And thinking so much about how you're going to improve just ends up making you feel worse about yourself, so what's the point of even trying to be better if you're such a screwup?"

PK: So: another way to talk to yourself could be: "I don't have to perfect. I just have to be trying. I don't have to know everything. I just have to be learning.

V: That's being compassionate with myself. And if I can be more that way, I can feel better about letting other people be close to me. And also, if I feel better about myself I don't have to be so angry at my mother for what she did. I don't have to *forgive her. But at some point, you have to accept your parents for who they are or were. And just live your life.*

As a child, Vince believed that his feelings "didn't matter", and he did his best to shut them down rather than risk his parent's displeasure or rebuke. As an adult, he has continued to employ this strategy. He feels uncomfortable being seen, and uncomfortable with expressions of positive regard, a problem that Leeds (2022) has described as a complicating factor in therapy with survivors of early abuse or neglect. In this exchange, Vince reflects on the ways in which he is still affected by what he experienced as a child. Vince's closing observation suggests a growing sense that if he can be less self-critical and more accepting of himself, he'll be better able to "just live" his life. I (PK) sit opposite Vince and ask him to look into my eyes, as I say the following in a gentle voice:

When we're young, we see ourselves the way that our caregivers see us. We see ourselves reflected in their eyes, we believe what their eyes tell us, and we carry that way of seeing ourselves long past childhood. What we need as children is to be seen with warmth, and tenderness. What we need is to see ourselves reflected in the eyes of someone who sees us as good, who sees us as loveable. That's what we need. If we don't get that as a child it's hard for us to believe that we are good, that we are loveable.

As I continue to look into Vince's eyes, I am conscious of communicating this simple truth: you are good. You are deserving of love. The following week Vince tells me that he carried this message with him through the week. He said: "What you did surprised me. I wasn't expecting that. But afterwards I felt like it was just the thing I needed – it let me feel what you were telling me, not just the words, but the *feeling* of what you were telling me."

I hesitate to call this interaction a "technique", because it was born of an in-the-moment felt sense of wanting to communicate this message directly, right brain to right brain. That being said, our use of interventions is always influenced by the degree of comfort and familiarity we have with a given approach, in this case an approach grounded in right brain to right brain psychotherapy (Schore) and compassion-based grief therapy (Harris & Ho, 2022). Readers interested in becoming more familiar with interventions to strengthen self-compassion will find detailed examples in Steindl & Matos (2022), among others (Harris & Ho, 2022).

SUMMARY

Our goal in this chapter has been to illustrate a number of approaches to helping clients develop core capacities for emotional self-regulation. In many ways, these overlap with, or are the same as the Core Capacities described in Chapter 8 for grief therapists. Implicit in this emphasis on these capacities is the belief that what a grieving person needs from a therapist is not to be healed, fixed, or even "treated", but to be helped in a gentle and attuned manner to be present with the experience of loss, and to access the internal resources needed to integrate that experience.

The clinical examples included here, it should be emphasized, illustrate only part of treatment with the clients presented. As in any grief-oriented intervention, treatment in these cases included many other elements, including exploration of the full range of emotions related to the person and the loss, discussion of the bereaved's self-blame in relation to how the person died, and reconstruction of the bereaved's identity. What we have tried to do here is to pick out one aspect of treatment that we find is not always given the attention it warrants in accounts of work with the bereaved: that is, the effect of problems with emotion regulation as a factor in problematic grief. We are suggesting that when a grief therapist helps a client develop resources for affect management, the result is that they are better able to tolerate the other work that is involved in addressing their loss. When people are taught skills such as mentalizing, they often find that they are less reactive to the people in their lives (like Audrey) and more able to understand, if not forgive, the behavior of the deceased (like Vince). The net result is that they are able to recapture emotional energy that has been diverted to an unhealthy continuing bond.

A person who is able to understand their own motivations and behaviors and those of others is less prone to confusion and hopelessness in life, and in grief. Sadness and yearning may be inescapable parts of loss, but terror is not - nor is unrelenting anger or self-blame. A capacity for flexible attention, which is associated with secure attachment, but which we believe can be cultivated in the context of secure relationships at any time in life, enables a person to have a respite from painful emotions, and in those periods of respite, to enjoy what is good in the present moment, to identify what possibilities in life still exist, and to plan for a future guided by an understanding of what they most value. In the following chapter we look at another important part of this process of self-discovery, the reconstruction of meaning, with an eye toward illustrating how this process is managed within the context of attachment informed grief therapy.

NOTE

1   The literature on emotion and self-regulation reflects the interests and methods of researchers and clinicians from many disciplines. Such diversity inevitably leads to a certain amount of difficulty in communication and integration of knowledge. For example, the terms "emotion" and "affect" and "emotion regulation" and "affect regulation" are used interchangeably by some writers (Mikulincer etal., 2009) but not others (Siegel, 2012). For simplicity's sake, we use the term "emotion regulation" throughout this discussion.

10

MEANING MAKING IN ADAPTATION TO LOSS

Give sorrow words; the grief that does not speak knits up the o-er wrought heart and bids it break.

William Shakespeare, *Macbeth* (1606)

Our focus in Chapter 9 was on the importance of strengthening self-capacities, and emotion regulation in particular, in work with the bereaved. In this chapter, we focus on meaning making, an element of adaptation to loss that, depending on the individual and the nature of their loss, can be equally or even more important than emotion regulation. In practice it is clear that the ability to make meaning and to regulate emotion are inextricably connected and mutually impactful. When we can make sense of what has happened to us we are more likely to be able to maintain a calm emotional state; when we are calm, we are more likely to be able to make sense of what is happening or has happened to us.

Coming, as it does, to all living things, the end of life is something we might suppose would be a reality that would be easy for us to understand. We might not like it, we might recoil at the thought of our own life or the life of someone we love coming to an end. But as inevitable as it is, as expected as it may be, death, when it comes, is at best unsettling, and at worst, devastating, a blow that leaves a gaping hole in our map of reality.

DOI: 10.4324/9781003204183-14

Incredulity is an element of many losses, even ones that have been expected. Moreover, when things fall apart, it is in our nature to try to put them back together. When nothing makes sense, we try to find a way back to coherence, to meaning. Reflecting an emphasis on this collapse of coherence in bereavement, Neimeyer proposes that a "central process in grieving is the attempt to reaffirm or reconstruct a world of meaning that has been challenged by loss" (Neimeyer, 2006).

Everything that we have said about the variations in how people grieve applies to our consideration of meaning making as a component of grief and of grief therapy. Meaning making is more or less of an issue for some grievers in the aftermath of some deaths, the loss of some relationships. When a bereaved person tells us, tearfully, that their loved one "had to go" to escape from the prison of pain that their life had become, we may infer that their struggle is not with the "why" of death, although this does not spare them from the agonizing question of "why this had to happen". When death ends a life suffused by suffering, we can forgive death, but not the illness that was the agent of that suffering.

Meaning making in bereavement can take many forms. For some grievers it is a struggle to understand something that is beyond their understanding; for others, it is the search for a fragment of value amongst the ruins of life after loss. For many, meaning making is nothing more or less than an attempt to find a way to make the unbearable bearable.

Although the term "meaning making" may bring to mind a process that is more cognitive than emotional, in practice can be a deeply emotionally affecting process for both the client and the therapist, one that at times relies on metaphor, poetry, and other non-linear forms of thinking and communication (Neimeyer, 2001, 2006a; Neimeyer et al., 2011; Neimeyer & Sands, 2011). It is a process that is facilitated within the context of a trusting, secure bond, the creation of which, we suggest, is aided by the therapist's awareness of the client's attachment history and attachment related needs.

The death of a significant person in one's life is not a singular loss, but one that can ripple into every aspect of the bereaved's identity, social relations, and mental and physical health. Death is an emotional blow, but it is also a violation of a precious, if unconscious conviction that the important people in our live will not disappear, will not be taken from us, and certainly, will not be taken from us without advance warning. It is as if we have learned that, since the person has continuously been in our life in the past, that this state of affairs will simply go on in the future, and that the end can be postponed more or less indefinitely.

Those left behind after significant loss must also accommodate to changes that include not only the loss of the person who has died, but also the loss of parts of themselves and the world as they knew it - what has been described as our "assumptive world" (Kaufman, 2002; Milman, Neimeyer et al., 2019a). Grievers after a sudden violent loss may envy those whose loved ones die after a long illness, assuming that the advance knowledge that the person is dying makes it easier for those left behind to cope with and accept their loss, and that a sufficient leave taking with the dying person was possible. But the reality is that an awareness of impending death often makes little difference in how people react when someone dies. In this sense, death more often than not involves an element of trauma for the bereaved, even if does not meet the criteria of what is generally considered "traumatic death" (Boelen et al., 2019; Perlman et al., 2014). That being said, clinical experience and findings from research do suggest that meaning making is likely to be more difficult to achieve in the wake of deaths that are unexpected, violent, or untimely (i.e., out of the perceived developmental order of life, such as the death of a child) (Boelen et al., 2019; Milman, Neimeyer, et al., 2019a).

THE ROLE OF MEANING-MAKING IN BEREAVEMENT

A number of theorists have conceptualized grieving as a process of meaning reconstruction (Attig, 2011; Neimeyer, 2001, 2019; Milman & Neimeyer, et al., 2019a). In particular, Robert Neimeyer and his colleagues have made this the center of their thinking about the mourning process, providing extensive evidence of the crucial role that meaning reconstruction plays in this process (Currier, Holland, & Neimeyer, 2009; Gillies et al., 2014; Lichtenthal et al., 2011; Neimeyer, 2019). They have also contributed innovative clinical techniques to help facilitate the practice of meaning reconstruction in grief therapy (Neimeyer et al., 2021).

In considering what it means to make meaning of a loss, Neimeyer and Thompson (2014) suggest that it involves two distinct narrative processes, the first related to the story of the death, and the second the story of the griever's relationship to the deceased (Neimeyer & Sands, 2011).

In the first instance, the griever is trying to find answers to questions about the loss: *"How could this happen? Why did this happen to me? What could I have done to prevent it?"* These questions are generally most pressing in the aftermath of a loss that is unexpected and/or traumatic, such as suicide (Jordan, 2012). The death of a child is raises similar, and often unanswerable, questions (Lichtenthal et al., 2013). The second meaning making process addresses the bereaved's relationship with the deceased (see Chapter 5). *"What was the relationship like before the death? Can I still have a relationship with this person? What meaning has become attached to the relationship since the death? What unfinished business or lingering questions do I have with this person?"*

Research over the past 20 years has provided support for the role of meaning making in bereavement, demonstrating that meaning related variables have significant predictive power in identifying individuals who will have greater difficulty in their bereavement recovery. Studies of meaning making have identified the importance of *sense-making, benefit finding, and identity reformation* in how people cope with loss (Gamino & Sewell, 2004; Gillies & Neimeyer, 2006; Holland et al., 2007; Lichtenthal et al., 2013; Neimeyer, 2021).

Sense-making is the ability of the mourner to organize the events of the loss into an understandable sequence (emplotment) and to find a purpose or reason for a loss, rather than to experience it as incomprehensible (thematic deconstruction) (Currier & Neimeyer, 2006). An example of this would be when a daughter bereaved after her father's suicide observes that her father was "always in danger" and "made his own decision that it was time for him to leave" (see Chapter 5). Benefit finding is the capacity to find positive outcomes in the loss experience, despite its painful and unwelcome nature, as when a young woman whose sister has died by suicide tearfully recognizes that while the loss "blew my world apart", it also served as the catalyst for her to the make significant, positive changes in our own life. Identity reformation refers to the reconstruction of the self, as the griever adjusts to the changes necessitated by loss. Identity reformation involves processes as diverse as the reconstruction of self after the loss of parents (*Am I still someone's daughter?*) to a widow's assuming responsibility for financial decisions that were always handled by her husband.

None of this work of meaning making can be done before a client is ready to undertake it. As much as we may wish to try to ease their suffering, premature attempts at meaning making will in all likelihood cause a breakdown of trust and a rupture of the therapeutic relationship. In the following vignette, a grieving grandfather who was a client of the second author struggles to come to terms with the loss of a child, and a role in that child's life, that he cherished.

Tom

Tom was a 64-year-old man who was raised in a conservative religious tradition, and continued to follow that tradition in his adult life. Tom's life-long conviction was that God rewards those who are obedient to his will and punishes those who ignore his commandments. The arrival of his first grandchild was experienced by Tom as a gift from God that filled him with love and gratitude. He was thus shocked, outraged, and deeply bereaved when, at four months of age, his grandchild developed a severe respiratory infection that eventually led to his death. This loss was shattering for Tom. It resulted in many symptoms of being dysregulated – his sleep was disrupted, he had trouble concentrating at work, and his mood alternated between being depressed and extremely irritable. The death of his grandson also forced Tom into an excruciating reevaluation of his religious faith. How could God take this child from him when his Grandson could not yet have sinned? How could he continue to believe that God was always just and righteous, when something this unjust could happen? Could this somehow be God's punishment of Tom for his own transgressions? These agonizing questions were the result of the shattering of Tom's assumptive world about how the universe operated, and the nature of the God who he believed ran the world. They were both a cause of and a result of the profound feelings of anger, sorrow, and grief that Tom felt about the death of his grandson.

This brief story about Tom conveys the pervasive emotional and spiritual damage that the loss of an important relationship can inflict. In working with someone like Tom, who has suffered both a painful loss, and a profound disruption of their assumptive world, meaning making becomes a requisite part of restoring self-regulatory capacity. In the absence of a revised understanding of such a sudden an untimely death, it will be difficult for many clients to let go of painful rumination and speculation about the disconnect between what they expected and believed, and what has actually occurred. To do this work, Tom will need the support of someone who sensitively and patiently accompanies him through the darkness and helps him consider what the implications of the loss are for his beliefs (in this case, his spiritual beliefs).

MENTALIZING, REFLECTIVE FUNCTIONING, COHERENCE, AND PERSPECTIVE-TAKING

One of our goals in this book is to make linkages between the theoretical domains of attachment theory and thanatology. As discussed in Chapters 2, 4, and 9, mentalizing theory is based on the recognition that as children develop, they gradually recognize that other people have minds that are separate from their own, with their own thoughts and feelings. These thoughts and feelings are expressed, implicitly or explicitly, through their behavior. The ability to make sense of one's own and other people's behavior in terms of their mental states – thoughts, intentions, beliefs – is what Fonagy and others describe as "mentalizing capacity" and is crucial to the development of a separate, differentiated identity in the developing child (Fonagy et al., 2002; Allen, 2013). In adulthood, this capacity, as illustrated in several of the cases discussed thus far, has a significant bearing on people's ability to form, and maintain mutually satisfying relationships with others.

As with affect regulation, the capacity for mentalizing develops through interaction with our early attachment figures. The parents of the growing child, through repeated, empathically attuned transactions with their offspring, mirror back the child's internal affective and cognitive states, and thereby help the child to recognize their own experience as separate from their parents' and unique to themselves. High levels of this capacity are related to the development of good mental health and emotional resilience in the face of stressor events in children and adults, and conversely, the failure to adequately develop these resources is related to a vulnerability to the impact of traumatic events and a propensity towards psychiatric disorder (Ensink et al., 2014; Fonagy et al., 2014b). It has also been postulated that helping with the restoration and strengthening of mentalizing in therapy may be a key element in reducing activation of the attachment system and reduction of the trauma response (Allen, 2013). As used in attachment theory, reflective functioning (RF), which is assessed through administration of the Adult Attachment Interview (AAI) is the operationalization of the construct of mentalization (Fonagy et al., 1991, 1998). Research regarding the role of mentalizing/reflective functioning in mental health is convergent with research concerning the significant role of meaning making in adaptation to loss. In both cases, a restored sense of coherence is seen as an indication of positive accommodation, and the absence of coherence as evidence of unresolved loss or trauma.

Another concept that resonates in both attachment theory and meaning making approaches to bereavement is the idea of the *coherence of a narrative* (Hesse, 2008; Main et al., 2008). Recall from Chapter 2 that the AAI is scored with regard to loss and trauma in terms of the linguistic coherence of the narrative given by the respondent to the probes about relationships with early attachment figures. A lack of coherence in a narrative is viewed as a reflection of unresolved trauma and loss in the respondent's attachment history (Steele & Steele, 2008). In a similar fashion, meaning reconstruction theorists have emphasized the disruption of the coherence of the self-narrative and assumptive world as a central impact of traumatic losses, as well as a prime focus of meaning reconstruction-oriented interventions (Armour, 2006; Hibberd, 2013; Landsman, 2002; Nadeau, 1998; Neimeyer & Sands, 2011; Owens et al., 2008; Sands, 2008). This convergence of thinking from these two very different intellectual traditions informs the conceptual foundation of this chapter.

Meaning making can also be understood as critical for the reregulation of an individual's emotional equilibrium after it has been disrupted by a loss. Jurist and Meehan have referred to the strengthening of "mentalized affectivity" as a goal in psychotherapy (Jurist & Meehan, 2009). This construct refers to the capacity to reflect, in particular, on the emotions that drive our behavior, as well as on the emotions and behavior of others (see Chapter 9). We can see the effects of this kind of learning in Audrey (introduced in Chapter 4) as she speaks of her newfound ability to understand the behavior of family members after her mother's death. In the following exchange with PK, Audrey reflects on the behavior of her sister's children, with whom she has always had a close and loving relationship, despite ongoing conflict with her sister. For months, Audrey has bitterly resented the breakdown in communication with her niece and nephew's and their absence from her life.

Audrey

A: It's hurt me so much, the feeling that I never really knew my sister's kids. The reason I'm saying that is: if the love I had for them – if it was reciprocated – there is no way that they would not have reached out to me when my mother died ... There was all that with the will and the money – my sister must have been screaming in the house – and my niece must have said to herself: I'm done with this – I'm sticking by my mom

In the last week I've been able to think about it in depth – and I say to myself – you know what? I would do the same thing. I would stick up for my mother. No matter what.

PK: That's Interesting, Audrey, very interesting.

A: I really believe that it is interesting, because I never thought about it this way before.

But I know my gut, and I know ... they are my sister's kids. They are the product of her parents. Just like I was the product of my parents. You are the product of your parents.

PK: Wow, Audrey. I think that that's a remarkably clear-headed way of looking at them. What it says to me is that you're able to think about them without being carried away by your feelings. That you're able to see them in terms of their experience and their reality, so that you don't get hurt by the way that they behave. Because you see it as an inevitable consequence of how they've been raised.

A: And I could tear up – out of happiness – because, truly, I don't have that pain in my heart anymore.

And I could also tear up out of happiness from hearing you say something positive like that.

Because we're in this together.

In this exchange we see how the capacity for mentalizing facilitates meaning making, which in turn strengthens affect regulation (Schwarzer et al., 2021). In the following exchange Audrey shares what for her is the greatest gift of her efforts to understand her family, a newfound appreciation of her mother and a felt sense of her continuing bond presence in Audrey's life.

A: I am proud of myself. And I don't know why or how this happened ... everything that I look at now I look into the eyes of my mother's eyes at my age. Everything that I see now I see through her eyes. And that just means that she's within. She's really, really within.

When someone dies, I don't know, maybe you appreciate them more?

Because my mother was such a badass. The more my life goes on the more I realize what a badass she was. She did the best she could, under the terrible circumstances. And she never wavered. And you know what – that's a badass!

So now – I'm going to be sixty – I think about how she was at 60. How did she act and what did she do? And you know what - she was a pretty cool lady.

PK: Wow. So it's like – you have internalized her – and also – it's like, when she was alive, most of how you perceived her was how she was at the end of her life. But now that she's gone, you're seeing her more as the way she was when she was the age you are now. It's like your vision of her has cleared because the old her isn't here. Does that make any sense?

A: Yes.

FACILITATING MEANING-MAKING AFTER LOSS

How does the process of grief therapy help a client whose assumptive world has been shattered by a death? What elements of the format and structure of therapy allow this vital repair work to proceed? Are their specific techniques that may be used during therapy that can enhance this activity? These questions will be the focus of the remainder of this chapter.

The Arc of Grief Therapy

Holmes (2010, 2013) proposes a simple but useful tripartite model of the "phases" of all psychotherapeutic activity: Attachment, Meaning Making, and Change. Respectively, these involve the building of a secure and trusting attachment relationship with the client, the exploration of the meaning and origins of the presenting problem(s), and the fostering of new ways of thinking, feeling, and behaving in response to those presenting problems. Much of what we have said in previous chapters about the role of attachment orientation in the response to loss is relevant here. Clients begin grief therapy with expectations about what kind of help they may receive in the context of an intimate relationship with a professional caregiver at a time of great distress in their life. These expectations directly reflect the attachment orientation (and secondary attachment strategies) that the client has developed as a result of their life experiences. (See Chapter 4 for a discussion of some of these factors and related consider-ations regarding the customization of treatment in grief therapy.)

Almost all people who seek grief therapy have, by definition, had their attachment system (or in the case of bereaved parents, their caregiving system) activated by the loss, i.e. they are experiencing acute separation distress. In addition, as noted previously, the activation of the attachment system creates a state of emotional arousal that can interfere with higher order processing, including the capacity to mentalize. In traumatic bereavement, the mourner may have developed alexithymia, the inability to put feelings into words. The experience of trauma can sometimes be so fragmented and dissociated that it cannot be processed with language (Van der Kolk, 2014). The progression from dysregulation to reregulation is represented below.

Reactive/Dysregulated → Reflective → Reintegrated/Reregulated

Most individuals seeking professional assistance have been thrust into a *Reactive* stance with regard to their loss, in which they are dysregulated on physical, emotional, cognitive, and behavioral levels. This dysregulation may take the form of hyper-arousal, usually associated with an anxious attachment style, hypo-arousal, generally found in people with an avoidant attachment style, or a complex mixture of the two that is associated with a disorganized attachment style. This last category is usually accompanied by an exacerbation of typically pre-existing psychiatric and personality disorders that have been intensified by the death.

One goal of grief therapy is to support and promote the bereaved person's progress from a dysregulated state to one in which the individual is able to reflect on and make sense of their loss. This process is accomplished in the context of a secure and trusted attachment relationship with the grief therapist and requires that the therapist help the client with both affect regulation and meaning making about the death. This process of integration also involves helping the client to change. In the context of bereavement, change means adapting to the inevitable alterations in life functioning, identity, and ways of being in the world that significant losses demand of a mourner. It also means the acquisition of new skills and ways of thinking that can promote psychological coherence, and even growth, in clients (Cozolino, 2010; Holmes, 2010, 2013).

In addition to being dysregulating and inhibiting the capacity for meaning making, the death of a loved one also acts to *constrain the exploratory system of the individual, which is the reciprocal of the attachment behavioral system.* As Sbarra and Hazen explain, a reciprocal relationship of co-regulation exists between people who are bonded to one another (Sbarra & Hazan, 2008), and the loss of this other (whether parent, child, partner, or friend) results in dysregulation. Thus, it is common to begin grief therapy with a newly bereaved client who has been "hibernating" or "hunkering down" in their life. This withdrawal can take many forms. Many severely or traumatically bereaved individuals, for example, will show emotional constriction, numbing, and sometimes full-blown dissociative responses (particularly when they are also traumatized by the mode of death), with little capacity to feel their normal range of emotions, or to put their experience into words. Likewise, bereaved persons may present with a cognitive constriction that entails ruminative thinking about a yearned for reunion with the loved one and a diminished ability to imagine or problem solve about a world without the deceased. In extreme cases, this diminished problem solving capacity may result in suicidality in the mourner, where ending one's life can appear to be the only option for the mourner to obtain relief from their suffering and end the separation from the deceased (Johnson et al., 2008; Latham & Prigerson, 2004; Szanto et al., 2006). Lastly, many mourners will also have withdrawn from their usual social relationships, avoiding engagement in their previous social roles involving work, family, and friendships. *All of these common signs of bereavement can be understood as manifestations of the deactivation of the mourner's exploratory system, and protracted hyperactivation of their attachment system as manifested in the psychological need to "search" for the lost individual.* A central goal of grief therapy, then, can be understood as the restoration of a healthier and more balanced equilibrium between the attachment and exploratory systems in the bereaved individual. This is also another way of stating what we have previously noted in the Dual Process Model: that the oscillation between grieving (seeking proximity to the deceased) and restoration (exploration of the changed world), needs to be reactivated when it has become frozen.

What Does Meaning Making Mean for This Client?

The core stance of the therapist in psychotherapy, particularly in exploratory therapies such as client-centered and psychodynamic approaches, has frequently been described as one of curiosity (Epstein, 2022). That is, therapy is an effort by a clinician to engage in a shared exploration of and conversation with the client about the origins of and their efforts to ameliorate the presenting problem(s) (Holmes, 2009, 2010). We believe that this is also the case in grief therapy. In one sense, the presenting problem in grief therapy seems obvious, i.e., the client has lost a loved one to death. Yet in another sense, the problem is not always so clear to either the therapist or the client until this type of mutual investigation has been conducted. Thus, the presentation by clients of seemingly similar presenting problems may reflect quite different core issues. Consider the following three case vignettes:

> *Susan entered therapy after the suicide of her husband. She had endured a verbally and occasionally physically abusive marriage to this man for almost 30 years. Finally, she announced to him that she was done with the marriage and moved out. After a week or two of pleading with her to return, and her persistence in saying "no", he shot himself. Susan simultaneously felt a sense of liberation, along with a deep feeling of*

guilt – one that was compounded by the anger of one of her adult children who blamed her mother for her father's death.

Carol sought grief therapy for herself after the suicide of her husband, who had been depressed after getting himself and the family into significant financial difficulty. Carol felt confused and worried about how to help their 3-year-old son deal with the death of his father. She also was furious with her husband for deserting the family and leaving her with what seemed to be overwhelming challenges as a single parent, including significant financial difficulties. She resented her mother-in-law, whom she believed blamed her for her son's death, and who laid strong claim to the raising of her grandson. Carol was unsure about how to deal with her mother-in-law's frequent intrusive visits, which were usually framed as efforts to "help out" after the death.

Jim was deeply bereaved by the suicide of his wife. She had been depressed on and off throughout much of their five-year marriage and had made a previous suicide attempt. But their relationship had been one of childhood sweethearts who befriended and supported each other in separating from their conflictual and hurtful families of origin. Without the one person whom he had come to trust in life, Jim found himself feeling lost, afraid, and unsure about how he could have a life without his wife. He wondered if suicide was now the only option for him as well and fantasized that death would reunite him with his missing partner.

All of these vignettes involve the suicide of a life partner, a similarity in presenting problem that might lead one to expect a similarity in the main issues faced by the bereaved spouse. Nonetheless, the core issues that will need to be addressed in grief therapy are quite different for each of these individuals. They range from guilt over feeling relief, to anger at being abandoned to intense fearfulness about being alone. Put differently, the meaning of these three losses was unique to each of these bereaved individuals.

THEMATIC QUESTIONS FOR MEANING-MAKING

The process of exploring the meaning of a loss for a particular client, and the ways in which the self-narrative of the client has been damaged or frozen by the death, has been termed "mapping the terrain of loss" by the first author (Kosminsky, 2012). It can be described in a series of broad, thematic questions that are revisited over and over again during the course of the therapeutic journey. Some version of these questions will be raised as part of almost every session, including the first session of grief therapy. In parallel fashion, over the course of treatment, as the individual moves from a reactive, to a reflective, to a reintegrated stance, these questions will occupy a varying portion of each session. Conversation about all of these thematic questions facilitate the psychological integration of the individual's experience into a coherent narrative, and quite likely help with integration on a neurological level as well, as the client uses higher order cortical functioning to process experiences that may previously have been processed mainly by the affective systems of the brain (i.e., the limbic system) (Cozolino, 2010; Schore, 2012).

- *How are you doing now?* Therapy must begin with an assessment of the client's objective functioning, as well as their subjective experience, in the here and now. This includes the client's physical functioning (disruption of bio-rhythms; health issues; concerns about the bodily impact of the loss; loss of energy and stamina; use of prescription and non- prescription drugs, etc.), social functioning (availability and quality of social connection and support; changes emerging in relationships both inside and outside the family; desire to connect with others vs. withdrawal into the self, etc.), and psychological functioning (symptoms of anxiety, PTSD, anhedonia; rumination about the death & particular aspects of the death; suicidal thoughts and/or behaviors, etc.). As we have previously discussed, getting a sense of the bereaved person's general attachment orientation, and their characteristic ways of dealing with psychological pain, is also crucial.
  This process can also include history talking about client's prior experience with other losses and traumatizing events (which will frequently have been retriggered by the current loss), as well as the nature of their history with other close relationships with attachment figures. Some approaches to grief therapy advocate the initiation of treatment with a careful and systematic assessment of the client before beginning treatment (Pearlman et al., 2014). We understand and appreciate the merits of such a method. However, we also believe that treatment begins with the first moment of therapy, and we do not view assessment as a discrete and separate process that precedes therapy. In our opinion, an excessive focus on assessment with a newly bereaved and traumatized client, to the exclusion of building safety and the feeling of being understood in the therapeutic relationship, runs the risk of empathic failure with clients. With the exception of certain information about the client's safety (e.g., suicidal ideation, use of addictive drugs, etc.), we generally prefer to allow the history gathering process to evolve in parallel with the growth of the therapeutic alliance during the early phases of treatment.
- *Can you tell me about the death/dying?* The "death narrative" or "event story" (Neimeyer, 2012e) almost always plays some role in the mourning process, though it may not be the most prominent or problematic aspect of the loss. In cases of traumatic bereavement, the nature of the of death, including the client's actual or imagined mental pictures of the suffering and death of the deceased, should always be a part of the conversation, and quite likely a major focus of treatment. However, the timing of an intensive confrontation with the horrifying

or terrifying aspects of the death is a matter of clinical judgment and experience. It should be viewed in the context of the client's preferred way of dealing with very disturbing thoughts and feelings, which is a function of their attachment orientation. Such exposure work usually should not be pursued in depth unless and until a solid therapeutic relationship with the client has been established, and both client and clinician agree that the time for such work is appropriate (Allen, 2013). The clinician needs to be particularly cautious with a client who could be categorized as having a disorganized frame of mind with regard to attachment. A client with this type of defensive style is particularly likely to become emotionally dysregulated when asked to relive traumatic memories, leading them to experience therapy as a threatening, rather than helpful experience.

- *Can you tell me about the life of the person?* The narrative or "back story" of the life of the deceased and the client's relationship with their loved one is a key part of the mourning process (Neimeyer, 2012e) and is often central to understanding complicated grief. The development of a coherent story of the life of the deceased is considered by Walter to be a principal task of mourning (Walter, 1996). Note that this parallels the emphasis placed on narrative coherence in the assessment of attachment styles in the AAI. From the story telling done at funerals, to the reminiscing and reflection about the person done years later, reviewing the life of the deceased is a necessary part of the work of internalizing the relationship with the deceased (Pearlman et al., 2014; Rando, 1993). This is particularly true if the deceased served as an attachment figure for the mourner, or, in the case of parents, was the recipient of caregiving from the mourner (see section below on Fostering and Repairing Continuing Bonds). The narrative of the life of the deceased is also typically intertwined with the larger life narrative of the mourner, including their family of origin experiences with caregivers, and the trajectory of their physical, psychological, and social development.

- *What have you lost?* This question is central to the work of *sense making* in grief therapy. This core thematic inquiry embodies a host of subordinate questions for exploration over the course of grief therapy: What are the tangible and symbolic aspects of the loss (e.g. the death of a spouse might involve the loss of a companion to have breakfast with each morning, and the dream of a happy retirement in Florida). How will the mourner's world change without this individual in it? What must be relearned to live in the world going forward? (Attig, 2011). What has been, to use Neimeyer's phrase, the life imprint of this individual on the client's life (Neimeyer, 2012c)? What must the individual let go of, and how will she be able to do that? What does she need to hold on to, and how will she bring that about? How does this loss evoke or connect with other losses in the mourner's life? (Kosminsky, 2012).

- *Who are you now?* This thematic question pertains to the *changes in identity* that can often accompany loss. To an extent that is often under-appreciated, our identity is deeply involved with our relational world. Bereaved parents often question "Am I still a parent?" when a child dies, and bereaved spouses will report that "I still feel married" for long periods of time after the death of their partner. Thus, loss often involves the reworking of identity for the mourner. Consideration of identity related questions such as "How do you think of yourself now?" "How have you changed?" "Has your purpose in life changed?" and "What have you learned from this experience?" allow the client to reflect on their view of themselves, and how the loss has altered their identity and purpose in life.

- *What do you need to hold on to?* These questions address the meaning of the continuing bond with the deceased. Embedded in this inquiry is the idea that people can and do maintain a connection with the dead (see Chapter 5). There are, of course, as many ways to stay connected to a dead loved one as there are mourners who wish to do so. Some mourners will cultivate memories of the deceased, others will pursue the bond through spiritual means such as prayer or meditation, and still others will maintain connection by honoring the values and the unfinished business of the deceased. And for mourners who have a partner with whom they have shared the care of children, continuing to look out for the well-being of those children can contribute to a sense of their partner continuing on in their shared progeny. In emphasizing the value of continuing bonds, it is important to keep in mind that some people may also benefit from allowing themselves to distance themselves from aspects of the relationship that may have been hurtful, and detract from, rather than enhance, their well-being and healing.

- *Has anything positive come out of this experience for you?* This question relates to the *benefit finding* component of meaning making. This is obviously a theme that should not be the focus of attention early in the grief therapy process, when the individual typically still views the death of a loved one as a uniformly negative experience. It is usually only when people have been able to move towards a more reflective and reintegrated stance that they begin to discern benefits in the bereavement experience. Benefit finding may also take different forms for different people. Some people will find a new resilience in themselves or an enhanced appreciation of life and of their relationships. Still others may find a new or renewed sense of purpose in their life.

- *What is the future that you want?* Nearly all models of the mourning process suggest that healthy mourning must end in a reinvestment by the griever in their own life trajectory (Attig, 2011; Pearlman et al., 2014; Worden, 2009). These are some of the questions that reflect a shift towards what the Dual Process Model calls a Restoration Orientation (see Chapter 4): What will the client's future be without this person? What do they want it to be like, and how can they move on with their life? What holds them back from moving on with their life? What lies unfinished and unaccepted about the loss for the mourner? What new skills must they learn to go forward? And who do they know themselves to be without this person in their life? Who will they be in the future? Who do they want to be?

GRIEF THERAPY TECHNIQUES

Therapeutic techniques are usually thought of as deliberate activities, engaged in by the therapist to help the client achieve a certain goal or goals. In the context of grief therapy, these goals can include saying good-bye to a loved one, making peace with someone from whom they were estranged, or reestablishing or repairing the connection with the deceased. Techniques can also be used to help a person come to terms with the reality of a death, find meaning in the loss, or reduce the symptoms associated with the loss.

While we understand the value of techniques in grief therapy, we also believe that like all tools, the efficacy of therapeutic techniques depends on the skill and clinical wisdom of the person using them. From the moment the client walks in the door, we are employing our best skills at engaging with and helping the bereaved person. At times, these skills will involve the explicit use of specific techniques. *But over the course of therapy, most of what we do is in direct response to what is happening in the moment with the client.* Our interventions emerge from the kind of attunement we have described in the therapeutic relationship in Chapter 8. In this sense, the therapeutic encounter is directed by the client and by what they seem to need from us in the here, and now. In our opinion, the application of technique, without this kind of therapeutic resonance and wisdom, is at best a hollow exercise, and at worst, has the potential to be actively harmful to the client.

The Therapeutic Conversation as Technique

While meaning making after a loss may seem to be primarily an intrapsychic process, in fact, it is also a transpersonal activity that is greatly facilitated (or hindered) by our dialogue with other people (Neimeyer & Jordan, 2001; Neimeyer et al., 2000). The careful exploration of variation after variation of the thematic questions noted above, with a supportive clinician, is central to our view of grief therapy. *Thus, the very process of asking good questions of the client and listening with skilled and empathic attunement to the answers – what Allen calls "plain old therapy"* (Allen, 2013) *– facilitates the entire progression of meaning making.*

There have been many debates within the psychotherapy literature about the merits or drawbacks of manualized and technique-oriented therapies versus a more relational and improvisational style of conducting treatment (Shear et al., 2011). It is beyond our scope or intention here to take a firm stand on one side of this debate or another. Even carefully designed approaches to grief therapy acknowledge the importance of a foundational therapeutic alliance and flexibility on the part of the therapist as necessary components of a successful treatment protocol (Pearlman et al., 2014). Likewise, even less structured approaches to therapy have implicit agendas and goals on the part of the clinician and the client, and skill sets on the part of the therapist that help clients to achieve these goals (Allen, 2013; Shear et al., 2021).

It is probably obvious from our earlier discussions that in our own work, we emphasize customization of the therapy to the needs of the client, both on a moment-to-moment basis in a given session, and over the whole course of the therapy. We believe that attachment theory offers one highly useful framework for doing that. And we have also argued that the foundation of attachment informed grief therapy is the therapeutic relationship itself, again based in our understanding of attachment dynamics. *In a sense, the cultivation of a safe haven and secure base through the medium of the therapist-client bond is the core "technique" of attachment informed grief therapy.* It is the medium of empathically attuned conversation that allows the development of this bond. And above all, it is to this factor that we encourage grief therapists of all therapeutic orientations to pay attention.

As an example of technique that is embedded in the context of the therapeutic conversation, recall that we earlier discussed the concept of "mentalized affectivity" (Jurist & Meehan, 2009) – the idea that gaining insight into emotions can be tremendously helpful to clients. This is particularly true in therapy with bereaved clients, many of whom must cope with feelings that are unfamiliar and more intense than any they have experienced in the past. The following case summary is from the practice of the second author.

Stewart

Stewart was stunned by the car skidding accident that took his wife from him on a snowy winter evening. Her death initially left Stewart disoriented and in shock. The intensity of his conflicting and powerful emotions was frighteningly unfamiliar to him. Moreover, as the initial shock wore off, he found himself starting to feel worse, as waves of grief began to alternate with surges of anxiety, so Stewart sought grief counseling. After some initial assessment, the clinician decided that his client needed help just understanding what was happening to him. Stewart's only other experience of loss had been the death of his best friend in high school in a reckless boating accident. By asking Stewart to reflect on what he was noticing in his emotions and in his bodily reactions, and by offering psychoeducation about normal grief and trauma responses, the therapist was able to help Stewart identify, label, and begin to gain a sense of control over his responses. He also taught Stewart some specific breathing exercises that helped him to stay calmer when the anxiety overtook him.

Later on in the treatment, Stewart and his therapist had an important, breakthrough session. Noticing that Stewart often looked tense and flushed when he spoke about the circumstances of his wife's death, the therapist asked Stewart whether some of what he might be feeling could be anger. Stewart initially rejected this idea, saying that he knew that his wife's death was "not anyone's fault." The therapist persisted however, noting that grief can sometimes bring up thoughts and emotions that seem irrational, until they are understood from a different perspective. He asked Stewart if he had ever had anything stolen from him, and Stewart recalled having a prized baseball glove stolen as a teenager. When asked how he felt, Stewart immediately said "angry – really furious." The therapist then noted that the Latin root of the word bereavement actually meant to be robbed of something – and a look of recognition immediately came over Stewart's face. He realized that while it may not have been anyone's fault that his wife died, it was still understandable that he might feel quite angry about having his wife "stolen" away from him. Further, when asked if he could recall ever feeling that way before, Stewart quickly remembered that he was also very angry when his best friend had died. He realized that he had felt furious with the friend for the reckless behavior that had needlessly cost him his life. With this discovery of what the loss of his wife, and his friend, had meant to him emotionally, Stewart began to notice a lighter, calmer feeling in his emotions. This also showed itself in his posture and facial expressions – like a heavy burden was beginning to lift from his shoulders.

By carefully using the security of the therapeutic bond, along with some well-timed questions and observations over the course of their conversation, the clinician was able to help his client reflect on (i.e., mentalize about) his own emotional reactions and gain a different perspective on his mourning experience. This process helped Stewart to make sense of his bereavement and to move towards a more reflective and eventually re-regulated and integrated stance towards his loss.

Writing Techniques

There are a number of specific writing or journaling techniques that directly ask the client to reflect on the meaning of a loss, or a particular aspect of a loss (Graybeal etal., 2002; Lichtenthal & Neimeyer, 2012; Neimeyer, 2012b; Neimeyer et al., 2008; Pennebaker et al., 2007). Writing seems to offer a number of possible benefits for the bereaved, ranging from emotional catharsis to an enhancement of perspective about the loss. Writing may also enhance the work of transforming the relationship with the deceased into an internalized continuing bond. These writing activities can range from simply asking the client to keep a journal about their thoughts and feelings to more directed writing exercises such as writing letters to the deceased, writing letters from the deceased to oneself, and letters from one part of the self to another part (Lichtenthal & Neimeyer, 2012).In his work with Nancy, a bereaved mother, the second author made effective use of writing techniques

Nancy

Nancy felt great guilt over the suicide death of her daughter. She believed that had she been more vigilant about her daughter's eating disorder and depression, she could have prevented the suicide. But another part of Nancy's mind knew that this was an unfair verdict about her functioning as a parent and her vigorous efforts to find help for her daughter. Nancy was asked to write out a dialogue between these two parts of herself, and then to read this out loud. In doing this exercise, Nancy began to see that there was some merit in what both of the voices had to say, and that they both came out of the same deep well sorrow at the loss of her daughter. Engaging in this activity seemed to help Nancy gain more perspective about her inner conflict, and well as to feel more kindheartedness towards herself.

In a sense, this technique helped Nancy to become more of a wise and compassionate attachment figure for herself. In addition to being emotionally cathartic, such writing facilitated the process of meaning-making about her loss and to gain insight into some of the distress that had been engendered by the loss – the strong feelings of failure and guilt that she felt, which were in conflict with her more reasonable sense that she had done all that she could to help her daughter.

Visualization and Enactment Techniques

This third category of technique involves asking the client to be more mentally and sometimes physically active with their grief by engaging in a specific kind of activity. Visualization, sometimes also called guided imagery (Brown, 1990; Creagh, 2005; Jordan, 2012), asks the client to summon mental images so that they can be confronted and mastered, or so that they can provide a different vision of the dying process or of the deceased loved one now.

One common use for these techniques is in the case of traumatic bereavement. When a death is sudden, unexpected, and/or violent, it is common for mourners to experience not only grief, but trauma (Litz, 2004; Pearlman et al., 2014). As we discussed in Chapter 6, this can lead to real complications in the mourning process and require attention by the clinician to both the separation distress *and* the traumatic distress of the client. Intrusive memories, re-experiencing of certain sensory aspects of the death, avoidance of stimuli associated with the death that trigger memories and physiological arousal, and amnesias regarding the event itself are all signs that the individual has likely been traumatized by the death. Since trauma intensifies emotional arousal while at the same time reducing the person's ability to engage in higher order processing, i.e., meaning making, this aspect of grief may need to be dealt with early in the treatment process. Nonetheless, we caution clinicians about prematurely encouraging clients to confront and re-live the horrifying or terrifying aspects of the death scene until a trusting therapeutic alliance has been established. The clinician and client must agree that going further into the death-related memories will be helpful (Allen, 2013). Note that this does *not* mean that the client has be free from any trepidation about confronting the traumatic components of their grief – usually, traumatized clients will be fearful of anything that asks them to "go back there." But the client must feel secure with the therapist and believe that doing the trauma work will be helpful to their recovery before it can safely begin. Lastly, it is important to recognize that although eyewitnesses are probably more likely to develop PTSD type symptomatology, a person does *not* need to have been a direct eyewitness to the death of their loved one to be traumatized by it – they simply must have developed a mental picture of the event.

Neimeyer (2019) describes his work with a bereaved father struggling to cope with his daughter's accidental death by drowning. Fearful that he will not be able to bear the pain of imagining her last moments, the father nevertheless believes that drawing closer to what he imagines was his daughter experienced is the only way he can hope to "integrate what happened to Sofie into my life." Client and therapist construct a metaphor that acknowledges the father's sense of danger while emphasizing the safety provided by the therapist's continuous, engaged presence. Imagining themselves as two technical climbers, they "explore the extremes" of the environment in a slow and steady manner, with Neimeyer taking responsibility for tracking the client's progress and making sure that he feels "securely anchored by ropes to solid ground." At the conclusion of the session Neimeyer acknowledges that he felt he had been "taken along" on the client's journey and had experienced "some of the same tension" as the grieving father. With emotion resonant with Neimeyer's own, the client responds: "Thank you for that. Thank you for coming along."

Restorative Retelling: Reworking the Death Narrative

A related category of techniques involves retelling and reworking the death narrative in a way that can also help with trauma reduction and the building of a continuing bond with the deceased. Rynearson, in particular, has done pioneering work in which bereaved clients not only retell the story of the death, but then rework the narrative in a fashion that makes it more bearable and less traumatizing (Rynearson, 2001, 2006; Rynearson & Salloum, 2011). After first learning self-soothing procedures, the mourner re-exposes themselves to the death scene and narrative, and/or changes that narrative in a fashion that "pacifies" the imagery, calms the physiological hyperarousal associated with their trauma response, and allows the emergence of a transformed continuing bond with the deceased and a revised perspective about the loss.

This is illustrated in work of Harriet, a client seen by the second author (Chapter 6).

Harriet

Harriet was deeply bereaved after the death of her young adult son in a hiking accident. Her son had been hiking with friends in the desert canyons of the American southwest and became separated from his companions at one point in the trip. It appeared that he fell and broke a leg, and was for a time at least, knocked unconscious by the fall. The body was not discovered until almost 72 hours later, where it was found at the bottom of a small ravine. Since the death, Harriet had been haunted by the fear that her son had died a protracted and painful death – alone, in great physical and psychological pain, and calling out for his mother. After exploring this image of the death, the therapist introduced the idea of being able to rework the imagery in a way that might make it more bearable. Harriet agreed to try this. After a brief relaxation procedure, Harriet was asked to imagine her son dying in the worst possible way – a painful, slow, frightening, and terribly isolated passage. This was, understandably, upsetting for her to do. Then, however, she was invited to reimagine the death under circumstances that would have been more tolerable for her. Harriet chose to imagine her son having access to pain medication, warm blankets, and water to drink. She also imagined her and her son's spirits meeting before he died. This allowed them to do a tender leave-taking before he fell unconscious again and died peacefully and quickly. Harriet reported significant comfort from this "version" of her son's passing, and has subsequently been able to "switch the channel" to this scene when troubling thoughts of his passing return, which they have tended to do with much less frequency since completing this exercise.

In imagining the details of an alternative ending to her son's life, Harriet was able to gain some sense of control over and some relief from the intrusive images of his death. What she envisioned was a scenario in which she was able to continue to be her son's caregiver and to express her love for him one last time. It also allowed her to move beyond the specific details of his dying, and on to greater reflection about his life, and the love that they felt in their relationship with one another.

Other forms of visualization and enactment techniques that promote meaning-making, particularly after traumatic loss, are worth consideration (see Pearlman, et al., 2014 for a rich compendium of such techniques). Almost all of the writing activities discussed previously can equally well be imagined in the mind's eye of the mourner and/or enacted, rather than written out. Thus, empty chair techniques, where the mourner speaks to an empty chair that represents the deceased, or some other person or aspect of their own self, are familiar techniques for many grief therapists (Neimeyer, 2012a). The case vignette of Nancy (above), for example, could have also been done as a guided imagery application, or an empty chair enactment in which Nancy had a conversation with her daughter, rather than parts of herself. The common element of all of these modalities is symbolic conversation with someone: the dead, a part of the self, or another living person. When done in the context of addressing the deceased, they can help greatly with repairing and consolidating an internal sense of connection to the deceased, i.e., a continuing bond.

ADJUNCTIVE TECHNIQUES: COGNITIVE BEHAVIORAL THERAPY (CBT) AND EYE MOVEMENT DESENSITIZATION AND REPROCESSING (EMDR)

Cognitive Behavioral Therapy has long been a treatment of choice for addressing maladaptive cognitions. In grief, cognitions concerning the loss, the manner of death or the relationship with the deceased can interfere with adaptation to loss (Kosminsky, 2017; Malkinson, 2007).

The most straightforward approach to differentiating between helpful and non-helpful cognitions is to ask: "Does this way of thinking (about the death, or your life now and in the future) make you feel better or worse?"

> A widow in her late sixties whose husband accidentally choked to death, and who found his body several hours later, declares that her life is over. She has withdrawn from friends and from her children and grandchildren. She blames herself for not being present when her husband died and continually revisits the memory of finding him and trying to revive him. Recalling all the times that she "could have made him happy but didn't", she is overwhelmed with regret for not having been a more loving and attentive spouse.
>
> (Kosminsky, 2017, p. 8)

The client in this case was trapped by a combination of memories related to the traumatic death nature of the death, and persistent rumination about her failure as a wife and what this perceived failure says about her as a person. Treatment involved a combination of CBT and EMDR, a technique developed by Shapiro (2012) that affords the client the opportunity to confront and become desensitized to a disturbing traumatic scene (Kosminsky & McDevitt, 2012; Shapiro, 2012; Solomon, 2019). EMDR begins by teaching people self-soothing activities to help down-regulate the arousal of mind and body. These also provide a tool which the client can use when away from the therapist to self-regulate their autonomic arousal when triggering events happen. After learning and practicing these self-soothing techniques in session, the client then deliberately attempts to recall the traumatic material, while simultaneously receiving bi-lateral stimulation from the therapist. This technique involves rhythmic and alternating sensory stimulation of the left and right hemispheres of the brain. In the original EMDR protocol, this was accomplished by having the client follow the therapist's fingers moving back and forth across their visual field. The range of techniques for producing bilateral stimulation has since been expanded to include devices that provide auditory or tactile bilateral stimulation instead. This process seems to amplify and "reprocess" the traumatic memories, allowing the client full access to the memories while also increasing their experience of catharsis and mastery over the disturbing (and often dissociated) recollections. Finally, time is spent integrating the experience by discussing and cognitively restructuring the self-perceptions that have been distorted by the trauma (e.g., it was entirely my fault; I am a failure or a bad person because my loved one died, etc.). This last segment of EMDR affords the client an opportunity for reflection and integrative meaning-making about the traumatic death.

Psychologist Roger Solomon has taken a leading role in demonstrating how EMDR can be used to address complications in traumatic and non-traumatic experiences of loss (Solomon, 2007; Solomon & Hensley, 2020). Solomon's approach is grounded in attachment theory, and proceeds from the assumption that obstacles to healing from loss are often linked to early attachment experience. In working with grieving clients Solomon explores the client's relationship with the deceased and facilitates the development of a new relationship, while addressing cognitions ("I should have done more; I should have saved him" that block healing.

A study by Cotter, Meysner and Lee (20 17) was designed to assess the treatment effects of EMDR and CBT in grief therapy. Nineteen participants received seven weekly therapy sessions and were interviewed two weeks after completing therapy. Based on a thematic analysis of these interviews, the authors found commonalities, and differences in treatment effects. Both groups reported a positive shift in emotions, increased activity, improved self-confidence and a healthier mental relationship to the deceased. Consistent with the divergent goals of EMDR and CBT, the authors report that participants receiving CBT described the acquisition of emotion regulation skills and "a shift from being in an ongoing state of grief to feeling that they were at a new stage in their lives." Participants who received EMDR reported that "distressing memories were less clear and felt more distant" following treatment.

Also along the lines of visualization techniques that may help with both trauma reduction and development of continuing bonds with the deceased, the second author of this book has–developed a technique called "In Heaven" (Jordan, 2012). In this technique, the client is led through a guided imagery in which they imagine their loved one as being in heaven, or a paradise like place. The client is told that they do not need to believe in an afterlife to do the activity, since its goal is not to affirm a belief in heaven, but rather to help the mourner feel better and to cultivate an alternative image of the deceased that differs from the actual death scene. The mourner is invited to view their loved one as in heaven or paradise as they imagine it to be, completely healed, both physically and psychologically. The technique can also be extended to include an imagined dialogue with the deceased about unfinished business and a transformation of the continuing bond with the loved one, as seen in the second author's work with Sarah.

Sarah

Sarah was devastated by the suicide of her son. She found his lifeless body hanging in the basement of their house. She was haunted by the remembered shock and horror of first discovering his body, and the attempt to cut him down, summon help, and futilely try to revive him. Three years later, the imagery still intruded on her consciousness, unbidden and alien. In an effort to provide some relief from the PTSD symptoms, two procedures were used by the therapist. The first was to do a single session of EMDR, which was quite powerful in producing a strong abreaction of tears and physical shaking as Sarah deliberately summoned the mental pictures that she had of the morning she discovered her son's body. However, she also reported a feeling of relief at the end of the procedure. Three sessions later, the "In Heaven" technique was also employed to strengthen the trauma reduction work. Sarah wrestled a great deal with the question of whether she should allow herself to believe in a "heaven" or an afterlife for her son. She agreed to try the technique, however, when it was explained that the goal of the activity was to help calm her agitated physical and emotional state with regard to the details of her son's death, and to give her an alternative picture that she could "switch to" when the bad memories returned. After doing a relaxation exercise, Sarah was guided to imagine her son as now being in heaven, whatever that meant to her. She proceeded to picture her son sitting in a dining room with his deceased grandparents, having a meal together and enjoying the classical music that was a favorite of them all. Sarah reported that this experience helped her to "maybe allow myself to believe that he is still alive, and that he is not lonely. I have worried that he somehow was lonely." The therapist affirmed that mothers are "wired" to continue to worry about the well-being of their children, even after they have died. Sarah has subsequently used this experience to slowly cultivate an internal connection with her son, finding herself comfortably talking with him, both in times of stress, and just as a way of feeling closer to him when she is missing him more intensely.

The combination of the EMDR and In Heaven exercises allowed Sarah to develop more soothing images of her son, while leaving her mostly free of intrusions of the distressing memories. She also reported feeling that her son is "with me now, everywhere," even though she remains unsure whether she actually believes in an afterlife. This shift from the traumatic details of the death has freed Sarah to reflect more on the experience of facing a life without her son, her beliefs about an after-life, and even to re-evaluating other aspects of her life unrelated to the death. She has adapted to significant changes in her marriage and work relationships, and has begun exploring new interests and ways of relating to people in her life. The evolution of the focus in her grief reflects Sarah's movement from a reactive to a more reflective and ultimately reintegrated stance, as well as an on-going shift from a loss to a Restoration Orientation and a re-awakening of her exploratory behavioral system.

MEANING-MAKING AS A LIFELONG PROCESS

Grieving is a developmental process in the sense that the significance of a loss unfolds over time. In the beginning, it is impossible to know everything that a loss will mean. Rather, the implications of living one's life without an important person reveal themselves to us only as we go through our life, continuing on without that individual. The process of making sense of a loss, and reflecting on the emerging meanings of living a life without the loved one, is actually a lifelong process that is at the very heart of meaning-reconstruction in mourning.

Jack

The Father of the second author (JRJ) died in 1974, while the author was a graduate student in psychology. His father had been a public-school teacher and then a school administrator for all of his professional life. At the time of his father's death, the author was not married, nor was he a parent. But in 1998, as the author was about to attend the graduation of his first-born child from high school and then send her off to college, he found himself experiencing a wave of missing his father – at this point in his life, a relatively rare occurrence. Reflecting on the significance of this unanticipated upsurge of grief, it occurred to him that "My Dad should be here for this – he would have loved this." He realized that this was an aspect of living his life without his father that he could not possibly have understood at the time of his father's death. He recognized that the meaning of his loss was still unfolding, even 25 years after his father's death.

Jordan's observation is echoed in Kathryn Schulz's memoir of her father's death (2022). Years have passed, and at times she feels that she is "over" her grief. But then, it comes around again, and she decides that the "periodicity of grief is too unreliable and the overall condition too chameleon-like to track with any certainty" (p. 74.). And maybe that's how it has to be. Memories of her father will always persist, and with them, her sense of loss. Reminders of her father's absence are everywhere: in photographs and books, in her own face and her words; and in things like his favorite chair.

> Collectively, all of them serve to make the world a little less incomplete than it would otherwise be. They are still here, unlike him, and I assume they always will be, as enduring as the love that made them.
>
> (p. 75)

We don't "recover" from loss; we accommodate it as best we can, in whatever ways we can: by maintaining connection, by finding meaning, by finding ourselves.

Audrey

My mother is steering my ship. Sometimes when I'm down I sit, and think of her, and just let her spirit into the room.

When my mother was alive, I tried, for her, to keep the peace in the family. But I can't do it anymore. And I feel like my mother understands that, and that she's saying to me: 'you have to take care of yourself now. And to do that, you have to let go of the people who weigh you down'.

Marie

People say relationships take work. But so does love. It takes working on yourself – opening yourself up to be able to do it. And it takes courage to need another person – to risk your happiness by needing another person. It was a risk to love that much.

So much of my independence, my community activities was grounded in having David.

It was like something was physically torn off of me when he died. It was like my ectoplasm, or whatever is in there kind of leaked out and now I'm gathering it back in.

That strength – it didn't die with him – the strength he gave me is a part of me now.

SUMMARY

The reconstruction of meaning is an inescapable part of rebuilding a life in the aftermath of significant loss. It is an emotional, as well as an intellectual process, and one that contributes to the bereaved individual's ability to gain a sense of mastery with respect to what can be unbearably painful thoughts and feelings. It is particularly relevant in the case of traumatic death, where the circumstances of the death increase the loss of coherence in the individual's assumptive world.

This process of discovering, and/or creating, layers of meaning in the loss is one that is greatly facilitated by the support of an attachment figure – an attuned and skilled "expert companion" who serves as a confidant, a guide, and an audience to bear witness to the journey of healing (Tedeschi & Calhoun, 2003). It is the complement of emotional reregulation in bereavement recovery and is a central focus of the process of attachment informed grief therapy. As we help individuals to reflect on and integrate their loss, we help them to put the loss in the wider perspective of their larger life narrative. The death of their loved one becomes an important part of their life story, but only a part – not, as it may have seemed when their loss occurred, the whole story. This enhanced capacity to make sense of the loss is central to the transition from the reactive stance towards the loss that comes at the beginning of the mourning process, to the reflective, and then eventually to the reregulated and reintegrated place where we hope our clients will be able to arrive with the help of grief therapy.

Every significant loss interrupts the flow of our lives. But as long as we are still here, we have a chance to find meaning in life, not only in what brings us joy, but also in what brings us sorrow. And sometimes, even in the midst of our sorrow, we can have moments of joy.

Marie

M: I've been feeling so weak lately. But then yesterday I was out hiking and I felt strong. Crossing flowing water on rocks. And I don't use a hiking stick, I just walk on the rocks. And I got to the water, and I thought, I can do this. I thought – if you fall in the water, so what.

PK: That's a wow. It gives me great pleasure to imagine you scrambling up and down the rocks

11

CONCLUSIONS

Our goal in writing this book, as in the previous edition, has been to bring together attachment theory, relevant neuroscience research, and contemporary models of bereavement in order to better understand how people respond to loss, how they heal, and how we can promote healing when the process has been disrupted. In this chapter we reflect on progress within, and among, these domains and consider avenues for future work. We also take the opportunity to comment on the implications of recent changes in the diagnosis and treatment of problematic grief.

AN ATTACHMENT PERSPECTIVE ON ADAPTATION TO LOSS

Attachment theorists, starting with Bowlby, Ainsworth, and Main, proposed that attachment behaviors are rooted in the biological dependency on caretakers in a child's infancy and early childhood, and reflect the child's best efforts to ensure that the attachment figure will remain available to them so as to ensure their survival. As children grow into adulthood, they continue to engage with people largely on the basis of assumptions and models developed in relation to these early attachment figures. These ways of relating carry over into the way people react when someone to whom they are deeply attached or bonded is taken from them

DOI: 10.4324/9781003204183-15

by death. In other words, an individual's attachment style will be a major determinant of how they grieve losses in their life, and those variations in attachment style help to account for variations in the human grief response. Those who experienced secure attachment in their early relationships, while no less saddened by a current loss, will be less likely to evoke earlier separations from and ruptures with attachment figures in their development. For the most part, "grief will just be grief", and in time, they will usually heal from the psychological wound of separation and loss. In contrast, those with an insecure attachment history and orientation may well have a more problematic adjustment to loss, and those problems may intensify over time. The types of issues they are likely to face will differ depending on the type of insecure attachment at the root of their suffering – avoidant, anxious, or disorganized.

In defense of the value of theory, Lewin (1951) asserted that there is "nothing as practical as a good theory". As we have done our best to demonstrate, attachment theory is, by this measure, a very good theory indeed. Attachment theory has practical value in that it helps to account for differences in early childhood development, particularly the development of affective regulatory capacity and the shaping of internal working models of relationship. It has value as a lens through which to view the trajectory of a person's life: what they've chosen, what they've feared, what and whom they've loved, and what kind of life problems have been particularly difficult for them It is practical in that it serves as a guide to the development of treatment approaches tailored to the individual, rather than to a formal diagnosis. As such it is practical as a tool for the refinement of support for people who grieve, and for anyone faced with change, loss, and other challenges that threaten to overwhelm their ability to carry on with life.

The basic outlines of attachment theory proposed by Bowlby have not been substantially altered over decades of research into attachment, though it has been significantly refined and expanded upon. Echoes of a child's earliest interactions with significant others persist throughout life. Security – the sense that one can explore the world around one safe in the knowledge that help will be available if needed – is a gift that keeps on giving. Much of the recent work reported in these pages substantiates this view and expands our understanding of early attachment experience as a persistent and pervasive influence on emotional and physical well-being. Attachment security has been linked to a catalog of neurological, psychological and social advantages, and insecure attachment, to disadvantages in each of these areas. The genesis and manifestation of problems associated with disorganized attachment have been demonstrated by neurological studies and researchers in the social and developmental branches of psychological inquiry (Beeney et al., 2017; Beauchaine & Cicchetti, 2019; Sekowski & Prigerson, 2022).

What does this new knowledge mean for the practice of grief therapy? What have we learned and what can practitioners do with this new knowledge?

EMOTION REGULATION

This is an area of research that has had a high yield in terms of useful findings. Emotion regulation has been identified as an essential building block of mental health. Difficulties in emotion regulation may go unnoticed or unattended to through much of a person's life, with many people making accommodations to these difficulties through avoidance of emotionally impactful relationships and experiences. Such strategies often prove inadequate in the face of significant loss. Problems with emotion regulation contribute to difficulty in coping with uncertainty, so frequently an aspect of grief. Uncertainty, in turn, limits behavioral flexibility and the oscillation that is associated with uncomplicated grief.

These findings give new weight to the importance of recognizing and addressing difficulties in emotion regulation, over and above those that are a part of the normal, expected response to significant loss, and in full recognition that "normal" is not a universal standard as applied to grief. In directing attention to emotion regulation we are in effect taking a strength-based approach to bereavement support: we assume that the client has the potential to develop strengths and skills that will ease the course of their grief. Sharing this perspective with the client, we offer hope: not the false hope that grief will vanish all on its own by simply waiting long enough for it to pass, but the hope, based on our experience and our faith in them – that with sufficient effort on their part, and skilled support on our part, they can grow stronger, learn to soothe themselves, and have moments of peace. We present them with the prospect of a time when they will not feel perpetually overwhelmed and progressively more bereft. Whether or not they believe it (and they probably won't initially), we ask them to regard it as a possibility. We ask them to suspend disbelief. Explicitly or implicitly, we ask them to trust us, and to trust that, having worked with many, many bereaved people, we are comfortable offering this kind of hope. In fact, many clients have told us, that planting these "seeds of hope" has over time turned out to be an exceedingly important component of their healing process.

TRUST

We are continually asking our grieving clients to take in what we say – to *consider it* – even if it goes against what they think, what they have always thought, and what they expect. *Trust is both the prerequisite for, and the product of, a secure therapeutic relationship. Without such a bond, therapy, and grief therapy in particular, is likely to be ineffective or even counterproductive.*

Studies of clinical effectiveness consistently demonstrate that the largest contributor to outcome variance involves therapist differences and the emergent therapeutic relationship Yet as Norcross and Wampold have reported, treatment guidelines have paid little or no attention to these factors. The net result, as in APA clinical practice guidelines released in 2019, is that what is offered is "empirically dubious, clinically suspect, and marginally useful …

> … Efforts to promulgate guidelines without including the relationship and responsiveness are seriously incomplete and potentially misleading.
>
> (Norcross & Wampold, 2018, p. 391)

Among those who have sought to address this deficit in how we think about clinical practice, Jon Allen has been a consistent voice of reason and practicality. Recall that Allen has questioned the value of the what he sees as an alphabet soup of therapies and is a proponent of what he has dubbed "plain old therapy," i.e., therapy that privileges the therapeutic relationship and identifies the interactions that take place between client and clinician as the most important factor in effecting change in psychotherapy, a finding supported by clinical research. Allen concludes that if we want to improve clinical results, we need to "shift the balance of our efforts from developing therapies to developing therapists" (Allen, 2021, p. xxvii).

> Therapists should take heed: For distrusting patients who struggle with serious problems in close relationships, developing a strong alliance will be challenging.
>
> (Allen, 2021, p. 10)

This position is very much in line with our view of needed modifications of training. Our special interest is in the training of grief therapists and our particular concern is that training paradigms (with some notable exceptions) continue to emphasize education about techniques and models and to exclude, or pay little attention to, education about the importance of trust, the challenges to building trust, and the need to sensitively address these challenges. We further endorse Allen's recommendation that more research be conducted to expand our understanding of individual differences in the ability to trust and "elucidating the quality of the caregiving relationship that shapes the development and employment of this trusting capacity" (p. 69). Recent advances in attachment-informed psychotherapy research have addressed these questions and offered some practical guidance for psychotherapist training (Talia et al., 2019).

Trust is also the subject of ongoing work by Fonagy and colleagues. Our discussion of this group's work illustrated the evolution of the concept of "epistemic trust," in effect, a biopsychosocial ripple effect that begins with the development of a trusting relationship between client and therapist. The trust cultivated in this relationship can gradually provide a corrective to negative models of relationships that have limited the client's interest in and ability to sustain healthy relationships with others. The concept of "epistemic trust" is meant to suggest that the client's trust in the therapist can be a conduit to engagement with the wider world of interpersonal relationships. We suggest that such engagement, or re-engagement, is necessary if a grieving person is to be able to live in a way that is not only about acknowledging what has been lost, but recognizing what can be built with that which remains.

NEUROSCIENCE AND ATTACHMENT

Research findings on brain development in the first two years of life are yet another lens through which to view the connection between attachment security and adaptation to loss.

Secure attachment supports the development of emotion regulatory capacities in the brain. The stress of insecure attachment, and the more profound impact of ongoing neglect or abuse, adversely affects the development of these capacities. Indeed, attachment figures throughout our lives serve a homeostatic and regulatory function for our psychological and physiological stability. Conversely, the loss of people to whom we are attached, and the absence of such figures in times of great stress in our life, can be understood as a profoundly dysregulating experience. In this sense, grief therapy, as we have described it, is a process that helps people to integrate the loss and reregulate themselves on a physiological, emotional, and cognitive level. Chapter 3 of this volume has been updated to include a review of research made possible by advances in technology that give us a clearer picture of the development, organization and functioning of the brain. Studies that suggest the manner in which humans communicate "brain to brain" with one another are of particular interest to us as clinicians.

Neuroscience research has also contributed to our understanding of brain development in infancy as a dyadic process involving the caregiver and child, with each party being influenced by the internal state of the other. Maternal stress has received particular attention as a factor in compromised neural development. Studies of maternal stress, in turn, have linked it to a constellation of environmental factors in *the mother's own early life*, foremost among them being poverty and all of its associated deficiencies and uncertainties. Poverty is thus an intergenerational factor in the stress affecting the developing brain (Kim, 2020). Reducing stress exposure and providing support to caregivers can strengthen their ability to cope with stress, regulate their own moods, build more positive, security enhancing relationships with their own infants and children. These findings are important for work with bereaved clients who are the parents of young children. These parents, we suggest, may benefit from a treatment approach that addresses the stresses of caregiving and strengthens their ability to confidently parent their child, an end result that is of benefit to both.

THE THERAPIST AS A TRANSITIONAL ATTACHMENT FIGURE

Bowlby was the first to draw attention to the parallels between the activation of the attachment system in childhood and the grief response of adults in the wake of the death of a loved one. This book is part of what has become a cross disciplinary, decades-long project to explore the implications of Bowlby's profound insight (Duschinsky, 2020). We have looked at the concept of grief as the loss of an attachment figure (or its reciprocal, the loss of a care-seeking figure, in the case of the death of a dependent child). In many cases, the death of a loved one takes away the very person to whom the mourner would have turned for help in surviving and making sense of a traumatic experience. It is a logical extension of Bowlby's premise that in order for a loss to be integrated and for re-regulation of the attachment system to occur, bereavement requires the support of other individuals who can serve as attachment figures, be they family member, friend, or a professional (e.g., a clergy person or a good therapist). This is why we have emphasized the crucial role of the therapist as a *transitional attachment figure* who is empathically attuned to the psychological needs, and limitations, of the mourner.

The therapist must carefully titrate the bereaved person's exposure to painful reality, and gradually help to increase the mourner's ability to tolerate painful emotions, thoughts, and memories – a process guided by the therapist in light of the client's attachment orientation and evolving capacities for emotion regulation. In this way, it becomes possible for a person to learn and grow through the experience of therapy. In the course of this kind of therapeutic work, the client's comfort zone and tolerance for separation experience gradually expands, and with it the potential for further psychological growth. The therapeutic bond thus becomes another way of activating the "broaden and build" cycle of growth that occurs when a person is embedded in a protective and nurturing attachment relationship (Mikulincer & Shaver, 2020).

PROMOTING INTEGRATION IN GRIEF THERAPY

Human beings and their emotions are infinitely variable, complex and resistant to deconstruction and classification. Despite the impossibility of getting to the core of who we are, we are compelled to dig, to prospect for elements of our identity. We are driven by a need - be it passing or unrelenting – to *make sense of ourselves.* The difficulty of making sense of ourselves is heightened in periods of loss and change. Yet this is when we most need to be careful about losing hope, of preemptively concluding that maybe the real answer is that we *don't* make sense. This is a feeling familiar to people who have recently lost a loved one: *My life made sense before, but now it doesn't. I understood who I was before, but not who am I now. Even thinking about who I am now is exhausting.* When a griever describes their sadness, their fear, their anger as "overwhelming," what does that mean? What is it that is being overwhelmed? For each individual, of course, there will be unique answers to this question. But generally speaking, on balance, what is overwhelmed *is* balance – psychological balance. By this, we mean the feeling that one is more or less in an upright position and is not in immediate danger of collapse. The restoration of balance comes up as a recurring theme in discussions of the goals of psychotherapy, and grief therapy in particular.

Losing a loved one is painful, and confronting that pain is something that people do not readily or easily accept. But to avoid the pain, a mourner also needs to avoid the truth. The result can be a kind of emotional purgatory, in which the mourner is suspended between the poles of pain and healing, between grief and reengagement in life. As clinicians, we do not like causing people pain – quite the opposite; we want to help alleviate their suffering. But to help them move toward integration, it is often necessary to bring people face to face with what is painful and frightening – the reality of their loved one's death. Many times, although people know the fact of their loved one's death, they are keeping themselves from confronting the reality of their loved one's death, and all that implies for their life going forward. As a result of this self-protective work by the client, we need to say things that direct their attention to what they want to avoid. *We can say these things, and people can hear them, but only if they feel safe with us.* This is what Porges (2011) tells us is the beauty of the evolved nervous system, i.e., we can decide that someone is safe, and we can decide to listen to them and be comforted by them. The feeling of safety is what makes relationships possible. and that includes the therapeutic relationship. And because fear is so often a part of grief, clinicians who work with the bereaved need to be particularly attuned to verbal and non-verbal expressions of anxiety and trepidation, as well as anger, helplessness, and despair. Directing attention to the body may help both the therapist and the client to better understand their emotional state, and therefore to facilitate movement towards the integration of experience.

The need for therapists to pay attention to these cues, while increasingly emphasized in the literature on psychotherapy (Danqueth & Berry, 2014; Holmes, 2013, 2022; Wallin, 2007) has been an underdeveloped idea in the literature on grief therapy. It is a part of psychotherapy that calls upon clinicians to use their whole brains in order to engage the whole brains of clients, paying attention to and stimulating the emotional brain as well as the thinking brain. Siegel has said that it is emotional experience that changes us. Emotions that engage mind and body have the power to trigger a higher level of awareness. This expanded vantage point enables us to see something new, or to see something old in a new way. While we might understand what Siegel is describing as moments of insight, we believe that this is more than insight, because it is more than an intellectual awareness. It is a change in the whole of our person, and it is what we experience when the physical synapses in our brain have changed to adapt to a new reality. Something inside has shifted and we are different than we were before.

Audrey

I know that I've changed. My father abused me, and I've abused myself. This is an eternal game I've been playing with myself. I could cry. But I'm not going to.

I've reached a new plateau, and I don't want to go back. I'm not going to fight with anybody anymore about who I am as a human being. Last week, you said something to me that was hard for me to hear, and I said: I'm tired of this. And I know you thought I was tired of therapy, tired of hearing things I don't want to hear. But I trust you, and I know why you said what you did. And during the week what I've realized I was saying was: I'm tired of myself. I've been fighting for people to see who I really am. Don't you see who I really am? I'm not doing that anymore. I can live with myself now. What I want now is to fill my soul. I want to fill my soul with love and light and happiness, with graciousness and kindness.

REFLECTING ON THE MEANING OF A NEW DIAGNOSIS FOR GRIEF

With this headline *The New York Times* announced that a professional consensus had been reached regarding the parameters of "normal" grief:

How long should it take to grieve? Psychiatry has come up with an answer.
(*The New York Times*, 3/18/22)

The formulation of a description of grief that exceeds these parameters, designated Prolonged Grief Disorder, the article explained, would be included in a revision of the 5th Diagnostic and Statistical Manual (DSM V-R). Comments on this article from readers – over 1500 of them within 24 hours – made it clear that a lot of people were not on board with the position taken by the American Psychiatric Association Task Force regarding the nature of "abnormal" grief. So, is prolonged grief disorder just one more "disease" dreamed up by psychiatrists, or it is a breakthrough in the proper diagnosis and treatment of problematic grief?

Questions concerning the definition of normal vs. problematic grief, how to differentiate problematic grief from depression, and whether sufficient evidence exits to justify the introduction of a diagnosis for complicated grief have been the subject of sustained (some might say "prolonged") inquiry and debate in the field. Over the 13 years spent compiling the original version of DSM V, the APA Task Force could not reach agreement on diagnostic criteria for problematic grief, and the matter was placed in an appendix for further study. Not until the 2021 revision of DSM V was this resolved, and prolonged grief disorder made part of the diagnostic canon.

Now that problematic grief has been identified as a psychiatric disorder, treatments for this disorder, which have been preparing to take center stage over the past ten years, are ready for their close up. The most prominent among the proposed treatments involve multiple components and are designed to address obstacles that have been found to interfere with adaptation to loss (Shear & Bloom, 2017; Iglewicz et al., 2020). Put another way, these approaches start from the position of "what does the client *have?*" where the answer is, "they have prolonged grief disorder."

But what happens when we shift our inquiry from "What does the client *have"* (essentially a question about the patient's formal diagnosis) to "what do they *need?*" (a question about what kind of help or treatment does the patient need?). Here our primary source of data is the person sitting opposite us and treatment unfolds according to the trajectory of their bereavement.

Let's be clear before we go on that we are not anti-diagnosis, and we certainly endorse the APA's recognition that there are forms of grief that, without professional intervention, may leave the griever at risk of long-term distress and reduced capacity to live a healthy life. But we cannot view this change as unambiguously positive. Something has been gained, but something has been lost.

Some of our concerns have to do with terminology. We regret the passing of the term "Complicated Grief" from the professional lexicon. It always seemed a useful term, one that captured the difficulties that many grievers face without classifying their difficulties as pathological. The labeling of grief, even *in extremis*, as pathological, is a step that many people in and outside of professional thanatology find unacceptable and even abhorrent. Also problematic, discussion of the new diagnosis seems to be contributing to a dichotomous view of grief: on the one hand, there is normal grief and on the other, there is prolonged grief disorder. This of course is a view that woefully misrepresents the true nature of grief. As clinicians we must continually speak out in response to mischaracterization and oversimplification of grief. In this case, the false dichotomy of "normal grief" vs. "prolonged grief disorder" has the potential to characterize clients' grief as pathological, even when it does not meet PGD criteria. These clients would then, presumably, be candidates for a type of grief therapy that may or may not be suitable for them. The longer-term possibility is that anything short of pathological grief, or "prolonged grief disorder," will come to be viewed as "normal" and distressed clients who could benefit from therapy will not seek, or not be encouraged to seek, the therapeutic help they may need to ease their suffering.

A DIFFERENT APPROACH

Given what we already know about the multiple factors that contribute to the experience of bereavement, it should not be hard to recognize that what we are talking about when we talk about grief is a continuous variable, not a categorical or dichotomous one. Paul Boelen and colleagues have advocated for an approach to bereavement support that does justice to the nuances, variations, and motility of grief (Boelen et al., 2020). The ever growing body of knowledge about grief should help us to distinguish between "uncomplicated, benign grief that does not require mental health care" and grief that presents as unlikely to resolve without such care (Boelen, 2016). The care model Boelen outlines is based a "staging approach" designed to identify and address problems in in grief *as they occur,* and with levels of care to address symptoms of persistent and pervasive distress. Boelen describes the advantages of this approach; among them, we will only mention here that it allows for a *dimensional view of grief.* Grief, unlike death, is not dichotomous: it is not either uncomplicated and normal or disturbed and prolonged.

Norcross and Wampold are also advocates for individualized treatment and for clinical guidelines that reflect what has been demonstrated to be a factor highly related to clinical effectiveness: the therapeutic relationship (Norcross & Wampold, 2018). This knowledge is a cornerstone of an attachment informed approach to grief therapy and we believe it should be a fundamental feature of education for grief therapists, whatever their methodological orientation. In all arenas where discussion of grief and grief therapy take place, we must continue to see to it that, when clinical effectiveness is our goal, we do not leave behind the person of the therapist nor the particular needs of a particular client.

THE FUTURE OF GRIEF THERAPY – WHAT COMES NEXT?

One of our goals in writing this second edition has been to bring attention to the considerable amount of work that has been done to apply findings in the rapidly advancing field of neuroscience to the field of thanatology. There has been a concerted effort to understand the neurobiological mechanisms of separation/grief and chart the course of healing after loss. Researchers are also beginning to explore the specific neurological impact of social connection on facilitating recovery from bereavement. These are, indeed, exciting times in terms of new discoveries in the brain sciences, and we strongly encourage thanatology researchers to include in their theoretical models and empirical studies the universal experience of loss and separation, as well as the neuro-physiological role of attachment relationships (or lack of thereof) in recovery from loss.

Related to this, we believe that more needs to be understood about the relationship between the trauma response, the bereavement response, and attachment. While there are likely differences in the neurobiology of trauma (which is fundamentally a fear/anxiety response) and bereavement (which is basically a response to separation), it is also clear that they have much in common (Currier et al., 2008; O'Connor, 2022). Both trauma and bereavement represent a psychological, and sometimes a physical, threat to human beings. They both can produce considerable distress and can lead to a crisis in meaning-making for the affected individual. Moreover, both trauma and bereavement have similar risk and protective factors, not the least of which is a history (or absence) of secure attachments, and the role of supportive attachment figures in recovery. And, as we noted in Chapter 6, when the death of a loved one evokes both the trauma and the bereavement response, the trajectory of mourning is likely to be made more complicated. We hope to see in the future much more cross-fertilization between the fields of traumatology and thanatology, since so many of the phenomena that are the focus of both disciplines are found together in traumatic bereavement situations.

Further, there remains much to be learned about the role of attachment style in the response to loss, and about our understanding of how a client's attachment style can be used to customize therapy. We have described ways in which we try to customize therapy in our own work, and in support of this approach, we have drawn on the extensive body of literature in attachment theory about attachment styles. Still, a great deal of refinement and testing lies ahead, and we urge others to join in this task.

CLOSING THOUGHTS

Jon Allen concludes his latest treatise, *Trusting in Psychotherapy* with this "parting thought" about the requisite attitude of the therapist:

> I am put off by therapists brimming with enthusiasm and confidence when they lecture about their methods. Have they never felt bewildered, helpless, and inadequate in their work?
>
> (Allen, 2021)

We have no hesitation about where we stand with regard to Allen's query: periodic bewilderment is to be expected in life, in relationships, and in our work. In relating to clients, we do neither the client nor ourselves any good if we present ourselves as knowing more than we do, or possibly can, know. Indeed, we have come to view the ability and willingness to tolerate feelings of uncertainty, doubt, and inadequacy in doing clinical work as a genuine marker of maturing professional growth in mental health professionals, including ourselves.

Healing from loss means different things to different people, and like any healing process, it is only partially subject to the intervention of those who would assist in that process. In our work, and in our own times of grief, we must recognize the need to be comfortable with our discomfort, especially our discomfort with uncertainty, an inescapable part of life and one of which our work serves as a constant and daily reminder.

We return, finally to Rumi, whose characterization of what it is to be human remains, to us, sublime in its accuracy and its consolation.

All day I think about it, then at night I say it.
Where did I come from, and what am I supposed to be doing?
I have no idea.
My soul is from elsewhere, I'm sure of that. And I intend to end up there.
                                                                    (Rumi,1995)

Anyone who, day after day, year after year, has conversations with people about death, is bound to become acutely aware of his or her own mortality. As grief therapists, we know better than most how fleeting and unpredictable life is, and how little control we ultimately have over what happens to us and to the people we love. Is there anyone among us who has not wondered, at the end of a long day filled with dark stories, where we ourselves have come from, and where we are going? Like each of our clients, we are all on an uncertain journey toward an unknown destination.

In the face of this existential truth, we have come to share with many of our colleagues a deep trust in the belief that human connection can help to bring relief from suffering. This is the belief that brought us to this work, and that continues to influence the way we relate to our clients and go about our work as grief therapists. We believe in the healing power of relationships, including the therapeutic relationship. We understand the fundamental, shared elements of human response to loss and that under-standing supports our ability to respond to the suffering of a bereaved person with openness, compassion, and empathy. Only someone who is grieving knows the weight of their grief. But we do not need to experience another person's burden to help them bear it.

To work with people who are grieving is to know both the fragility of human life and the strength of the human spirit. We hope that what we have shared here of our own ideas and work will be of use to those who read this book in their role as grief therapists and healers.

                                        Phyllis Kosminsky and Jack Jordan

References

Aaron, R., Finan, P., Wegener, S., Keefe, F. J., & Lumley, M. (2020). *Emotion regulation as a transdiagnostic factor underlying pain and problematic opioid use*. American Psychological Association.

Agee, J. (1958/2009). *A Death in the Family*. Penguin Classics.

Ainsworth, M. D. S. (1967). *Infancy in Uganda: Infant care and the growth of love*. Johns Hopkins University Press.

Ainsworth, M. D. S., Blehar, M. C., Waters, E., & Wall, S. (1978). *Patterns of attachment: A psychological study of the strange situation*. Erlbaum.

Albertini, D., Lanzilotto, M., Maranesi, M., & Bonini, L. (2021). Largely shared neutral codes for biological and nonbiological observed movements but not for executed actions in monkey premotor areas. *Journal of Neurophysiology*, 126(3), 906–912.

Albom, M. (2002). *Tuesdays with Morrie: An old man, a young man, and life's greatest lesson*. Broadway Books.

Allen, J. G. (2001). *Traumatic relationships and serious mental disorders*. John Wiley & Sons Ltd.

Allen, J. G. (2003). Mentalizing. *Bulletin of the Menninger Clinic*, 67(2: Special Issue), 91–112.

Allen, J. G. (2013). *Restoring Mentalizing in Attachment Relationships: Treating Trauma with Plain Old Therapy*. American Psychiatric Publishing.

Allen, J. (2021). *Trusting in Psychotherapy*. American Psychiatric Publishing.

Allen, J. G., Fonagy, P., & Bateman, A. (2008). *Mentalizing in clinical practice*. American Psychiatric Publishing.

Allumbaugh, D. L., & Hoyt, W. T. (1999). Effectiveness of grief therapy: A meta-analysis. *Journal of Counseling Psychology*, 46(3), 370–380.

Ammaniti, M., & Gallese, V. (2014). *The birth of intersubjectivity: Psychodynamics, neurobiology, and the self*. WW Norton & Company.

Andriessen, K., Mowll, J., Lobb, E., Draper, B., Dudley, M., & Mitchell, P. B. (2018). "Don't bother about me." The grief and mental health of bereaved adolescents. *Death Studies*, 42(10), 607–615.

Aoun, S., Breen, L., White, I., Rumbold, B., & Kellehear, A. (2018). What sources of bereavement support are perceived helpful by bereaved people and why? Empirical evidence for the compassionate communities approach. *Palliative Medicine, 32*(8), 1378–1388.

Archer, J. (1999). *The nature of grief: The evolution and psychology of reactions to loss.* Taylor & Frances/Routledge.

Armour, M. (2006). Meaning making for survivors of violent death. In E. K. Rynearson (Ed.), *Violent death: Resilience and intervention beyond the crisis* (pp. 101–121). Routledge.

Arriaga, X. B., & Kumashiro, M. (2019). Walking a security tightrope: relationship-induced changes in attachment security. *Current Opinion in Psychology, 25*, 121–126.

Arriaga, X. B., Kumashiro, M., Simpson, J., & Overall, C. (2018). Revising working models across time: relationship situations that enhance attachment security. *Personality and Social Psychology Review, 22*(1), 71–96.

Attig, T. (2011). *How we grieve: Relearning the world* (revised ed.). Oxford University Press.

Atzil, S., Gao, W., Fradkin, I., & Barret, L. (2018). Growing a social brain. *Nature Human Behaviour, 2*, 624–636.

Authier, J. (2022). Personal communication from Dr. Authier to P. Kosminsky.

Azevedo, F., Carvalho, L., Grinberg, L., Farfel, J., Ferretti, R., Leite, R., ...Herculano-Houzel, S. (2009). Equal numbers of neuronal and nonneuronal cells make the human brain an isometrically scaled-up primate brain. *Journal of Comparative Neurology, 513*(5), 532–541.

Bakermans-Kranenburg, M. J., & van IJzendoorn, M. H. (2009). The first 10,000 Adult Attachment Interviews: Distributions of adult attachment representations in clinical and non-clinical groups. *Attachment & Human Development, 11*(3), 223–263.

Bakkum, L., Verhage, M. L., Schuengel, C., Duschinsky, R., van Klaveren, C. et.al. (2022). Exploring the meaning of unresolved loss and trauma in more than 1,000 adult attachment interviews. *Development and Psychopathology, 35*(2), 587–603.

Balk, D. E. (2013). Life span issues and loss, grief, and mourning: Adulthood. In D. K. Meagher & D. E. Balk (Eds.), *Handbook of Thanatology: The Essential Body of Knowledge for the Study of Death, Dying, and Bereavement: The Essential Body of Knowledge for the Study of Death, Dying, and Bereavement* (pp. 157–169). Routledge.

Barlé, N., Wortman, C. B., & Latack, J. A. (2017). Traumatic bereavement: Basic research and clinical implications. *Journal of Psychotherapy Integration, 27*(2), 127–139.

Bartholomew, K., & Horowitz, L. M. (1991). Attachment styles among young adults: a test of a four-category model. *Journal of Personality and Social Psychology, 61*(2), 226–244.

Baumann, M., Frank, D. L., Liebenstein, M., Kiffer, J., Pozuelo, L., Cho, L., ...Hatipoglu, B. (2011). Biofeedback in Coronary Artery Disease, Type 2 Diabetes, and Multiple Sclerosis. *Cleveland Clinic Journal of Medicine, 78*(Suppl 1), S80–S80.

Baumeister, D., Akhtar, R., Ciufolini, S., et. al. (2016). Childhood trauma and adulthood inflammation: a meta-analysis of peripheral C-reactive protein, interleukin-6 and tumor necrosis factor-α. *Molecular Psychiatry, 21*, 642–649.

Beauchaine, T. P., & Cicchetti, D. (2019). Emotion dysregulation and emerging psychopathology: A transdiagnostic, transdisciplinary perspective. *Development and Psychopathology, 31*(3), 799–804.

Beeney, J. E., et. al. (2017). Disorganized attachment and personality functioning in adults: A latent class analysis. *Personality Disorders: Theory, Research, and Treatment, 8*(3), 206–216.

Benbassat, N. (2020). Reflective function: A move to the level of concern. *Theory & Psychology, 30*(5) 657–673.

Berant, E., Mikulincer, M., & Shaver, P. R. (2008). Mothers' Attachment Style, Their Mental Health, and Their Children's Emotional Vulnerabilities: A 7-Year Study of Children With Congenital Heart Disease. *Journal of Personality, 76*(1), 31–66.

Bergman, A. S., Axberg, U. & Hanson, E. (2017). When a parent dies – a systematic review of the effects of support programs for parentally bereaved children and their caregivers. *BMC Palliative Care, 16*, 39.

Berking, M., Poppe, C., Wupperman, P., Luhmann, M., Ebert, D., & Seifritz, E. (2011). Emotion-regulation skills and psychopathology: Is the ability to modify one's negative emotions the ultimate pathway by which all other skills affect symptoms of mental disorders. *Journal of Behavior Therapy and Experimental Psychiatry, 43,* 931–937.

Berry, K., & Danquah, A. (2015). Attachment-informed therapy for adults: Towards a unifying perspective on practice. *Psychology and Psychotherapy: Theory, Research and Practice,* 89(1), 15–32.

Birkeland, M., Skar, A., & Jensen, T. K. (2021). Do different traumatic events invoke different kinds of post-traumatic stress symptoms?, *European Journal of Psychotraumatology,* 12(sup1). DOI: 10.1080/20008198.2020.1866399.

Black, J., Belicki, K., Emberley-Ralph, J., & McCann, A. (2022). Internalized versus externalized continuing bonds: Relations to grief, trauma, attachment, openness to experience, and posttraumatic growth. *Death Studies,* 46(2), 399–414.

Bodhi, B. (2005). *In the Buddha's words. An Anthology of Discourses from the Pāli Canon.* Wisdom Publications.

Boelen, P. A. (2016). Improving the understanding and treatment of complex grief: an important issue for psychotraumatology. *European Journal of Psychotraumatology,* 7(1), 32609.

Boelen, P. A., & Klugkist, I. (2011). Cognitive behavioral variables mediate the associations of neuroticism and attachment insecurity with prolonged grief disorder severity. *Anxiety Stress Coping,* 24(3), 291–307. doi: 10.1080/10615806.2010.527335929457485.

Boelen, P. A., & Lenferink, L. I. M. (2020). Symptoms of prolonged grief, posttraumatic stress, and depression in recently bereaved people: Symptom profiles, predictive value, and cognitive behavioural correlates. *Social Psychiatry and Psychiatric Epidemiology, 55,* 765–777.

Boelen, P. & Lenferink, L. I. M. (2021). Prolonged grief disorder in DSM-5-TR: Early predictors and longitudinal measurement invariance. *Australian & New Zealand Journal of Psychiatry,* 56(6), 667–674.

Boelen, P. A., Stroebe, M. S., Schut, H. A. W., & Zijerveld, A. M. (2006). Continuing bonds and grief: A prospective analysis. *Death Studies,* 30(8), 767–776. doi:10.1080/07481180600852936.

Boelen, P. A., de Keijser, J., van den Hout, M. A., & van den Bout, J. (2011). Factors associated with outcome of cognitive–behavioural therapy for complicated grief: A preliminary study. *Clinical Psychology & Psychotherapy,* 18(4), 284–291.

Boelen, P., Reijintjes, A., & Carleton, N. (2014). Tolerance of uncertainty and adult separation anxiety. *Cognitive Behaviour Therapy,* 43(2), 133–144.

Boelen, P. A., de Keijser, J., & Smid, G. (2015). Cognitive-behavioral variables mediate the impact of violent loss on post-loss psychopathology. *Psychological Trauma,* 7(4), 382–390.

Boelen, P. A., Olff, M., & Smid, G. E. (2017). Traumatic loss: Mental health consequences and implications for treatment and prevention. *European Journal of Psychotraumatology,* 8(Suppl 6), Article 159133.

Boelen, P., Eisma, M., Smid, G., & Lenferink, L. I. M. (2020). Prolonged grief disorder in section II of DSM-5: a commentary. *European Journal of Psychotraumatology, 11,* 1771008.

Bonanno, G. A. (2009). *The Other Side of Sadness: What the New Science of Bereavement Tells Us About Life After Loss.* Basic Books.

Bonanno, G. A., & Boerner, K. (2008). Trajectories of grieving. In C. B. Wortman, M. S. Stroebe, R. O. Hansson, H. Schut & W. Stroebe (Eds.), *Handbook of bereavement research and practice: Advances in theory and intervention* (pp. 287–307). American Psychological Association.

Bonanno, G. A., Wortman, C. B., & Nesse, R. M. (2004). Prospective Patterns of Resilience and Maladjustment During Widowhood. *Psychology and Aging,* 19(2), 260–271. doi:10.1037/0882-7974.19.2.260.

Borelli, J. L., Cohen, C., Pettit, C., Normandin, L., Target, M., Fonagy, P., & Ensink, K. (2019). Maternal and child sexual abuse history: An intergenerational exploration of children's adjustment and maternal trauma-reflective functioning. *Frontiers in Psychology, 10,* 1062. 10.3389/fpsyg.2019.01062.

Bornstein, M. H. (2014). Human Infancy ... and the Rest of the Lifespan. *Annual Review of Psychology, 65*, 121–158.

Bowlby, J. (1944). Forty-four juvenile thieves: Their characters and home life. International *Journal of Psychoanalysis, 25*(19–52), 107–127.

Bowlby, J. (1951). *Maternal care and mental health* (Vol. 2): World Health Organization.

Bowlby, J. (1960). Grief and mourning in infancy and early childhood. *Psychoanalytic Study of the Child, 15*(1), 9–52.

Bowlby, J. (1977). The making and breaking of affectional bonds. I. Aetiology and psychopathology in the light of attachment theory. An expanded version of the Fiftieth Maudsley Lecture, delivered before the Royal College of Psychiatrists, 19 November 1976. *British Journal of Psychiatry, 130*, 201–210.

Bowlby, J. (1980). *Attachment and loss: Loss, sadness and depression.* Basic Books.

Bowlby, J. (1982). *Attachment and loss: Attachment* (Vol. 1). Basic Books.

Bowlby, J. (2005). *A secure base: Clinical applications of attachment theory.* Taylor & Francis.

Bowlby, J. (2008). *A secure base: Parent-child attachment and healthy human development.* Basic Books.

Bowlby, J., & Parkes, C. M. (1970). Separation and loss within the family. In E. J. Anthony (Ed.), *The Child in his family I* (pp. 197–216). Wiley.

BRAIN Initiative Cell Census Network (BICCN) (2021). A multimodal cell census and atlas of the mammalian primary motor cortex. *Nature, 598*, 86–102.

Braun, K. (2011). The prefrontal-limbic system: development, neuroanatomy, function, and implications for socioemotional development. *Clinics in Perinatology, 38*(4), 685–702.

Bretherton, I. (1992). Social referencing, intentional communication, and the interfacing of minds in infancy. In S. Feinman (Ed.), *Social referencing and the social construction of reality in infancy* (pp. 57–77). Plenum Press.

Briere, J., Godbout, N., & Runtz, M. (2012). The Psychological Maltreatment Review (PMR): Initial Reliability and Association with Insecure Attachment in Adults. *Journal of Aggression, Maltreatment & Trauma, 21*(3), 300–320. doi:10.1080/10926771.2012.659801.

Brown, J. C. (1990). Loss and grief: An overview and guided imagery intervention model. *Journal of Mental Health Counseling, 12*(4), 434–445.

Buckle, J. L., & Fleming, S. J. (2011). Parenting challenges after the death of a child. In R. Neimeyer, D. Harris, & H. Winoker, *Grief and bereavement in contemporary society: Bridging research and practice* (pp. 93–105). Routledge/Taylor & Francis Group.

Buehner, Carl (1971). Selected from the 'Spoken Word' and 'Thought for the Day' and from many inspiring thought-provoking sources from many centuries. In Richard Evans, *Quote Book* (p. 244). Publishers Press. (Attributed to many others, notably Maya Angelou.) https://quoteinvestigator.com/2014/04/06/they-feel/.

Bureau, J. F., Martin, J., & Lyons-Ruth, K. (2010). Attachment dysregulation as hidden trauma in infancy: Early stress, maternal buffering and psychiatric morbidity in young adulthood In R. Lanius, E. Vermette, E., & C. Pain, *The impact of early life trauma on health and disease: The hidden epidemic* (pp. 48–56). Cambridge University Press.

Burke, L. A., & Neimeyer, R. A. (2013). Prospective risk factors for complicated grief: A review of the empirical literature. In M. S. Stroebe, H. Schut & J. van den Bout (Eds.), *Complicated grief: Scientific foundations for health care professionals* (pp. 145–161). Routledge/Taylor & Francis Group.

Burke, L. A., Neimeyer, R. A., & McDevitt-Murphy, M. E. (2010). African American homicide bereavement: Aspects of social support that predict complicated grief, PTSD, and depression. *Omega: Journal of Death and Dying, 61*(1), 1–24. doi: 10.2190/OM.61.1.a.

Burki, T. (2019). Post-traumatic stress in the intensive care unit. *The Lancet, 7*(10), 842–844.

Bylund-Grenklo, T., et. al. (2021). Acute and long-term grief reactions and experiences in parentally cancer-bereaved teenagers. *BMC palliative care, 20*(1), 75. 10.1186/s12904-021-00758-7.

Byrne, G. J. A., & Raphael, B. (1997). The psychological symptoms of conjugal bereavement in elderly men over the first 13 months. *International Journal of Geriatric Psychiatry, 12*(2), 241–251.

Cacciatore, J., & Flint, M. (2011). ATTEND: Toward a Mindfulness-Based Bereavement Care Model. *Death Studies, 36*(1), 61–82. doi: 10.1080/07481187.2011.591275.

Cacciatore, J., Thieleman, K., Fretts, R., & Jackson, L. B. (2021). What is good grief support? Exploring the actors and actions in social support after traumatic grief. *PloS One, 16*(5), e0252324. 10.1371/journal.pone.0252324.

Campbell, L., and Stanton, S. C. (2019). Adult attachment and trust in romantic relationships. *Current Opinion in Psychology, 25*, 148–151.

Candel, O.-S., & Turliuc, M. N. (2019). Insecure attachment and relationship satisfaction: A meta-analysis of actor and partner associations. *Personality and Individual Differences, 147*, 190–199.

Cantwell-Bartell A. (2018). Grief and coping of parents whose child has a constant life-threatening disability, hypoplastic left heart syndrome with reference to the Dual-Process Model. *Death Studies, 42*(9), 569–578.

Carr, D., & Jeffreys, J. S. (2011). Spousal bereavement in later life. In *Grief and bereavement in contemporary society. Bridging research and practice* (pp. 81–92). Routledge/Taylor & Francis Group.

Carr, D., Nesse, R. M., & Wortman, C. B. (Eds.). (2006). *Spousal Bereavement in Late Life.* Springer Publishing.

Caserta, M. S., & Lund, D. A. (2007). Toward the development of an inventory of daily widowed life (IDWL): guided by the dual process model of coping with bereavement. *Death Studies, 31*(6), 505–535.

Cassidy, J. (2021). In the Service of Protection from Threat. In: Thompson, J., Simpson, A. & Berlin, J. (Eds.). *Attachment: The fundamental questions* (pp. 103–110). Guilford.

Cassidy, J. & Shaver, P. R. (Eds.) (2008). *Handbook of Attachment: Theory, Research, and Clinical Application* (2nd ed.). Guilford Press.

Cassidy, J. & Shaver, P. R. (Eds.) (2016). *Handbook of Attachment: Theory, Research, and Clinical Application* (3rd ed.). Guilford Press.

Cassidy, J., & Kobak, R. R. (1988). Avoidance and its relation to other defensive processes. In J. Belsky & T. Nezworski (Eds.), *Clinical implications of attachment* (pp. 300–323). Lawrence Erlbaum Associates, Inc.

Cassidy, J., & Shaver, P. R. (Eds.). (2008). *Handbook of Attachment: Theory, Research, and Clinical Applications.* Guilford.

Cesario, J., Johnson, D. J., & Eisthen, H. L. (2020). Your Brain Is Not an Onion With a Tiny Reptile Inside. *Current Directions in Psychological Science, 29*(3), 255–260.

Cesur-Soysal G, Durak-Batıgün A. (2022). Prolonged grief, emotion regulation and loss-related factors: An investigation based on cognitive and behavioral conceptualization. *Death Studies, 46*(6), 1316–1328.

Chami, J. & Pooley, J. (2019). Widowed Young: The Role of Stressors and Protective Factors for Resilience in Coping with Spousal Loss. *OMEGA-Journal of Death and Dying.* Advance online publication. 10.1177/00302228211047088.

Charles, D. R., & Charles, M. (2006). Sibling loss and attachment style: An exploratory study. *Psychoanalytic Psychology, 23*(1), 72–90.

Charles, M., & Devon, C. (2006). Sibling loss and attachment style. *Psychoanalytic Pscyhology, 23*(1), 72–90.

Chen, L., Fu, F., Sha, W., Chan, C. L. W., & Chow, A. Y. M., (2017). Mothers Coping with Bereavement in the 2008 China Earthquake: A Dual Process Model Analysis. *Omega, 80*(1), 69–86.

Cheng, H.-L., McDermott, R. C., & Lopez, F. G. (2015). Mental health, self-stigma, and help-seeking intentions among emerging adults: An attachment perspective. *The Counseling Psychologist, 43*(3), 463–487.

Child Welfare Information Gateway (2023). Child Maltreatment and Brain Development: A Primer for Child Welfare Professionals. Children's Bureau/ACYF/ACF/HHS.

Chisholm, J. S., Quinlivan, J. A., Petersen, R. W., & Coall, D. A. (2005). Early stress predicts age at menarche and first birth, adult attachment, and expected lifespan. *Human Nature*, *16*(3), 233–265.

Chopik, W. J., Edelstein, R. S., & Grimm, K. J. (2019). Longitudinal changes in attachment orientation over a 59-year period. *Journal of Personality and Social Psychology*, *116*(4), 598–611.

Cisneros-Franco, J. M., Voss, P., Thomas, M.E., & de Villers-Sidani, E. (2020). Critical periods of brain development. *Handbook of Clinical Neurology*, *173*, 75–88.

Coan, J. A. (2008). Toward a neuroscience of attachment. In J. Cassidy & P. R. Shaver (Eds.), *Handbook of Attachment: Theory, Research, and Clinical Applications*. Guilford.

Cockle-Hearne, J., et. al. (2021).Support interventions provided during palliative care to families with dependent children when a parent has terminal illness: a scoping review protocol. *JBI Evidence Synthesis*, *19*(11), 3163–3173.

Coleman, R. A., & Neimeyer, R. A. (2010). Measuring meaning: Searching for and making sense of spousal loss in late-life. *Death Studies*, *34*(9), 804–834. doi:10.1080/07481181003761625.

Collins, N. L., & Feeney, B. C. (2004). Working models of attachment shape perceptions of social support: evidence from experimental and observational studies. *Journal of Personality and Social Psychology*, *87*(3), 363.

Conway, J. K. (1989). *The Road from Coorain*. Knopf.

Corr, C. A. (2022). Elisabeth Kübler-Ross and the Five Stages Model in Selected Social Work Textbooks. *Illness, Crisis & Loss*, *30*(2), 320–332.

Costello, P. C. (2013). *Attachment-based Psychotherapy: Helping Patients Develop Adaptive Capacities*. American Psychological Association.

Cotter, P., Meysner, L., & Lee, C. W. (2017). The effectiveness of Cognitive Behavioral Therapy as a component of grief therapy. *European Journal of Psychotraumatology*, *8*(sup6: Traumatic Loss).

Cozolino, L. J. (2010). *The neuroscience of psychotherapy: healing the social brain* (1st ed.). W.W. Norton & Co.

Cozolino, L. J. (2014). *The neuroscience of human relationships: Attachment and the developing social brain* (2nd ed.). WW Norton & Company.

Cozolino, L. (2017). *The Neuroscience of Psychotherapy: Healing the Social Brain* (3rd ed). Norton.

Cozolino, L. J., & Santos, E. N. (2014). Why we need therapy – and why it works: A neuro-scientific Perspective. *Smith College Studies in Social Work*, *84*(2–3), 155–157.

Creagh, B. A. (2005). Transformative Mourning:The Bonny Method of Guided Imagery and Music for widowed persons. Unpublished doctoral dissertation, Union Institute and University.

Currier, J. M., & Neimeyer, R. A. (2006). Fragmented stories: The narrative integration of violent loss. In E. K. Rynearson (Ed.), *Violent death: Resilience and intervention beyond the crisis* (pp. 85–100). Routledge/Taylor & Francis Group.

Currier, J. M., Holland, J. M., & Neimeyer, R. A. (2006). Sense-Making, Grief, and the Experience of Violent Loss: Toward a Mediational Model. *Death Studies*, *30*(5), 403–428.

Currier, J. M., Holland, J. M., Coleman, R. A., & Neimeyer, R. A. (2008). Bereavement following violent death: An assault on life and meaning. In R. G. Stevenson & G. R. Cox (Eds.), *Perspectives on violence and violent death* (pp. 177–202): Baywood Publishing Co.

Currier, J. M., Neimeyer, R. A., & Berman, J. S. (2008). The effectiveness of psychotherapeutic interventions for bereaved persons: A comprehensive quantitative review. *Psychological Bulletin*, *134*(5), 648–661. doi:10.1037/0033-2909.134.5.648.

Currier, J. M., Holland, J. M., & Neimeyer, R. A. (2009). Assumptive Worldviews and Problematic Reactions to Bereavement. *Journal of Loss and Trauma*, *14*(3), 181–195.

Danquah, A. N., & Berry, K. (2013). *Attachment Theory in Adult Mental Health: A Guide to Clinical Practice*. Routledge.

Danqueth, A. N., & Berry, K. (Eds.) (2014). *Attachment Theory in Adult Mental Health*. Routledge.

Davidson, D. (2018) Sibling loss – Disenfranchised grief and forgotten mourners. *Bereavement Care, 37*(3), 124–130.

Davis, D., Shaver, P. R., & Vernon, M. L. (2003). Physical, emotional, and behavioral reactions to breaking up: The roles of gender, age, emotional involvement, and attachment style. *Personality and Social Psychology Bulletin, 29*(7), 871–884.

Davis, J. P., Dumas, T. M., & Roberts, B. W. (2018). Adverse Childhood Experiences and Development in Emerging Adulthood. *Emerging Adulthood, 6*(4), 223–234.

De Leo, D., Cimitan, A., Dyregrov, K., Grad, O., & Andriessen, K. (2014). *Bereavement After Traumatic Death: Helping the Survivors*. Hogrefe.

Decety, J. (2012). *Empathy: From Bench to Bedside*. MIT Press.

Decety, J., & Ickes, W. (Eds.). (2009). *The Social Neuroscience of Empathy*. MIT Press.

Delespaux, E., Ryckebosch-Dayez, A.-S., Heeren, A., & Zech, E. (2013). Attachment and severity of grief: the mediating role of negative appraisal and inflexible coping. *OMEGA Journal of Death and Dying, 67*(3), 269–289.

Denckla, C. A., Mancini, A. D., Bornstein, R. F., & Bonanno, G. A. (2011). Adaptive and Maladaptive Dependency in Bereavement: Distinguishing Prolonged and Resolved Grief Trajectories. *Personality and Individual Differences, 51*(8), 1012–1017. doi:10.1016/j.paid. 2011.08.014.

Deno, M., Miyashita, M., Fujisawa, D., Nakajima, S., & Ito, M. (2013). The influence of alexithymia on psychological distress with regard to the seriousness of complicated grief and the time since bereavement in the Japanese general population. *Journal of Affective Disorders, 149*(1), 202–208.

DeOliveira, C. A., Moran, G., & Pederson, D. R. (2005). Understanding the link between maternal adult attachment classifications and thoughts and feelings about emotions. *Attachment & Human Development, 7*(2), 153–170.

Didion, J. (2005). *The Year of Magical Thinking*. Random House.

Didion, J. (2007). *The year of magical thinking*. Random House LLC.

Djelantik, A., Smid, G. E., Mroz, A., Kleber, R. J., & Boelen, P. A. (2020). The prevalence of prolonged grief disorder in bereaved individuals following unnatural losses: Systematic review and meta regression analysis. *Journal of Affective Disorders, 265*, 146–156.

Doherty, N. A., & Feeney, J. A. (2004). The composition of attachment networks throughout the adult years. *Personal Relationships, 11*(4), 469–488.

Dozier, M., Stovall-McClough, C. K., & Albus, K. E. (2008). Attachment and psychopathology in adulthood. In J. a. S. Cassidy, P. (Ed.), *Handbook of Attachment* (2nd ed.). Guilford Press.

Duncan, B. L., Miller, S. D., Wampold, B. E., & Hubble, M. A. (2010). *The Heart & Soul of Change: Delivering What Works in Therapy* (2nd ed.). American Psycholological Association.

Duncan, B. L., Miller, S. D., Wampold, B. E., & Hubble, M. A. (2010). *The heart and soul of change: Delivering what works in therapy*. American Psychological Association.

Duschinsky, R., Collver, J., & Carel, H. (2019). Trust comes from a sense of feeling one's self understood by another mind: An interview with Peter Fonagy. *Psychoanalytic Psychology, 36*(3), 224–227.

Duschinsky, R. (2020). *Cornerstones of Attachment Research*. Oxford University Press.

Dykas, M. J., & Cassidy, J. (2011). Attachment and the processing of social information across the life span: theory and evidence. *Psychological Bulletin, 137*(1), 19.

Dyregrov, K. (2005). Experiences of social networks supporting traumatically bereaved. *OMEGA: Journal of Death and Dying, 52*(4), 339–358. doi: 10.2190/claa-x2lw-jhqj-t2dm.

Dyregrov, K., & Dyregrov, A. (2008). *Effective Grief and Bereavement Support: The Role of Family, Friends, Colleagues, Schools, and Support Professionals*. Jessica Kingsley Publishers.

Ein-Dor, T., & Doron, G. (2015). Psychopathology and attachment. In J. A. Simpson & W. S. Rholes (Eds.), *Attachment theory and research: New directions and emerging themes* (pp. 346–373). The Guilford Press.

Eisma, M. C., & Stroebe, M. S. (2021). Emotion Regulatory Strategies in Complicated Grief: A Systematic Review. *Behavior Therapy, 52*(1), 234–249.

Eisma, M., de Lang, T. & Stroebe, S. (2022) Restoration-oriented stressors of bereavement. *Anxiety, Stress, & Coping, 35*(3), 339–353.

Elliott, R., Bohart, A. C., Watson, J. C., & Greenberg, L. S. (2011). Empathy. In J. C. Norcross (Ed.), *Psychotherapy Relationships That Work: Evidence-Based Responsiveness* (2nd ed.). Oxford University Press.

Elwert, F. & Christakis, N.A. (2008). The effect of widowhood on mortality by the causes of death of both spouses. *American Journal of Public Health, 98*, 2092–2098.

Ensink, K., Berthelot, N., Bernazzani, O., Normandin, L., & Fonagy, P. (2014). Another step closer to measuring the Ghosts in the Nursery: Preliminary Validation of the Trauma Reflective Functioning Scale. *Frontiers in Psychology, 5*.

Epstein, Mark (2022). *The Zen of Therapy: Uncovering a Hidden Kindness in Life*. Penguin Press.

Epstein, R., Kalus, C., & Berger, M. (2006). The continuing bond of the bereaved towards the deceased and adjustment to loss. *Mortality, 11*(3), 253–269. doi:10.1080/13576270600774935.

Erickson, M. H., & Rossi, E. L. (1979). *Hypnotherapy, an exploratory casebook*. Irvington Publishers.

Esbjørn, B. H., Bender, P. K., Reinholdt-Dunne, M. L., Munck, L. A., & Ollendick, T. (2012). The Development of Anxiety Disorders: Considering the Contributions of Attachment and Emotion Regulation. *Clinical Child and Family Psychology Review, 15*(2), 129–143.

Eubanks, C. F., Muran, J. C., & Safran, J. D. (2018). Alliance rupture repair: A meta-analysis. *Psychotherapy, 55*(4), 508–519.

Euler, S., et. al. (2019). Interpersonal Problems in Borderline Personality Disorder: Association with Mentalizing, Emotion Regulation and Impulsiveness. *Journal of Personality Disorders, 35*(12), 1–17.

Excerpts from *Lincoln in the Bardo: A Novel* by George Saunders, copyright 2017 by George Saunders. Used by permission of Random House, an imprint division of Penguin Random House L.L.C. All rights reserved.

Eyetsemitan, F. E. (2022). *The Deceased-focused Approach to Grief, An Alternative Model*. Springer.

Fanos, J. (1996). *Sibling Loss*. Psychology Press.

Fávero, M., Lemos, L., Moreira, D., Ribeiro, F. & Sousa-Gomes, V. (2021). Romantic attachment and emotion regulation. *Frontiers in Psychology, 13*. Doi:10.3389/fpsyg.2021.723823.

Feigelman, W., Cerel, J., McIntosh, J. L., Brent, D., & Gutin, N. (2018). Suicide exposures and bereavement among American adults: Evidence from the 2016 General Social Survey. *Journal of Affective Disorders, 227*, 1–6.

Feigelman, W. & Cerel, J. (2020). Feelings of blameworthiness and their associations with the grieving process in suicide mourning. *Frontiers in Psychology, 11*, 610.

Feigelman, W., Jordan, J. R., McIntosh, J. L., & Feigelman, B. (2012). *Devastating Losses: How Parents Cope With the Death of a Child to Suicide or Drugs*. Springer.

Feldman R. (2015). The adaptive human parental brain: implications for children's social development. *Trends in Neuroscience, 38*(6), 387–399.

Felitti, V. J., et al., (1998). Relationship of childhood abuse and household dysfunction to many of the leading causes of death in adults: The Adverse Childhood Experiences (ACE) Study. *American Journal of Preventive Medicine, 14*(4), 245–258.

Fernandez-Rodriguez, C., Paz-Caballero, D., Gonzalez-Fernandez & Perez-Alvarez (2018). Activation vs. Experiential Avoidance as a Transdiagnostic Condition of Emotional Distress: An Empirical Study. *Frontiers in Psychology, 3*(9).

Field, N. P. (2006). Unresolved grief and continuing bonds: An attachment perspective. *Death Studies, 30*(8), 739–756.

Field, N. P. (2008). Whether to relinquish or maintain a bond with the deceased. In M. S. Stroebe, R. O. Hansson, H. Schut & W. Stroebe (Eds.), *Handbook of bereavement research and practice: Advances in theory and intervention* (pp. 113–132). American Psychological Association.

Field, N. P., & Filanosky, C. (2010). Continuing bonds, risk factors for complicated grief, and adjustment to bereavement. *Death Studies, 34*(1), 1–29. doi:10.1080/07481180903372269.

Field, N. P., & Friedrichs, M. (2004). Continuing bonds in coping with the death of a husband. *Death Studies, 28*(7), 597–620. doi:10.1080/07481180490476425.

Field, N. P., & Wogrin, C. (2011). The changing bond in therapy for unresolved loss: An attachment theory perspective. In R. Neimeyer, D. L. Harris, H. R. Winokuer & G. F. Thompson (Eds), *Grief and bereavement in contemporary society: Bridging research and practice.* (pp. 37–46). Routledge/Taylor & Francis Group.

Field, N. P., Gal-Oz, E., & Bonanno, G. A. (2003). Continuing bonds and adjustment at 5 years after the death of a spouse. *Journal of Consulting and Clinical Psychology, 71*(1), 110–117. doi:10.1037/0022-006x.71.1.110.

Field, N. P., Gao, B., & Paderna, L. (2005). Continuing Bonds in Bereavement: An Attachment Theory Based Perspective. *Death Studies, 29*(4), 277–299. doi:10.1080/07481180590923689.

Field, N. P., Nichols, C., Holen, A., & Horowitz, M. J. (1999). The relation of continuing attachment to adjustment in conjugal bereavement. *Journal of Consulting and Clinical Psychology, 67*(2), 212–218. doi: 10.1037/0022-006x.67.2.212

Field, N. P., Packman, W., Ronen, R., Pries, A., Davies, B., & Kramer, R. (2013). Type of Continuing Bonds Expression and Its Comforting Versus Distressing Nature: Implications for Adjustment Among Bereaved Mothers. *Death Studies, 37*(10), 889–912. doi: 10.1080/07481187.2012.692458.

Fiore, J. (2021). A Systematic Review of the Dual Process Model of Coping With Bereavement (1999–2016). *Omega, 84*(2), 414–458.

Fischer-Kern, M., Tmej, A., Naderer, A., Zimmerman, J., Nolte, T. (2022). Failure to resolve loss and compromised mentalizing in female inpatients with major depressive disorder. *Attachment & Human Development, 24*(4), 503–524.

Fitter, M. H., Stern, J. A., Straske, M. D., Allard, T., Cassidy, J. & Riggins, T. (2022). Mothers' Attachment Representations and Children's Brain Structure. *Frontiers in Human Neuroscience, 16*(16), 740195.

Foa, E. B., Keane, T. M., Friedman, M. J., & Cohen, J. A. (2009). *Effective treatments for PTSD: Practice guidelines from the International Society for Traumatic Stress Studies* (2nd ed.). Guilford Press.

Fonagy, P., Steele, M., Steele, H., Moran, G. S., & Higgitt, A. C. (1991). The capacity for understanding mental states: The reflective self in parent and child and its significance for security of attachment. *Infant Mental Health Journal, 12*(3), 201–218.

Fonagy, P., Steele, M., Leigh, H., Kennedy, R., & Mattoon, G. (1995). Attachment, the reflective self, and borderline states: The predictive specificity of the Adult Attachment Interview and pathological emotional development. In S. Goldberg, R. Muir, & J. Kerr (Eds.), *Attachment Theory. Social, Developmental and Clinical Perspectives* (pp. 233–278). Analytic Press.

Fonagy, P., Target, M., Steele, H., & Steele, M. (1998). *Reflective-functioning manual, version 5.0, for application to adult attachment interviews.* University College, London.

Fonagy, P., Gergeley, G., Jurist, E., & Target, M. (2002). *Affect Regulation, Mentalization, and the Development of the Self.* Other Press.

Fonagy, P., Steele, M., Steele, H., Leigh, T., & Kennedy, R. (2013). The Predictive Specificity of the Adult Attachment Interview and Pathological Emotional Development. *Attachment theory: Social, developmental, and clinical perspectives, 233.*

Fonagy, P., Bateman, A. W., Lorenzini, N., & Campbell, C. (2014). Development, attachment, and childhood experiences. In J. M. Oldham, Skodol, Andrew E., Bender, Donna S. (Ed.), *The American Psychiatric Publishing Textbook of Personality Disorders* (pp. 55–77). American Psychiatric Publishing.

Fonagy, P., Luyten, P., Allison, E. et al. (2017). What we have changed our minds about: Part 2. Borderline personality disorder, epistemic trust and the developmental significance of social communication. *Borderline Personality Disorder and Emotion Dysregulation, 4*, 9. doi:10.1186/s40479-017-0062-8.

Fraley, R. C., & Bonanno, G. A. (2004). Attachment and loss: A test of three competing models on the association between attachment-related avoidance and adaptation to bereavement. *Personality and Social Psychology Bulletin, 30*(7), 878–890.

Fraley, C., & Hudson, N. (2017). The development of attachment styles. In J. Specht (Ed.), *Personality Development Across the Lifespan* (pp. 275–292). Elsvier.

Fraley, C. R., Fazzari, D. A., Bonanno, G. A., & Dekel, S. (2006). Attachment and psychological adaptation in high exposure survivors of the September 11th attack on the World Trade Center. *Personality and Social Psychology Bulletin, 32*(4), 538–551.

Fraley, C. R., Roisman, G. I., & Haltigan, J. D. (2013). The legacy of early experiences in development: Formalizing alternative models of how early experiences are carried forward over time. *Developmental Psychology, 49*(1), 109–126. doi:10.1037/a0027852.

Fraley, R. C., & Shaver, P. R. (2016). Attachment, loss, and grief: Bowlby's views, new developments, and current controversies. In J. Cassidy & P. R. Shaver (Eds.), *Handbook of attachment: theory, research, and clinical applications* (3rd ed., pp. 40–62). Guilford Press.

Fraley, R. C. & Roisman, G. (2019). The development of adult attachment styles: four lessons. *Current Opinion in Psychology, 25*, 26–30.

Fraley, C., & Shaver, P. (2020). Adult Romantic Attachment: Theoretical Developments, Emerging Controversies, and Unanswered Questions. *Review of General Psychology, 4*(2), 132–154.

Fraley, R. C., & Dugan, K. A. (2021). The consistency of attachment security across time and relationships. In R. A. Thompson, J. A. Simpson, & L. J. Berlin (Eds), *Attachment: The Fundamental Questions* (pp. 147–153). Guilford Press.

Frank, J. D. (1991). *Persuasion and Healing: A Comparative Study of Psychotherapy* (3rd ed.). Johns Hopkins University Press.

Funk, A. M., Jenkins, S., Astroth, K. S., Braswell, G., & Kerber, C. (2018). A narrative analysis of sibling grief. *Journal of Loss and Trauma, 23*(1), 1–14.

Gallo, L. C., Smith, T. W., & Ruiz, J. M. (2003). An Interpersonal Analysis of Adult Attachment Style: Circumplex Descriptions, Recalled Developmental Experiences, Self-Representations, and Interpersonal Functioning in Adulthood. *Journal of Personality, 71*(2), 141–182.

Gamino, L. A., & Sewell, K. W. (2004). Meaning Constructs As Predictors of Bereavement Adjustment: A Report From The Scott & White Grief Study. *Death Studies, 28*(5), 397–421. doi:10.1080/07481180490437536.

Gaudet, C. (2010). Pregnancy after perinatal loss: Association of grief, anxiety and attachment. *Journal of Reproductive and Infant Psychology, 28*(3), 240–251. doi:10.1080/02646830903487342.

Gegieckaite, G., & Kazlauskas, E. (2022). Do emotion regulation difficulties mediate the association between neuroticism, insecure attachment, and prolonged grief? *Death Studies, 46*(4), 911–919.

George, C., Kaplan, N., & Main, M. (1985). Attachment interview for adults. Unpublished manuscript, University of California, Berkeley.

George, C., & Solomon, J. (2008). The Caregiving System: A Behavioral Systems Approach to Parenting. In J. Cassidy & P. R. Shaver (Eds.), *Handbook of Attachment: Theory, Research, and Clinical Applications* (pp. 833–856). Guilford.

Germer, C. K., Siegel, R. D., & Fulton, P. R. (2013). *Mindfulness and psychotherapy*. Guilford Press.

Gilbert, L. (2022). Emotion Coaching in relation to triune brain, polyvagal theory & hand brain model. Research Lead, Emotion Coaching UK. louisegilbert.ec@outlook.com.

Gillath, O., Bunge, S. A., Shaver, P. R., Wendelken, C., & Mikulincer, M. (2005). Attachment-style differences in the ability to suppress negative thoughts: exploring the neural correlates. *Neuroimage, 28*(4), 835–847.

Gillies, J., & Neimeyer, R. A. (2006). Loss, grief, and the search for significance: Toward a model of meaning reconstruction in bereavement. *Journal of Constructivist Psychology, 19*(1), 31–65.

Gillies, J., Neimeyer, R. A., & Milman, E. (2014). The meaning of loss codebook: Construction of a system for analyzing meanings made in bereavement. *Death Studies, 38*(4), 207–216.

Gilligan, S. G. (2012). *Generative Trance: The Experience of Creative Flow.* Crown House Publishing.

Gilligan, S. G. (2013). *Therapeutic trances: The co-operation principle in Ericksonian hypnotherapy.* Routledge.

Gilligan, S. G., & Price, R. (1993). *Therapeutic conversations.* WW Norton.

Gilligan, S., & Dilts, R. (2022). *Generative Coaching,* Vol. 2. International Association for Generative Change.

Girme, Y., Jones, R. E., Fleck, C., Simpson, J. A., & Overall, N. C. (2021). Infants' attachment insecurity predicts attachment-relevant emotion regulation strategies in adulthood. *Emotion, 2,* 260–272.

Goldin, P., Ziv, M., Jazaieri, H., & Gross, J. J. (2012). Randomized controlled trial of Mindfulness-Based Stress Reduction versus aerobic exercise: effects on the self-referential brain network in social anxiety disorder. *Frontiers in Human Neuroscience, 6.*

Goldstein, R. D., Lederman, R. I., Lichtenthal, W. G., Morris, S.E., ...PASS Network (2018). The Grief of Mothers After the Sudden Unexpected Death of Their Infants. *Pediatrics, 141*(5), e20173651. doi:10.1542/peds.2017-3651.

Granqvist, P., Sroufe, A., et. al. (2017). Disorganized attachment in infancy: a review of the phenomenon and its implications for clinicians and policymakers. *Attachment and Human Development, 19*(6), 534–558.

Gratz, K. L., & Roemer, L. (2004). Multidimensional assessment of emotion regulation and dysregulation: Development, factor structure, and initial validation of the difficulties in emotion regulation scale. *Journal of Psychopathology and Behavioral Assessment, 26*(1), 41–54.

Graybeal, A., Sexton, J. D., & Pennebaker, J. W. (2002). The role of story-making in disclosure writing: The psychometrics of narrative. *Psychology & Health, 17*(5), 571–581. doi:10.1080/0887044029002578.

Greenberg, M. (2004). *Healing Through the Dark Emotions.* Shambhala.

Groh, A., Pasco, F., van IJzendoorn, H., Bakerman-Kranenburg, M., & Roisman, G. (2017). Attachment in the Early Life Course: Meta-Analytic Evidence for Its Role in Socioemotional Development. *Child Development Perspectives, 11*(1), 70–76.

Gross, J. J. (2014). *Handbook of Emotion Regulation* (2nd ed.). Guilford Press.

Gross, J. J., & Muñoz, R. F. (1995). Emotion Regulation and Mental Health. *Clinical Psychology: Science and Practice, 2*(2), 151–164.

Gross, J. J., & John, O. P. (2003). Individual differences in two emotion regulation processes: implications for affect, relationships, and well-being. *Journal of Personality and Social Psychology, 85*(2), 348.

Grossmann, K., Grossmann, K. E., & Kindler, H. (2005). Early care and the roots of attachment and partnership representation: The Bielefeld and Regensburd Longitudinal Studies. In K. Grossman, E. Grossman, & H. Kindler (Eds.), *Attachment from infancy to adulthood* (pp. 98–136). Guilford Press.

Grossmann, K, Grossmann, K. E., Kindler, H., & Zimmermann, P. (2008). A wider view of attachment and exploration: The influence of mothers and fathers on the development of psychological security from infancy to young adulthood. In Cassidy J. & Shaver P., *Handbook of Attachment: Theory, research, and clinical applications* (pp. 857–874). Guilford Publications.

Gunnar, M. R. (2017). Social Buffering of Stress in Development: A Career Perspective. *Perspectives on Psychological Science, 12*(3), 355–373.

Haim-Nachum, S., Sopp, M. Bonanno, G., & Levy-Gigi, E. (2022). The Lasting Effects of Early Adversity and Updating Ability on the Tendency to Develop PTSD Symptoms Following Exposure to Trauma in Adulthood. *Cognitive Therapy and Research*. 10.1007/s10608-022-10328-7.

Hall, C. (2014). Bereavement theory: recent developments in our understanding of grief and bereavement. *Bereavement Care, 33*(1), 7–12.

Hankin, B. L., Kassel, J. D., & Abela, J. R. Z. (2005). Adult attachment dimensions and specificity of emotional distress symptoms: Prospective investigations of cognitive risk and interpersonal stress generation as mediating mechanisms. *Personality and Social Psychology Bulletin, 31*(1), 136–151.

Hanson, J. & Nacewicz, B. (2021). Amygdala Allostasis and Early Life Adversity: Considering Excitotoxicity and Inescapability in the Sequelae of Stress. *Frontiers in Human Science*, 10.3389/fnhum.2021.624705.

Hanson, R. (2009). *Buddha's brain: The practical neuroscience of happiness, love, and wisdom*. New Harbinger Publications.

Hanson, R. (2013). *Hardwiring happiness*. Random House, Incorporated.

Harlow, H. F., & Zimmermann, R. R. (1959). Affectional responses in the infant monkey. *Science, 130*, 421–432.

Harris, D. (2021) Compassion-focused grief therapy. *British Journal of Guidance & Counselling, 49*(6), 780–790.

Harris, D. & Winokuer, H. (2021). *Principles and Practice of Grief Therapy*. Springer.

Harris, D. L. & Ho, A. H. Y. (2022). *Compassion Based Approaches in Loss and Grief*. Routledge.

Harrop, E., Morgan, F., Longo, M., et al. (2020). The impacts and effectiveness of support for people bereaved through advanced illness: A systematic review and thematic synthesis. *Palliative Medicine, 34*(7), 871–888.

Hart, H., & Rubia, K. (2012). Neuroimaging of child abuse: A critical review. *Frontiers in Human Neuroscience, 6*. doi:10.3389/fnhum.2012.00052.

Hayes, S. C., Strosahl, K. D., & Wilson, K. G. (2011). *Acceptance and commitment therapy: The process and practice of mindful change*. Guilford Press.

Hazan, C., & Shaver, P. R. (1987). Romantic love conceptualized as an attachment process. *Journal of Personality and Social Psychology, 52*(3), 511–524. doi: 10.1037/0022-3514.52.3.511.

Hazan, C., & Selcuk, E. (2015). Normative processes in romantic attachment: Introduction and overview. In V. Zayas & C. Hazan (Eds.), *Bases of adult attachment: Linking brain, mind and behavior* (pp. 3–8). Springer Science + Business Media.

Heeke, C., Kampisiou, H., Niemeyer R., & Knaevelsrud, C. (2017) A systematic review and meta-analysis of correlates of prolonged grief disorder in adults exposed to violent loss, *European Journal of Psychotraumatology, 8*(sup6), 1583524. doi:10.1080/20008198.2019.1583524.

Heller, D. P. (2019). *The Power of Attachment*. Sounds True.

Herman, J. L. (1992). *Trauma and Recovery*. Basic Books.

Herman, J. L. (1995). Complex PTSD: A syndrome in survivors of prolonged and repeated trauma Psychotraumatology. In *Key papers and core concepts in post-traumatic stress* (pp. 87–100). Plenum Press.

Herman, J. L. (2008). Craft and science in the treatment of traumatized people. *Journal of Trauma & Dissociation, 9*(3), 293–300. doi:10.1080/15299730802138966.

Herzog, J. I., & Schmahl, C. (2018). Adverse childhood experiences and the consequences on neurobiological, psychosocial, and somatic conditions across the lifespan. *Frontiers in Psychiatry, 9*, Article 420. 10.3389/fpsyt.2018.00420.

Hesse, E. (2008). The Adult Attachment Interview: Protocol, method of analysis, and empirical studies. In J. Cassidy & P. R. Shaver (Eds.), *Handbook of Attachment: Theory, Research, and Clinical Applications* (2nd ed., pp. 552–598). Guilford.

Hesse, E., & Main, M. (2000). Disorganized infant, child, and adult attachment: collapse in behavioral and attentional strategies. *Journal of the American Psychoanalytic Association,* *48*(4), 1097–1127.

Hibberd, R. (2013). Meaning Reconstruction in Bereavement: Sense and Significance. *Death Studies, 37*(7), 670–692. doi:10.1080/07481187.2012.692453.

Hickok, G. (2014). *The Myth of Mirror Neurons: The Real Neuroscience of Communication and Cognition.* W. W. Norton & Company

Hill, D. (2016). *Affect Regulation:A Clinical Model.* W.W. Norton & Company.

Ho, S. M. Y., Chan, I. S. F., Ma, E. P. W., & Field, N. P. (2012). Continuing Bonds, Attachment Style, and Adjustment in the Conjugal Bereavement Among Hong Kong Chinese. *Death Studies,* *37*(3), 248–268. doi:10.1080/07481187.2011.634086.

Hodges, S. D., & Wegner, D. M. (1997). Automatic and controlled empathy. In W. Ickes (Ed.), *Empathic Accuracy* (pp. 311–339). Guilford.

Hofer, M. A. (1996). On the nature and consequences of early loss. *Psychosomatic Medicine,* *58*(6), 570–581.

Holland, J. & Rozalski, V. (2017). Clinical issues related to sibling loss in older adults. In: Marshall, B., & Winokuer, H. (Eds.) *Sibling Loss Across the Lifespan: Research, Practice, and Personal Stories* (pp. 129–140). Routledge.

Holland, J. M., Currier, J. M., & Neimeyer, R. A. (2006). Meaning reconstruction in the first two years of bereavement: The role of sense-making and benefit-finding. *Omega: Journal of Death and Dying, 53*(3), 175–191.

Holland, J. M., Neimeyer, R. A., Currier, J. M., & Berman, J. S. (2007). The efficacy of personal construct therapy: A comprehensive review. *Journal of Clinical Psychology, 63*(1), 93–107.

Hollinger, Dorothy (2020). *The Anatomy of Grief.* Yale University Press.

Holm, A. L., Berland, A. K., & Severinsson, E. (2019). Factors that influence the health of older widows and widowers – A systematic review of quantitative research. *Nursing Open, 6*(2), 591–611.

Holmes, J. (2001). *The search for the secure base: Attachment theory and psychotherapy.* Psychology Press.

Holmes, J. (2010). From Attachment Research to Clinical Practice: Getting It Together. In J. H. Obegi & E. Berant (Eds.), *Attachment theory and research in clinical work with adults* (pp. 490–514). Guilford.

Holmes, J. (2010). *Exploring in Security: Towards and Attachment-Informed Psychoanalytic Psychotherapy.* Routledge.

Holmes, J. (2013). Attachment Theory in Therapeutic Practice. In A. N. Danqueth & K. Berry (Eds.), *Attachment Theory in Adult Mental Health* (pp. 16–32). Routedge.

Holmes, J. (2022). Attachment, Neurobiology and the New Science of Psychotherapy. *The Weekend University,* 18 March. https://www.youtube.com/watch?v=2M6Z3XgdCVE.

Holmes, J. & Slade, A. (2018). *Attachment in Adult Psychotherapy.* Sage.

https://Cancer.net/coping-with-cancer/managing-emotions/grief-and-loss/grieving-loss-sibling

https://copefoundation.org/sibling-support-group/2022.

Huber, C. (2001). *There is nothing wrong with you: Going beyond self-hate A compassionate process for learning to accept yourself exactly as you are.* Keep It Simple Books.

Huh, H. J., Kim, K. H., Lee, H. K., & Chae, J. H. (2017). Attachment Style, Complicated Grief and Post-Traumatic Growth in Traumatic Loss: The Role of Intrusive and Deliberate Rumination. *Psychiatry Investing, 17*(7), 636–644.

Huh, H. J., Kim, K. H., Lee, H. K., & Chae, J. H. (2017). Attachment styles, grief responses, and the moderating role of coping strategies in parents bereaved by the Sewol ferry accident, *European Journal of Psychotraumatology, 8*(sup6), 1424446. doi:10.1080/20008198.201 8.1424446.

Hunter, A. & Flores, G. (2021). Social determinants of health and child maltreatment: a systematic review. *Pediatric Research, 89,* 269–274.

Hybholt L. et. al. (2020). Older Adults' Conduct of Everyday Life After Bereavement by Suicide: A Qualitative Study. *Frontiers in Psychology*, *19*(11), 1131.

Iglewicz, A., Shear, M. K., Reynolds, C. F., Simon, N., Lebowitz, B., & Zisook, S. (2020). Complicated grief therapy for clinicians: An evidence-based protocol for mental health practice. *Depression and anxiety*, *37*(1), 90–98.

Innamorati, M., Pompili, M., Amore, M., Vittorio, C. D., Serafini, G., Tatarelli, R., & Lester, D. (2011). *Suicide prevention in late life: Is there sound evidence for practice?* In M. Pompilli & R. Tatarelli (Eds.), *Evidence-based practice in suicidology: A source book* (pp. 211–232). Hogrefe Publishing.

Iob, E., Lacey, R., Giunchiglia, V. et al. (2022). Adverse childhood experiences and severity levels of inflammation and depression from childhood to young adulthood: a longitudinal cohort study. *Molecualr Psychiatry*, *27*(4), 2255–2263.

Ivengar, U., Rajhans, P., Fonagy, P., Strathearn, L./& Solve, K. (2019). Unresolved Trauma and Reorganization in Mothers: Attachment and Neuroscience Perspectives. *Frontiers in Psychology*, *30*, 10110.

Jacobvitz, D., Hazen, N., Zaccagnino, M., Messina, S., & Beverung, L. (2011). Frightening maternal behavior, infant disorganization, and risks for psychopathology. In D. Cicchetti & G. I. Roisman (Eds.), *The origins and organization of adaptation and maladaptation* (pp. 283–322). John Wiley & Sons, Inc.

Jacobvitz, D. & Reisz (2018) Disorganized and Unresolved States in Adulthood. *Current Opinion in Psychology*, *25*,172–176.

James, W. (1890). *The Principles of Psychology*. Rinehart.

Jerga, A. M., Shaver, P. R., & Wilkinson, R. B. (2011). Attachment insecurities and identification of at-risk individuals following the death of a loved one. *Journal of Social and Personal Relationships*, *28*(7), 891–914. doi:10.1177/0265407510397987.

Johnson, J. G., Zhang, B., & Prigerson, H. G. (2008). Investigation of a developmental model of risk for depression and suicidality following spousal bereavement. *Suicide and Life-Threatening Behavior*, *38*(1), 1–12. doi:10.1521/suli.2008.38.1.1.

Jones, J. D., Cassidy, J., & Shaver, P. R. (2015). Parents' Self-Reported Attachment Styles A Review of Links with Parenting Behaviors, Emotions, and Cognitions. *Personality and Social Psychology Review*, *19*(1), 44–76.

Jordan, J. R. (2000). Introduction: Research that matters: Bridging the gap between research and practice in thanatology. *Death Studies*, *24*(6), 457–467. doi:10.1080/07481180050121444.

Jordan, J. R. (2012). Guided imaginal conversations with the deceased. In R. A. Neimeyer (Ed.), *Techniques of Grief Therapy: Creative Practices for Counseling the Bereaved* (pp. 262–265). Routledge.

Jordan, J. (2020). Lessons Learned: Forty Years of Clinical Work with Suicide Survivors. *Frontiers in Psychology*, *11*, 766, doi: 10.3389/fpsyg.2020.00766.

Jordan, J. R., & Ware, E. S. (1997). Feeling like a motherless child: A support group model for adults grieving the death of a parent. *Omega: Journal of Death and Dying*, *35*(4), 361–376.

Jordan, J. R., & Neimeyer, R. A. (2003). Does grief counseling work? *Death Studies*, *27*(9), 765–786.

Jordan, J. R., Kraus, D. R., & Ware, E. S. (1993). Observations on loss and family development. *Family Process*, *32*(4), 425–440.

Juffer, F., Bakermans-Kranenburg, M. J., & van IJzendoorn, M. H. (2012). *Promoting positive parenting: An attachment-based intervention*. Routledge.

Jurist, E. L., & Meehan, K. B. (2009). Attachment, Mentalization, and Reflective Functioning. In J. H. Obegi & E. Berant (Eds.), *Attachment theory and research in clinical work with adults* (pp. 71– 93). Guilford.

Kagan, R. (2004). *Rebuilding attachments with traumatized children: Healing from losses, violence, abuse, and neglect*. Haworth Maltreatment and Trauma Press/The Haworth Press.

Kalia, V., & Knauft, K. (2020). Emotion regulation strategies modulate the effect of adverse childhood experiences on perceived chronic stress with implications for cognitive flexibility. PLoS ONE, 15(6), e0235412.

Kampling H, et. al., (2022). Epistemic trust and personality functioning mediate the association between adverse childhood experiences and posttraumatic stress disorder and complex posttraumatic stress disorder in adulthood. Frontiers in Psychiatry, 13, 919191.

Kandel, E. R. (1998). A new intellectual framework for psychiatry. American Journal of Psychiatry, 155(4), 457–469.

Kandel, E. R., Markram, H., Matthews, P. M., Yuste, R., & Koch, C. (2013). Neuroscience thinks big (and collaboratively). Nature Reviews Neuroscience, 14(9), 659–664.

Kaniasty, K. (2012). Predicting social psychological well-being following trauma: The role of postdisaster social support. Psychological Trauma: Theory, Research, Practice, and Policy, 4(1), 22.

Kastenbaum R. (1969). Death and bereavement in later life. In A. H. Kutscher (Ed.), Death and bereavement (pp. 28–54). Charles C Thomas.

Kato, P. M., & Mann, T. (1999). A synthesis of psychological interventions for the bereaved. Clinical Psychology Review, 19(3), 275–296.

Katz, M., Liu, C., Schaer, M., Parker, K. J., Ottet, M.-C., Epps, A., ... Schatzberg, A. F. (2009). Prefrontal plasticity and stress inoculation-induced resilience. Developmental Neuroscience, 31(4), 293.

Kauffman, J. (2002). Loss of the assumptive world: A theory of traumatic loss. Brunner-Routledge.

Kauffman, J. (2012). The Empathic Spirit in Grief Therapy. In R. A. Neimeyer (Ed.), Techniques of Grief Therapy: Creative Practices for Counseling the Bereaved (pp. 12–15). Routledge.

Kealy, D. & Ogrodniczuk, J. (Eds.). (2019). Contemporary Psychodynamic Psychotherapy: Evolving Clinical Practice. Elsevier.

Keesee, N. J., Currier, J. M., & Neimeyer, R. A. (2008). Predictors of grief following the death of one's child: The contribution of finding meaning. Journal of Clinical Psychology, 64(10), 1145–1163. doi:10.1002/jclp.20502.

Keysers, C. (2011). The Empathic Brain: How the Discovery of Mirror Neurons Changes Our Understanding of Human Nature. Kindle Edition.

Keysers, C., & Perrett, D. I. (2004). Demystifying social cognition: a Hebbian perspective. Trends in Cognitive Sciences, 8(11), 501–507.

Kiecolt-Glaser, J. K., McGuire, L., Robles, T. F., & Glaser, R. (2002). Emotions, morbidity, and mortality: new perspectives from psychoneuroimmunology. Annual Review of Psychology, 53(1), 83–107.

Kim, B.-R., Stifter, C. A., Philbrook, L. E., & Teti, D. M. (2014). Infant emotion regulation: Relations to bedtime emotional availability, attachment security, and temperament. Infant Behavior and Development, 37(4), 480–490.

Kissane, D. & Kasparian, N. (2017). Theoretical models guiding our understanding of bereavement. In: Marshall, B., & Winokuer, H. (Eds.), Sibling Loss Across the Lifespan: Research, Practice, and Personal Stories (pp. 1–14). Routledge.

Klass, D. (1997). The deceased child in the psychic and social worlds of bereaved parents during the resolution of grief. Death Studies, 21(2), 147–175. doi: 10.1080/074811897202056.

Klass, D. (1999). The Spiritual Lives of Bereaved Parents. Brunner/Mazel.

Klass, D. (2006). Continuing conversation about continuing bonds. Death Studies, 30(9), 843–858. doi:10.1080/07481180600886959.

Klass, D. & Steffen, E. M. (Eds.) (2018). Continuing bonds in bereavement: New directions for research and practice. Routledge.

Klass, D., Silverman, P. R., & Nickman, S. L. (1996). Continuing bonds: New understandings of grief. Taylor & Francis: Philadelphia.

Klingspon, K. L., Holland, J. M., Neimeyer, R. A., & Lichtenthal, W. G. (2015). Unfinished business in bereavement. Death Studies, 39(7), 387–398.

Kobylińska, D., & Kusev, P. (2019). Flexible Emotion Regulation: How Situational Demands and Individual Differences Influence the Effectiveness of Regulatory Strategies. *Frontiers in Psychology, 10,* 72.

Konig, N., et. al. (2019). How Therapeutic Tapping Can Alter Neural Correlates of Emotional Prosody Processing in Anxiety. *Brain Sciences, 9*(8), 206.

Kooiman, C. G., van Rees Vellinga, S., Spinhoven, P., Draijer, N., Trijsburg, R. W., & Rooijmans, H. G. M. (2004). Childhood adversities as risk factors for alexithymia and other aspects of affect dysregulation in adulthood. *Psychotherapy and Psychosomatics, 73*(2), 107–116.

Kosminsky, P. S. (2012). Mapping the Terrain of Loss. In R. A. Neimeyer (Ed.), *Techniques in Grief Therapy: Creative Practices for Counseling the Bereaved* (pp. 30–32). Routledge.

Kosminsky, P. (2017). CBT for grief: Clearing cognitive obstacles to healing from loss. *Journal of Rational-Emotive & Cognitive-Behavior Therapy, 35*(1), 26–37.

Kosminsky, P. (2018). Working with continuing bonds from an attachment theoretical perspective. In D. Klass, & E. M. Steffen (Eds.), *Continuing bonds in bereavement: New directions for research and practice* (pp. 112– 128). Routledge.

Kosminsky, P. S., & McDevitt, R. (2012). Eye Movement Desensitization and Reprocessing (EMDR). In R. A. Neimeyer (Ed.), *Techniques of Grief Therapy: Creative Practices for Counseling the Bereaved* (pp. 95–98). Routledge.

Kosminsky, P. S., & Jordan, J. R. (2016). *Attachment-informed grief therapy, The clinician's guide to foundations and applications.* Routledge.

Kraiss, J. T., ten Klooster, P. M., Moskowitz, J. T., & Bohlmeijer, E.T. (2020). The relationship between emotion regulation and well-being in patients with mental disorders: A meta-analysis. *Comprehensive Psychiatry, 102,*152189.

Kübler-Ross, E. (1997). *On death and dying.* Simon and Schuster.

Kumashiro, M. & Arriaga, X. (2020) Attachment security enhancement model: Bolstering attachment securing through close relationships. In A. Brent, K. Mattingly, P. McIntyre, & G. Lewandowski (Eds.), *Interpersonal Relationships and the Self-Concept* (pp. 69–88). Springer.

Landsman, I. (2002). Crises of Meaning in Trauma and Loss. In J. Kauffman (Ed.), *Loss of the assumptive world: A theory of traumatic loss* (pp. 13–30). Brunner-Routledge.

Lanius, R. A., Vermetten, E., & Pain, C. (2010). *The impact of early life trauma on health and disease: The hidden epidemic.* Cambridge University Press.

Larson, Dale G. (2020). *The Helper's Journey: Empathy, Compassion, and the Challenge of Caring* (2nd ed.) Faculty Book Gallery.

Latham, A. E., & Prigerson, H. G. (2004). Suicidality and Bereavement: Complicated Grief as Psychiatric Disorder Presenting Greatest Risk for Suicidality. *Suicide and Life-Threatening Behavior, 34*(4), 350–362.

Leahy, R. L., Tirch, D. D., & Napolitano, L. A. (2012). *Emotion regulation in psychotherapy: A practitioner's guide.* Guilford Press.

Leblanc, É., Dégeilh, F., Daneault, V., Beauchamp, M. H., & Bernier, A. (2017). Attachment security in infancy: a preliminary study of prospective links to brain morphometry in Late Childhood. *Frontiers in Psychologyi, 8,* 2141.

Leeds, A., (2022). The Positive Affect Tolerance and Integration Protocol: A Novel Approach to Help Survivors of Early Emotional Neglect Learn to Tolerate and Assimilate Moments of Appreciation, Praise and Affection. *Journal of EMDR Practice and Research, 16*(4), 202–214.

LeRoy, A., et. al. (2020). Attachment orientations and loss adjustment among bereaved spouses. *Psychoneuroendocrinology, 112,* 104401.

LeRoy, A. S., Knee, C. R., Derrick, J. L., & Fagundes, C. P. (2019). Implications for Reward Processing in Differential Responses to Loss: Impacts on Attachment Hierarchy Reorganization. *Personality and Social Psychology Review, 23*(4), 391–405.

Letkiewicz, A., Funkhouser, C. J., & Shankman, S. (2021). Childhood maltreatment predicts poorer executive functioning in adulthood beyond symptoms of internalizing psychopathology. *Child Abuse & Neglect, 118,* 105140.

Levi-Belz, Y. (2015) Stress-related growth among suicide survivors: The role of inter-personal and cognitive factors. *Archives of Suicide Research*, 19(3), 305–320.

Levi-Ari, L. & Levi-Belz, Y. (2018). Interpersonal theory dimensions facilitate posttraumatic growth among suicide-loss survivors: An attachment perspective. *Death Studies*, 43(9), 582–590.

Levi-Belz, Y., & Lev-Ari, L. (2019). Attachment styles and posttraumatic growth among suicide-loss survivors: The mediating role of interpersonal factors. *The Journal of Crisis Intervention and Suicide Prevention*, 40(3), 186–195.

Levi-Belz, Y. & Lev-Ari, L. (2019). Is there anybody out there? Attachment style and interpersonal facilitators as protective factors against complicated grief among suicide-loss survivors. *Journal of Nervous Mental Disorders*, 207, 131–136.

Levine, L. & Heller, R. (2019). *Attached: How the science of adult attachment can help you find and keep love*. Bluebird Publishers.

Levy, K. N., & Kelly, K. M. (2009). Using interviews to assess adult attachment. In J. H. a. B. Obegi, E. (Ed.), *Attachment theory and research in clinical work with adults* (pp. 121–152). Guilford.

Levy, K. N., Ellison, W. D., Scott, L. N., & Bernecker, S. L. (2011). Attachment Style. In J. C. Norcross (Ed.), *Psychotherapy Relationships That Work* (2nd ed., pp. 279–300). Oxford University Press.

Lewin, K. (1951). Problems of research in social psychology. In D. Cartwright (Ed.), *Field theory in social science: Selected theoretical papers* (pp.155–169). Harper & Row.

Lewis, T., Amini,F., &Lannon, R. (2020). *A General Theory of Love*. Random House.

Li, J., Li, M., & Reid, J.K. (2022). Social support in bereavement: Developing and validating a new scale. *International Journal of Psychology*, 57(2): 306–313.

Li, W., Xiaoqin M., & Liu, C. (2014). The default mode network and social understanding of others: what do brain connectivity studies tell us. *Frontiers in human neuroscience*, 8, 74.

Lichtenthal, W. G., & Neimeyer, R. A. (2012). Directed writing to facilitate meaning making. In R. A. Neimeyer (Ed.), *Techniques of Grief Therapy: Creative Practices for Counseling the Bereaved* (pp. 165–168). Routledge.

Lichtenthal, W. G., Currier, J. M., Neimeyer, R. A., & Keesee, N. J. (2010). Sense and significance: a mixed methods examination of meaning making after the loss of one's child. *Journal of Clinical Psychology*, 66(7), 791–812.

Lichtenthal, W. G., Burke, L. A., & Neimeyer, R. A. (2011). Religious coping and meaning-making following the loss of a loved one. *Counselling and Spirituality/Counseling et spiritualité*, 30(2), 113–135.

Lichtenthal, W. G., Neimeyer, R. A., Currier, J. M., Roberts, K., & Jordan, N. (2013). Cause of Death and the Quest for Meaning After the Loss of a Child. *Death Studies*, 37(4), 311–342. doi:10.1080/07481187.2012.673533.

Linehan, M. M. (1993). *Skills training manual for treating borderline personality disorder*. Guilford Press.

Linehan, M. M. (2015). *DBT Skills Training Manual*. The Guilford Press.

Liotti, G. (2014). Disorganised attachment in the pathogenesis and the psychotherapy of bor-derline personality disorder. In A. N. Danquah, & K. Berry (Eds.), *Attachment Theory in Adult Mental Health: A Guide to Clinical Practice* (pp. 113–128). Routledge.

Litz, B. T. (2004). *Early intervention for trauma and traumatic loss*. Guilford Press.

Livingston, G. (2018). Stay-at-home moms and dads account for about one-in-five U.S. parents. https://www.pewresearch.org/fact-tank/2018/09/24/stay-at-home-moms-and-dads-account-for-about-one-in-five-u-s-parents/.

Lobb, E. A., Kristjanson, L. J., Aoun, S. M., Monterosso, L., Halkett, G. K. B., & Davies, A. (2010). Predictors of Complicated Grief: A Systematic Review of Empirical Studies. *Death Studies*, 34(8), 673–698.

Logan, E., Thornton, J., & Kane, R. (2018). Social support following bereavement: The role of beliefs, expectations, and support intentions. *Death Studies*, 42(8), 471–482.

Loman, M. M., & Gunnar, M. R. (2010). Early experience and the development of stress reactivity and regulation in children. *Neuroscience & Biobehavioral Reviews, 34*(6), 867–876.

Lopez, F. (2009). Clinical Correlates of Adult Attachment Organization. In O. A. Berant (Ed.), *Attachment theory and research in clinical work with adults* (pp. 94–117). Guilford Press.

Lopez, F. G. (2019). Adult attachment security. In M. W. Gallagher & S. J. Lopez (Eds.), *Positive psychological assessment: A handbook of models and measures* (pp. 267–283). American Psychological Association.

Lorenz, K. (1957). Companionship in bird life. In C. H. Schiller (Ed.), *Instinctive behavior: the development of a modern concept* (pp. 83–128). Internaitonal Universities Press.

Luby, J. L., Tillman, R., & Barch, D. M. (2019). Association of timing of adverse childhood experiences and caregiver support with regionally specific brain development in adolescents. *JAMA Network Open, 2*(9), e1911426–e1911426.

Luecken, L. J. (2008). Long-term consequences of parental death in childhood: Psychological and physiological manifestations. In M. S. Stroebe, R. O. Hansson, H. Schut & W. Stroebe (Eds.), *Handbook of bereavement research and practice: Advances in theory and intervention* (pp. 397–416). American Psychological Association.

Lund, D., Caserta, M., Utz, R., & de Vries, B. (2010). Experiences and Early Coping of Bereaved Spouses/Partners in an Intervention Based on the Dual Process Model (DPM). *OMEGA – Journal of Death and Dying, 61*(4), 291–313.

Lundberg, T., Forinder, U., Olsson, M., Fürst, C., Årestedt, K. & Alvariza, A. (2020) Poor Psychosocial Well-Being in the First Year-and-a-Half After Losing a Parent to Cancer. *Journal of Social Work in End-of-Life & Palliative Care, 16*(4), 330–345.

Lundorff, M., Holmgren, H., Zachariae, R., Farver-Vestergaard, I., O'Connor, M. (2017). Prevalence of prolonged grief disorder in adult bereavement: A systematic review and meta-analysis. *Journal of Affective Disorders, 212*, 138–149.

Luyten, P., Campbell, C., Allison., E., & Fonagy, P. (2020). The Mentalizing Approach to Psychopathology: State of the Art and Future Directions. *Annual Review of Clinical Psychology, 7*(16), 297 –325.

MacCallum, F. (2021). Normal and Pathological Mourning: Attachment Processes in the Development of Prolonged Grief. In J. Thompson, J. Simpson, & L. Berlin (Eds.), *Attachment: The Fundamental Questions* (pp. 289–295). The Guilford Press.

MacCallum, F., & Bryant, R. A. (2018). Prolonged grief and attachment security: A latent class analysis. *Psychiatry Research, 268*, 297–302.

MacLean, P. D. (1990). *The triune brain in evolution: Role in paleocerebral functions.* Springer.

Main, M. (1996). Introduction to the special section on attachment and psychopathology: 2. Overview of the field of attachment. *Journal of Consulting and Clinical Psychology, 64*(2), 237–243.

Main, M. (2000). The Organized Categories of Infant, Child, and Adult Attachment: Flexible Vs. Inflexible Attention Under Attachment-Related Stress. *Journal of the American Psychoanalytic Association, 48*(4), 1055–1096. doi:10.1177/00030651000480041801.

Main, M., & Solomon, J. (1986). *Discovery of an insecure-disorganized/disoriented attachment pattern.* In T. B. Brazelton & M. Yogman (Eds.), *Affective Development in Infancy* (pp. 95–124). Ablex.

Main, M., & Hesse, E. (1990). Parents' unresolved traumatic experiences are related to infant disorganized attachment status: Is frightened and/or frightening parental behavior the linking mechanism? In M. T. E. C. Greenberg, D. Cicchetti, & E.M. Cummings (Eds), *Attachment in the preschool years: Theory, research, and intervention.* The John D. and Catherine T. MacArthur Foundation series on mental health and development (pp. 161–182). University of Chicago Press.

Main, M., Kaplan, N., & Cassidy, J. (1985). Security in infancy, childhood, and adulthood: A move to the level of representation. *Monographs of the Society for Research in Child Development*, 66–104.

Main, M., Goldwyn, R., & Hesse, E. (1998). Adult attachment scoring and classification system. Unpublished manuscript, University of California at Berkeley.

Main, M., Hesse, E., & Goldwyn, R. (2008). Studying differences in language usage in recounting attachment history: An introduction to the AAI. In H. S. M. Steele (Ed.), *Clinical applications of the Adult Attachment Interview* (pp. 31–68). Guilford Press.

Malik, S., Wells, A., & Wittkowski, A. (2014). Emotion regulation as a mediator in the relationship between attachment and depressive symptomatology: A systematic review. *Journal of Affective Disorders 172*, 428–444.

Malkinson, R. (2012). The ABC of Rational Response to Loss. *Techniques of Grief Therapy, 129.*

Malkinson, R., Rubin, S. S., & Witztum, E. (2006). Therapeutic issues and the relationship to the deceased: working clinically with the two-track model of bereavement. *Death Studies, 30*(9), 797–815. doi:10.1080/07481180600884723.

Mallinckrodt, B., Daly, K., & Wang, C.-C. D. C. (2009). An Attachment Approach to Adult Psychotherapy. In J. H. Obegi & E. Berant (Eds.), *Attachment theory and research in clinical work with adults* (pp. 234–268). Guilford.

Mancini, A. D., & Bonanno, G. A. (2009). Predictors and parameters of resilience to loss: Toward an individual differences model. *Journal of Personality, 77*(6), 1805–1832.

Mancini, A. D., Pressman, D. L., & Bonanno, G. A. (2006). Clinical interventions with the Bereaved: What clinicians and counselors can learn from the changing lives of older couples study. In D. Carr, R. M. Nesse & C. B. Wortman (Eds.), *Spousal bereavement in late life* (pp. 255–278). Springer.

Mancini, A. D., Robinaugh, D., Shear, K., & Bonanno, G. A. (2009). Does attachment avoidance help people cope with loss? The moderating effects of relationship quality. *Journal of Clinical Psychology, 65*(10), 1127–1136. doi:10.1002/jclp.20601.

Mancini, A. D., Griffin, P., & Bonanno, G. A. (2012). Recent trends in the treatment of prolonged grief. *Current Opinion in Psychiatry, 25*(1), 46–51.

Manevich, A., Rubin, S. S., Katz, M., Ben-Hayun, R., Aharon-Peretz, J. (2022). Spousal mourning for partners living with cognitive impairment: The Interplay of Attachment and the Two-Track Model of Dementia Grief. *Omega: Online First*, 10.1177/00302228221142632.

Marganska, A., Gallagher, M., & Miranda, R. (2013). Adult attachment, emotion dysregulation, and symptoms of depression and generalized anxiety disorder. *American Journal of Orthopsychiatry, 83*(1), 131–141.

Mars, R. B., et. al (2012). On the relationship between the "default mode network" and the "social brain." *Frontiers in Human Neuroscience,* 6, Article 189.

Marsh, A. A. (2013). What can we learn about emotion by studying psychopathy? *Frontiers in Human Neuroscience, 7.*

Marshall, B., & Davies, B. (2011). Bereavement in children and adults following the death of a sibling. In R. Neimeyer, D. L. Harris, H. R. Winokuer & G. F. Thompson (Eds), *Grief and bereavement in contemporary society: Bridging research and practice* (pp. 107–116). Routledge/Taylor & Francis Group.

Martínez-García, M., Cardenas, S. I., Pawluski, J., Carmona, S., Saxbe, D. E. (2022). Recent Neuroscience Advances in Human Parenting. In G. González-Mariscal (Ed.), *Patterns of Parental Behavior*. Advances in Neurobiology, vol 27. Springer.

McEwen, B., & Akil, Huda (2020). Revisiting the Stress Concept: Implications for Affective Disorders. *Journal of Neuroscience, 40*(1), 12 –21.

McEwen, B. S., & Stellar, E. (1993). Stress and the individual. Mechanisms leading to disease. *Archives of Internal Medicine, 153*(18), 2093–3101.

McIntosh, J. L. (1992). Epidemiology of suicide in the elderly. *Suicide and Life-Threatening Behavior, 22*(1), 15–35.

Meert, K. L., et.al. (2010). Complicated grief and associated risk factors among parents following a child's death in the pediatric intensive care unit. *Archives of Pediatric and Adolescent Medicine, 164*(11), 1045–1051.

Meichsner, F., O'Connor, M., Skritskaya, N., & Shear, M. åK. (2020). Grief Before and After Bereavement in the Elderly: An Approach to Care. *American Journal of Geriatric Psychiatry, 28*(5) 560 –569.

Meier, A. M., Carr, D. R., Currier, J. M., & Neimeyer, R. A. (2013). Attachment Anxiety and Avoidance in Coping with Bereavement: Two Studies. *Journal of Social and Clinical Psychology* (In press).

Meij, L. W.-d., Stroebe, M. S., Schut, H., Stroebe, W., van den Bout, J., van der Heijden, P., & Dijkstra, I. (2007). Neuroticism and attachment insecurity as predictors of bereavement outcome. *Journal of Research in Personality, 41*(2), 498–505. doi:10.1016/j.jrp.2006.06.001.

Meisenhelder, J. B. (2021). Maternal grief: analysis and therapeutic recommendations. *BMJ Supportive & Palliative Care, 11*, 101 –106.

Melitta Fischer-Kern, M., Tmei, A., Naderer, A., Zimmerman, J., & Nolte, T. (2022). Failure to resolve loss and compromised mentalizing in female inpatients with major depressive disorder. *Attachment & Human Development, 24*(4), 503–524.

Mennin, D. S., & Fresco, D. M. (2009). Emotion regulation as an integrative framework for understanding and treating psychopathology. In A. M. Kring & D. M. Sloan (Eds.), *Emotion regulation and psychopathology: A transdiagnostic approach to etiology and treatment* (pp. 356–379). Guilford Press.

Mennin, D. S., & Fresco, D. M. (2014). Emotion regulation therapy. *Handbook of Emotion Regulation, 2,* 469–490.

Merwin, W.S. (1993). "Separation" from The Second Four Books of Poems (Port Townsend, Washington: Copper Canyon Press, 1993). Copyright © 1993 by W. S. Merwin. Reprinted with the permission of The Wylie Agency, Inc.

Michaels, T., Stone, E., Singal, S. I., Michaels, T. & Stone, E. (2021). Brain reward circuitry: The overlapping neurobiology of trauma and substance use disorders. *World Journal of Psychiatry, 11*(6), 222–231.

Mickelson, K. D., Kessler, R. C., & Shaver, P. R. (1997). Adult attachment in a nationally representative sample. *Journal of Personality and Social Psychology, 73*(5), 1092.

Mikulincer, M., & Orbach, I. (1995). Attachment styles and repressive defensiveness: the accessibility and architecture of affective memories. *Journal of Personality and Social Psychology, 68*(5), 917.

Mikulincer, M., & Florian, V. (1998). The relationship between adult attachment styles and emotional and cognitive reactions to stressful events. *Attachment theory and close relationships, 143,* 165.

Mikulincer, M., & Shaver, P. R. (2007). *Attachment in adulthood: Structure, dynamics, and change.* Guilford Press.

Mikulincer, M., & Shaver, P. R. (2008a). Adult attachment and affect regulation. In J. C. P. R. Shaver (Ed.), *Handbook of attachment: Theory, research, and clinical applications* (2nd ed.) (pp. 503–531). Guilford Press.

Mikulincer, M., & Shaver, P. R. (2008b). An attachment perspective on bereavement. In J. Cassidy & P. R. Shaver (Eds.), *Handbook of bereavement research and practice: Advances in theory and intervention* (pp. 87–112). Routldedge.

Mikulincer, M., & Shaver, P. R. (2009). An attachment and behavioral systems perspective on social support. *Journal of Social and Personal Relationships, 26*(1), 7–19. doi:10.1177/02654 07509105518.

Mikulincer, M., & Shaver, P. R. (2012). An attachment perspective on psychopathology. *World Psychiatry, 11*(1), 11–15.

Mikulincer, M., & Shaver, P. R. (2013). Attachment insecurities and disordered patterns of grief. In M. Stroebe, H. Schut & J. van den bout (Eds.), *Complicated grief: Scientific foundations for health care professionals* (pp. 190–203). Routledge.

Mikulincer, M., & Shaver, P. R. (2014). *Mechanisms of social connection: From brain to group.* American Psychological Association.

Mikulincer, M., & Shaver, P. R. (2017). *Attachment in adulthood: structure, dynamics, and change* (2nd ed.). Guilford Press.

Mikulincer, M., & Shaver, P. (2019). Attachment orientations and emotion regulation. *Current Opinion in Psychology, 25,* 6–10.

Mikulincer, M., & Shaver, P. R. (2020). Broaden-and-Build Effects of Contextually Boosting the Sense of Attachment Security in Adulthood. *Current Directions in Psychological Science, 29*(1), 22–26.

Mikulincer, M., & Shaver, P. (2021). Attachment theory: A behavioral systems approach for studying species-universal and individual-differences aspects of the social mind. In T. K. Shackleford (Ed.), *The SAGE handbook of evolutionary psychology: Foundations of evolutionary psychology* (pp. 260–282). Sage Publications.

Mikulincer, M. & Shaver, P. (2022) An attachment perspective on loss and grief. *Current Opinion in Psychology, 45,* 101283.

Mikulincer, M., Shaver, P. R., & Pereg, D. (2003). Attachment theory and affect regulation: The dynamics, development, and cognitive consequences of attachment-related strategies. *Motivation and emotion, 27*(2), 77–102.

Mikulincer, M., Shaver, P. R., Cassidy, J., & Berant, E. (2009). Attachment-related defensive processes. *Attachment theory and research in clinical work with adults,* 293–327.

Mikulincer, M., Shaver, P., Sapir-Lavid, Y. & Ayib Abu-Kansa, N. (2009). What's inside the minds of securely and insecurely attached people? The secure base script and its associations with attachment style dimensions. *Journal of Personal Social Psychology, 97,* 615–622.

Mikulincer, M., Shaver, P. R., Bar-On, N., & Ein-Dor, T. (2010). The pushes and pulls of close relationships: Attachment insecurities and relational ambivalence. *Journal of Personality and Social Psychology, 98*(3), 450–468. doi: 10.1037/a0017366.

Mikulincer, M., Shaver, P. R., & Berant, E. (2013). An attachment perspective on therapeutic processes and outcomes. *Journal of Personaliy, 81*(6), 606 –616.

Milman, E., Neimeyer, R., et. al., (2019a). Prolonged grief and the disruption of meaning: Establishing a mediation model. *Journal of Counseling Psychology, 66*(6), 714–725.

Milman, E., Neimeyer, R., et. al. (2019b). Rumination moderates the role of meaning in the development of prolonged grief symptomatology. *Journal of Clinical Psychology, 75*(6), 1047–1065.

Montgomery, A. (2013). *Neurobiology Essentials for Clinicians: What Every Therapist Needs to Know* (Norton Series on Interpersonal Neurobiology). WW Norton & Company.

Morris, S. Fletcher, K. & Goldstein, R. (2019) The grief of parents after the death of a young child. *Journal of Clinical Psychology in Medical Settings, 26*(3), 321–338.

Moss, M. S., Moss, S. Z., & Hansson, R. O. (2001). Bereavement and old age. In M. S. Stroebe, R. O. Hansson, W. Stroebe & H. Schut (Eds.), *Handbook of bereavement research: Consequences, coping, and care* (pp. 241–260). American Psychologcial Association.

Moutsiana C, et. al. (2014). Making an effort to feel positive: insecure attachment in infancy predicts the neural underpinnings of emotion regulation in adulthood. *Journal of Child Psychology and Psychiatry, 55*(9), 999–1008.

Muller, R. T. (2010). *Trauma and the avoidant client: Attachment-based strategies for healing.* WW Norton & Company.

Murray, H., Grey, N., Wild, J.,et. al. (2020). Cognitive therapy for post-traumatic stress disorder following critical illness and intensive care unit admission. *The Cognitive Behaviour Therapist, 13,* e13.

Nadeau, J. (1998). *Families making sense of death.* Sage Publications.

Naidu, M. (2012). Belief and Bereavement: The Notion of "Attachment" and the Grief Work Hypothesis. *Journal for the Study of Religion, 25*(2), 71–88.

Naragon-Gainey, K., McMahon, T. P., & Park, J. (2018). The contributions of affective traits and emotion regulation to internalizing disorders: Current state of the literature and measurement challenges. *American Psychologist, 73*(9), 1175–1186.

Neimeyer, R. A. (2001). *Meaning reconstruction & the experience of loss*. American Psychological Association.

Neimeyer, R. A. (2004). Research on grief and bereavement: Evolution and revolution. *Death Studies, 28*(6), 489–490.

Neimeyer, R. A. (2006a). Bereavement and the quest for meaning: Rewriting stories of loss and grief. *Hellenic Journal of Psychology, 3*(3), 181–188.

Neimeyer, R. A. (2006b). Complicated Grief and the Reconstruction of Meaning: Conceptual and Empirical Contributions to a Cognitive-Constructivist Model. *Clinical Psychology: Science and Practice, 13*(2), 141–145.

Neimeyer, R. A. (2009). *Constructivist psychotherapy: Distinctive features*. Routledge/Taylor & Francis Group.

Neimeyer, R. A. (2012a). Chairwork. In R. A. Neimeyer (Ed.), *Techniques of Grief Therapy: Creative Practices for Counseling the Bereaved* (pp. 266–273). Routledge.

Neimeyer, R. A. (2012b). Correspondence with the Deceased. In R. A. Neimeyer (Ed.), *Techniques of Grief Therapy: Creative Practices for Counseling the Bereavement* (pp. 259–260). Routledge.

Neimeyer, R. A. (2012c). The Life Imprint. In R. A. Neimeyer (Ed.), *Techniques of Grief Therapy: Creative Practices for Counseling the Bereaved* (pp. 274–276). Routledge.

Neimeyer, R. A. (2012d). Presence, Process, and Procedure: A Relational Frame for Technical Proficiency in Grief Therapy. In R. A. Neimeyer (Ed.), *Techniques of Grief Therapy: Creative Practices for Counseling the Bereaved* (pp. 3–11). Routledge.

Neimeyer, R. A. (2012e). Retelling the Narrative of the Death. In R. A. Neimeyer (Ed.), *Techniques of Grief Therapy: Creative Practices for Counseling the Bereaved* (pp. 86–94). Routledge.

Neimeyer, R. A. (Ed.). (2012f). *Techniques of Grief Therapy: Creative Practices for Counseling the Bereaved*. Routledge.

Neimeyer, R. A. (2015). Treating complicated bereavement: The development of grief therapy. In J. M. Stillion & T. Attig (Eds.), *Death, Dying, and Bereavement: Contemporary Perspectives, Institutions, and Practices* (pp. 307–320). Springer.

Neimeyer, R. A. (Ed.) (2016). *Techniques of grief therapy: Assessment and intervention*. Routledge.

Neimeyer, R. A. (2019). Meaning reconstruction in bereavement: Development of a research program. *Death Studies, 43*(2), 79–91.

Neimeyer, R. A., & Raskin, J. D. (2000). *Constructions of disorder: Meaning-making frameworks for psychotherapy*. American Psychological Association.

Neimeyer, R. A., & Jordan, J. R. (2001). Disenfranchisement as empathic failure: Grief therapy and the co-construction of meaning. In K. J. Doka (Ed.), *Disenfranchised Grief: New Directions, Challenges, and Strategies for Practice*. Research Press.

Neimeyer, R. A., & Sands, D. C. (2011). Meaning reconstruction in bereavement: From principles to practice. In R. Neimeyer, D. L. Harris, H. R. Winokuer & G. F. Thompson, (Eds), *Grief and bereavement in contemporary society: Bridging research and practice* (pp. 9–22). Routledge.

Neimeyer, R. A., & Jordan, J. R. (2013). Historical and contemporary perspectives on assessment and intervention. In D. Meager, and Balk, D. (Ed.), *Handbook of Thanatology* (2nd ed., pp. 219–237). Routledge.

Neimeyer, R. A., Keesee, N. J., & Fortner, B. V. (2000). Loss and meaning reconstruction: Propositions and procedures. In R. Malkinson, S. S. Rubin & E. Witztum (Eds.), *Traumatic and nontraumatic loss and bereavement: Clinical theory and practice* (pp. 197–230). Psychosocial Press.

Neimeyer, R. A., Prigerson, H. G., & Davies, B. (2002). Mourning and meaning. *American Behavioral Scientist, 46*(2), 235–251.

Neimeyer, R. A., Baldwin, S. A., & Gillies, J. (2006). Continuing bonds and reconstructing meaning: Mitigating complications in bereavement. *Death Studies, 30*(8), 715–738.

Neimeyer, R. A., van Dyke, J. G., & Pennebaker, J. W. (2008). Narrative medicine: Writing through bereavement. In H. C. W. Breitbart (Ed.), *Handbook of psychiatry in palliative medicine* (pp. 454–469). Oxford University Press.

Neimeyer, R. A., Burke, L. A., Mackay, M. M., & van Dyke Stringer, J. G. (2010). Grief therapy and the reconstruction of meaning: From principles to practice. *Journal of Contemporary Psychotherapy, 40*(2), 73–83. doi:10.1007/s10879-009-9135-3.

Neimeyer, R. A., Harris, D. L., Winokuer, H. R., & Thornton, G. (2011). *Grief and bereavement in contemporary society: Bridging research and practice.* Routledge/Taylor & Francis Group.

Nelson, & Gabard-Durnam (2020). Early adversity and critical periods: neurodevelopmental consequences of violating the expectable environment. *Trends in Neuroscience, 43,* 133–143.

Nelson, E. E., & Panksepp, J. (1998). Brain substrates of infant–mother attachment: contributions of opioids, oxytocin, and norepinephrine. *Neuroscience & Biobehavioral Reviews, 22*(3), 437–452.

Neves, I., Dinis-Oliveira, R. J., & Magalhães, T. (2021). Epigenomic mediation after adverse childhood experiences: a systematic review and meta-analysis. *Forensic Sciences Research, 6*(2), 103–114.

Nicholson, W. (1993). Screenwriter, Shadowlands, United International Pictures.

Norcross, J. C. (2011). *Psychotherapy relationships that work: Evidence-based responsiveness* (2nd ed.). Oxford University Press.

Norcross, J. C., & Lambert, M. J. (2006). The therapy relationship. In J. Norcross, L. Beutler, & R. Levant (Eds.), *Evidence-based practices in mental health,* (pp. 208–218). Oxford University Press.

Norcross, J. C., & Lambert, M. J. (2011). Evidence-based therapy relationships. In J. C. Norcross (Ed.), *Psychotherapy relationships that work: Evidence-based responsiveness* (2nd ed., pp. 3–21). Oxford University Press.

Norcross, J. C., & Wampold, B. E. (2011a). Evidence-based therapy relationships: Research conclusions and clinical practices. *Psychotherapy, 48*(1), 98–102. doi:10.1037/a0022161.

Norcross, J. C., & Wampold, B. E. (2011b). What works for whom: Tailoring psychotherapy to the person. *Journal of Clinical Psychology, 67*(2), 127–132. doi:10.1002/jclp.20764.

Norcross, J. C., & Lambert, M. J. (2018). Psychotherapy relationships that work III. *Psychotherapy, 55*(4), 303–315.

Norcross, J. C. & Wampold, B. E. (2018). A new therapy for each patient: Evidence-based relationships and responsiveness. *Journal of Clinical Psychology, 74,* 1889–1906.

Norcross, J. C. & Wampold, B. E. (2019). Relationships and Responsiveness in the Psychological Treatment of Trauma: The Tragedy of the APA Clinical Practice Guideline. *Psychotherapy, 56*(3), 391–399.

Nuttall, A., Ballinger, A. Levendosky, A. & Borkov, J. (2021). Maternal parentification history impacts evaluative cognitions about self, parenting, and child. *Infant Mental Health Journal, 42*(3), 315–330.

O'Connor, M-F. (2005). Bereavement and the Brain: Invitation to a Conversation between Bereavement Researchers and Neuroscientists. *Death Studies, 29*(10), 905–922. doi:10.1080/07481180500299063.

O'Connor, M-F. (2013). Physiological mechanisms and the neurobiology of complicated grief. In M. Stroebe, H. Schut & J. van den Bout (Eds.), *Complicated grief: Scientific foundations for health care professionals* (pp. 204–218). Routledge/Taylor & Francis Group.

O'Connor, M. (2019). Grief: A Brief History of Research on How Body, Mind, and Brain *Adapt. Psychosomatic Medicine, 81*(8), 731–738.

O'Connor, M-F. (2022). *The Grieving Brain.* HarperOne.

O'Connor, M-F., & Seeley, S.H. (2022). Grieving as a form of learning: Insights from neuroscience applied to grief and loss. *Current Opinion in Psychology, 43,* 317–322.

Obegi, J., & Berant, E. (2010). *Attachment Theory and Research in Clinical Work With Adults.* Guilford Publication.

Ogden, P. (2009). Emotion, Mindfulness, and Movement. In D. Fosha, D. J. Siegel, & M. F. Solomon (Eds), *The Healing Power of Emotion: Affective Neuroscience, Development & Clinical Practice* (pp. 204–231). Norton Series on Interpersonal Neurobiology.

Ogden, P., & Fisher, J. (2015). *Sensorimotor psychotherapy: Interventions for trauma and attachment*. Norton.

Ogden, P., Minton, K., & Pain, C. (2006). *Trauma and the Body: A Sensorimotor Approach to Psychotherapy*. NY: Norton.

Ohashi, K., Anderson, C. M., Bolger, E. A., Khan, A., McGreenery, C. E., & Teicher, M. H. (2019). Susceptibility or Resilience to Maltreatment Can Be Explained by Specific Differences in Brain Network Architecture. *Biological Psychiatry, 85*(8), 690 −702.

Okamoto, A., Dattilio, F. M., Dobson, K. S., & Kazantzis, N. (2019). The therapeutic relationship in cognitive–behavioral therapy: Essential features and common challenges. *Practice Innovations, 4*(2), 112–123.

Olsson, C. A. (2021). Early childhood attachment stability and change: a meta-analysis. *Attachment and Human Develoment, 23*(6), 897 −930.

Opie, J. E., McIntosh, J. E., Esler, T. B., Duschinsky, R., George, C., Schore, A., Kothe, E. J., Tan, E. S., Greenwood, C. J., & Olsson, C. A. (2021). Early childhood attachment stability and change: a meta-analysis. *Attachment & Human Development, 23*(6), 897 −930.

Orange, D. M. (2010). Recognition as: Intersubjective Vulnerability in the Psychoanalytic Dialogue. *International Journal of Psychoanalytic Self Psychology, 5*(3), 227–243. doi:10.1080/15551024.2010.491719.

Ott, C. H., Lueger, R. J., Kelber, S. T., & Prigerson, H. G. (2007). Spousal bereavement in older adults: Common, resilient, and chronic grief with defining characteristics. *Journal of Nervous and Mental Disease, 195*(4), 332–341.

Owens, C., Lambert, H., Lloyd, K., & Donovan, J. (2008). Tales of biographical disintegration: how parents make sense of their sons' suicides. *Sociology of Health & Illness, 30*(2), 237–254.

Ozeren, G.S. (2021). The correlation between emotion regulation and attachment styles in undergraduates. *Perspective of Psychiatric Care, 58*(2), 482–490.

Paetzold, R. L., & Rholes, S. (2017).Disorganized Attachment Style. In V. Zeigler-Hill, & T. K. Shackelford (Eds.), *Encyclopedia of Personality and Individual Differences*. Springer.

Paetzold, R. L., Rholes, S., & Kohn, J. L. (2015). Disorganized attachment in adulthood: Theory, measurement, and implications for romantic relationships. *Review of General Psychology, 19*(2), 146–156.

Palmieri, A., Pick, E., Grossman-Giron, A. & Tzur Bitan, D. (2021). Oxytocin as the Neurobiological Basis of Synchronization: A Research Proposal in Psychotherapy Settings. *Frontiers in Psychology, 12*, 628011.

Panksepp, J. (2011). The neurobiology of social loss in animals: Some keys to the puzzle of psychic pain in humans. In G. MacDonald & L. A. Jensen-Campbell (Eds.), *Social pain: Neuropsychological and health implications of loss and exclusion* (pp. 11−51). American Psychological Association.

Panksepp, J., & Biven, L. (2012). *The archaeology of mind: Neuroevolutionary origins of human emotion*. W. W. Norton.

Panksepp, J., Solms, M., Schläpfer, T. E., & Coenen, V. A. (2014). Primary-process separation-distress (PANIC/GRIEF) and reward eagerness (SEEKING) processes in the ancestral genesis of depressive affect. In M. Mikulincer & P. R. Shaver (Eds.), *Mechanisms of social connection: From brain to group* (pp. 33–53). American Psychological Association.

Parens, E., & Johnston, J. (2014). Neuroimaging: Beginning to Appreciate Its Complexities. *Hastings Center Report, 44*(s2), S2–S7. doi:10.1002/hast.293.

Parker, A. M., Sricharoenchai, T., Raparla, S., Schneck, K. W., Bienvenu, O. J., & Needham, D. M. (2015). Posttraumatic stress disorder in critical illness survivors: a meta-analysis. *Critical Care Medicine, 43*, 1121–1129.

Parkes, C. M. (1972). *Bereavement: Studies of Grief in Adult Life*. International Universities Press.

Parkes, C. M. (2013). *Love and loss: The roots of grief and its complications*. Routledge.

Parkes, C. M., & Prigerson, H. G. (2013). *Bereavement: Studies of grief in adult life* (4th ed.). Routledge.

Parnell, L. (2008). Tapping In: *A Step b y Step Guide to Activating Healing Resources Through Bilateral Stimulation*. Boulder, CO.: Sounds True.

Pearlman, L. A., & Courtois, C. A. (2005). Clinical applications of the attachment framework: Relational treatment of complex trauma. *Journal of Traumatic Stress, 18*(5), 449–459.

Pearlman, L. A., Wortman, C. B., Feuer, C. A., Farber, C. H., & Rando, T. A. (2014). *Treating traumatic bereavement: A practitioner's guide*. Guilford Press.

Pediatric E Journal Workgroup of National Hospice & Palliative Care Organization (NHPCO) (2022). *Pediatric E Journal, 68*, Supporting Siblings.

Pennebaker, J. W., Violanti, J. M., Paton, D., & Dunning, C. (2000). The effects of traumatic disclosure on physical and mental health: The values of writing and talking about upsetting events. In R. Ricciardelli, S. Bornstein, A. Hall & N. Carleton (Eds), *Posttraumatic stress intervention: Challenges, issues, and perspectives*. (pp. 97–114): Charles C. Thomas Publisher.

Pennebaker, J. W., Chung, C. K., Friedman, H. S., & Silver, R. C. (2007). *Expressive Writing, Emotional Upheavals, and Health Foundations of health psychology*. Oxford University Press.

Perlini, C., et.al.. (2019). Disentangle the neural correlates of attachment style in healthy individuals. *Epidemiology and psychiatric sciences, 28*(4), 371–375.

Pietromonaco, P. R., Barrett, L. F., & Powers, S. A. (2006). Adult attachment theory and affective reactivity and regulation. In J. Simpson, D. Snyder, & J. Hughes (Eds.), *Emotion regulation in families and close relationships: Pathways to dysfunction and health* (pp. 57–74). American Psychological Association.

Popova, M. (2021). Marginalia. 2021/06/18/sylvia-plath-journals-loneliness-love/.

Porges, S. W. (2009). Reciprical influences between body and brain in the perception of affect: A polyvagal perspective. In D. Fosha, Siegel, D., Solomon, M. (Ed.), *The Healing Power of Emotion Affective neuroscience, development and clinical practice*. Norton.

Porges, S. W. (2011). *The Polyvagal Theory: Neurophysiological foundations of emotions, attachment, communication and self regulation*. Norton.

Porges, S. W. (2017). *The Pocket Guide to Polyvagal Theory*. W. W. Norton & Company.

Porges, S.W. (2021). Polyvagal Theory: A biobehavioral journey to sociality. *Comprehensive Psychoneuroendocrinology, 7*, 100069.

Porges, S. (2021). *Polyvagal Safety: Attachment, Communication, Self-Regulation*. W.W. Norton.

Porter, N., & Claridge, A. M. (2021). Unique grief experiences: The needs of emerging adults facing the death of a parent. *Death Studies, 45*(3), 191–201.

Putnam, F. W., Berlin, L. J., Ziv, Y., Amaya-Jackson, L., & Greenberg, M. T. (2005). The Developmental Neurobiology of Disrupted Attachment: Lessons from Animal Models and Child Abuse Research. In L. Berlin, Y. Zev, L. Amaya-Jackson & M. T. Greenberg (Eds.), *Enhancing early attachments: Theory, research, intervention, and policy* (pp. 79–99). Guilford Press.

Rajhans, P., Goin-Kochel, R. P., Strathearn, L., & Kim, S. (2019). It takes two! Exploring sex differences in parenting neurobiology and behaviour. *Journal of Neuroendocrinology. 31*(9), e12721. doi:10.1111/jne.12721.

Rando, T. A. (1993). *Treatment of complicated mourning*. Research Press.

Rando, T. A., Papadatou, D., & Papadatos, C. (1991). Parental adjustment to the loss of a child. In D. Papdatou, & C. Papadatos, C. (Eds), *Children and death*. (pp. 233–253): Hemisphere Publishing Corp.

Reed, M. D. (1998). Predicting grief symptomatology among the suddenly bereaved. *Suicide and Life-Threatening Behavior, 28*(3), 285–301.

Reiner, A. (1990). *The triune brain in evolution. Role in paleocerebral functions*. Paul D. MacLean: Plenum.

Reisz, S., Duschinsky, R., & Siegel, D. (2018) Disorganized attachment and defense: exploring John Bowlby's unpublished reflections. *Attachment & Human Development, 20*(2), 107–134.

Rigon, A., Duff M., & Voss M. (2016). Structural and functional neural correlates of self-reported attachment in healthy adults: evidence for an amygdalar involvement. *Brain Imaging Behavior*, *10*(4), 941 –952.

Ringel, S. (2019). Developmental Trauma and Unresolved Loss in the Adult Attachment Interview. *New Directions in Relational Psychoanalysis and Psychotherapy*, *13*(1), 1–14.

Ringel, S. & Brandell, J., (Eds). (2019). *Trauma: Contemporary Directions in Trauma Theory, Research, and Practice*. Columbia University Press.

Riva, D., Njiokiktjien, C., & Bulgheroni, S. (2011). *Brain Lesion Localization and Developmental Functions: Frontal lobes, Limbic system, Visuocognitive system* (Vol. 25): John Libbey Eurotext.

Rizzolatti, G., Fadiga, L., Gallese, V., & Fogassi, L. (1996). Premotor cortex and the recognition of motor actions. *Cognitive Brain Research*, *3*(2), 131–141. doi:10.1016/0926-6410(95)00038-0.

Rogers, C. R. (1951). *Client-centered therapy*. Houghton-Mifflin.

Rogers, C. R. (1957). The necessary and sufficient conditions of therapeutic personality change. *Journal of Counseling Psychology*, *21*, 95–103.

Roisman, G. I. (2009). Adult Attachment Toward a Rapprochement of Methodological Cultures. *Current Directions in Psychological Science*, *18*(2), 122–126.

Rothschild, B. (2000). *The body remembers: The psychophysiology of trauma and trauma treatment*. WW Norton & Company.

Rothschild, B. (2006). *Help for the helper: The psychophysiology of compassion fatigue and vicarious trauma*. W.W. Norton & Co.

Rowe Jr, C. E., & Mac Isaac, D. S. (1989). *Empathic attunement: The "technique" of psychoanalytic self psychology*. Jason Aronson.

Rubin, S. S. (1981). A two-track model of bereavement: Theory and application in research. *American Journal of Orthopsychiatry*, *51*(1), 101–109.

Rubin, S. S. (1999). The Two Track Model of Bereavement: Overview, Retrospect and Prospect. *Death Studies*, *23*(8), 681–714. doi:10.1080/074811899200731.

Rubin, S. S., Malkinson, R., & Witztum, E. (2011). The two-track model of bereavement: The double helix of research and clinical practice. In R. Neimeyer, D. L. Harris, H. R. Winokuer & G. F. Thompson (Eds), *Grief and bereavement in contemporary society: Bridging research and practice* (pp. 47–56). Routledge/Taylor & Francis Group.

Rubin, S. S., Malkinson, R., & Witztum, E. (2012). *Working with the bereaved: multiple lenses on loss and mourning*. Routledge.

Rubin, S. S., Stroebe, M. S., Stroebe, W., & Hansson, R. O. (1993). The death of a child is forever: The life course impact of child loss. In M. Stroebe (Ed.), *Handbook of bereavement: Theory, research, and intervention*. (pp. 285–299). Cambridge University Press.

Rubin, S. S., Malkinson, R., Stroebe, M. S., Hansson, R. O., Stroebe, W., & Schut, H. (2001). Parental response to child loss across the life cycle: Clinical and research perspectives. In M. S. Stroebe, R. O. Hansson, W. Stroebe & H. Schut (Eds.), *Handbook of bereavement research: Consequences, coping, and care* (pp. 219–240): American Psychological Association.

Rubin, S., Malkinson, R. & Witztum, E. (2020). Traumatic Bereavements: Rebalancing the Relationship to the Deceased and the Death Story Using the Two-Track Model of Bereavement. *Frontiers in Psychiatry*, *15*(11), 537–596.

Rumi, Jalāl al-Dīn Muhammad Balkhī, & Coleman Barks (1995). *The Essential Rumi*. Harper.

Rynearson, E. K. (2001). *Retelling Violent Death*. Brunner-Routledge.

Rynearson, E. K. (Ed.). (2006). *Violent death: Resilience and intervention beyond the crisis*. Routledge/Taylor & Francis Group.

Rynearson, E. K., & Salloum, A. (2011). Restorative retelling: Revising the narrative of violent death. In R. Neimeyer, D. L. Harris, H. R. Winokuer & G. F. Thompson (Eds), *Grief and bereavement in contemporary society: Bridging research and practice* (pp. 177–188). Routledge/Taylor & Francis Group.

Sands, D. C. (2008). Suicide grief: Meaning making and the griever's relational world. PhD, University of Technology, Sydney, Australia. http://epress.lib.uts.edu.au/dspace/handle/2100/777<https://webmail.lib.uts.edu.au/exchweb/bin/redir.asp?URL=http://epress.lib.uts.edu.au/dspace/handle/2100/597.

Sands, D. C., Jordan, J. R., & Neimeyer, R. A. (2011). The meanings of suicide: A narrative approach to healing. In J. Jordan & J. McIntosh (Eds.), *Grief after suicide: Understanding the consequences and caring for the survivors.* (pp. 249–282). Routledge/Taylor & Francis Group.

Saunders, G. (2017). *Lincoln in the Bardo.* Penguin/Random House.

Savi Çakar, F., Burden, M., Yerleşkesi,, I. (2020). The Role of Social Support in the Relationship Between Adolescents' Level of Loss and Grief and Well-Being. *International Education Studies, 13*(12), 27–40.

Sbarra, D. A., & Hazan, C. (2008). Coregulation, Dysregulation, Self-Regulation: An Integrative Analysis and Empirical Agenda for Understanding Adult Attachment, Separation, Loss, and Recovery. *Personality and Social Psychology Review, 12*(2), 141–167.

Sbarra, D. A., & Manvelian, A. (2021). The psychological and biological correlates of separation and loss. In R. A. Thompson, J. A. Simpson, & L. J. Berlin (Eds.), *Attachment: The fundamental questions* (pp. 275–281). The Guilford Press.

Scheidt, C., Hasenburg, A., Kunze, M., Waller, E., Pfeifer, R., Zimmermann, P., ...Waller, N. (2012). Are individual differences of attachment predicting bereavement outcome after perinatal loss? A prospective cohort study. *Journal of Psychosomatic Research, 73*(5), 375–382.

Scholtes D., & Browne M. (2015). Internalized and externalized continuing bonds in bereaved parents: their relationship with grief intensity and personal growth. *Death Studies, 39*(1–5), 75–83.

Schopenhauer, A. (1974). Parerga and Paralipomena: Short Philosophical Essays (trans. E. F. J. Payne). Clarendon.

Schore, A. N. (2001a). Effects of a secure attachment relationship on right brain development, affect regulation, and infant mental health. *Infant Mental Health Journal, 22*(1–2), 7–66. doi: 10.1002/1097-0355(200101/04)22:1<7::aid-imhj2>3.0.co;2-n.

Schore, A. N. (2001b). The effects of early relational trauma on right brain development, affect regulation, and infant mental health. *Infant Mental Health Journal, 22*(1–2), 201–269. doi:10.1002/1097-0355(200101/04)22:1<201::aid-imhj8>3.0.co;2-9.

Schore, A. N. (2002a). Advances in neuropsychoanalysis, attachment theory, and trauma research: Implications for self psychology. *Psychoanalytic Inquiry, 22*(3), 433–484. doi:10.1080/07351692209348996.

Schore, A. N. (2002b). Dysregulation of the right brain: a fundamental mechanism of traumatic attachment and the psychopathogenesis of posttraumatic stress disorder. *Australian and New Zealand Journal of Psychiatry, 36*(1), 9–30. doi:10.1046/j.1440-1614.2002.00996.x.

Schore, A. N. (2002c). The Neurobiology of Attachment and Early Personality Organization. *Journal of Prenatal & Perinatal Psychology & Health, 16*(3), 249–263.

Schore, A. N. (2003a). *Affect dysregulation and disorders of the self.* W W Norton & Co.

Schore, A. N. (2003b). *Affect regulation and the repair of the self.* W W Norton & Co.

Schore, A. N. (2009). Right-brain affect regulation. In D. Fosha, Siegel, D., Solomon, M. (Ed.), *The Healing Power of Emotion: Affective Neuroscience, Development & Clinical Practice* (pp. 112–144): W.W. Norton.

Schore, A. N. (2012). *The Science of the Art of Psychotherapy.* W.W. Norton.

Schore, A. N. (2013). Regulation Theory and the Early Assessment of Attachment and Autistic Spectrum Disorders: A Response to Voran's Clinical Case. *Journal of Infant, Child, and Adolescent Psychotherapy, 12*(3), 164–189. doi:10.1080/15289168.2013.822741.

Schore, A. N. (2019). *Right brain psychotherapy.* New York: W. W. Norton & Company.

Schore, A. (2021). The Interpersonal Neurobiology of Intersubjectivity. *Frontiers in Psychology, 12,* 648616.

Schore, J. R., & Schore, A. N. (2008). Modern attachment theory: The central role of affect regulation in development and treatment. *Clinical Social Work Journal, 36*(1), 9–20. doi:1 0.1007/s10615-007-0111-7.

Schore, J. R., & Schore, A. N. (2014). Regulation Theory and Affect Regulation Psychotherapy: A Clinical Primer. *Smith College Studies in Social Work, 84*(2–3), 178–195.

Schulz, K. (2022). *Lost and Found: A Memoir.* Random House.

Schut, H. A. W., Stroebe, M. S., Boelen, P. A., & Zijerveld, A. M. (2006). Continuing relationships with the deceased: Disentangling bonds and grief. *Death Studies, 30*(8), 757–766. doi:10.1080/07481180600850666.

Schuurman, D., (2022). Don't forget us! Voices of youth after the death of a sibling. *Pediatric E Journal, 68,* Supporting Siblings, 10–13.

Schwarzer, N., Nolte, T., Fonagy, P. & Gingelmaier, S. (2021) Mentalizing and emotion regulation: Evidence from a nonclinical sample. *International Forum of Psychoanalysis, 30*(1), 34–45.

Seaward, B. L. (2009). *Managing Stress: Principles and Strategies for Health and Well-Being.* Jones and Bartlett.

Sekowski, M., & Prigerson, H. (2021). Associations between interpersonal dependency and severity of prolonged grief disorder symptoms in bereaved surviving family members. *Comprehensive Psychiatry, 108,* 152242.

Sekowski, M., & Prigerson, H. G. (2022a). Conflicted or close: Which relationships to the deceased are associated with loss-related psychopathology? *British Journal of Clinical Psychology, 61*(2), 510–552.

Sekowski, M. & Prigerson, H. (2022b). Disorganized attachment and prolonged grief. *Journal of Clinical Psychology, 78*(9),1806–1823.

Shaffer, P. A., Vogel, D. L., & Wei, M. (2006). The mediating roles of anticipated risks, anticipated benefits, and attitudes on the decision to seek professional help: An attachment perspective. *Journal of Counseling Psychology, 53*(4), 442.

Shapiro, R. (2005). *EMDR solutions: Pathways to healing.* WW Norton & Company.

Shapiro, F. (2012). *Getting past your past: take control of your life with self-help techniques from EMDR therapy.* Rodale.

Shapiro, F., & Forrest, M. S. (2004). *EMDR: The breakthrough therapy for overcoming anxiety, stress, and trauma.* Basic Books.

Sharp, C., & Fonagy, P. (2008). The parent's capacity to treat the child as a psychological agent: Constructs, measures and implications for developmental psychopathology. *Social Development, 17*(3), 737–754.

Shaver, P. R., & Fraley, C. R. (2008). Attachment, loss, and grief: Bowlby's views and current controversies. In J. Cassidy & P. Shaver (Eds.), *Handbook of attachment: Theory, research, and clinical applications* (2nd ed., pp. 48–77). Guilford Press.

Shaver, P. R., & Mikulincer, M. (2009). *Attachment styles Handbook of individual differences in social behavior* (pp. 62–81). Guilford Press.

Shaver, P. R., & Mikulincer, M. (2010). New directions in attachment theory and research. *Journal of Social and Personal Relationships, 27*(2), 163–172. doi:10.1177/0265407509360899.

Shaver, P. R., & Mikulincer, M. (2012). *Attachment theory Handbook of theories of social psychology* (Vol. 2, pp. 160–179). Sage Publications Ltd.

Shaver, P. R., & Mikulincer, M. (2014). Attachment bonds in romantic relationships. In *Mechanisms of social connection: from brain to group* (pp. 273–290). American Psychological Association.

Shaver, P. & Mikulincer, M. (2021). Defining Attachment Relationships and Attachment Security from a Personality-Social Perspective on Adult Attachment. In J. Thompson, A. Simpson, & J. Berlin (Eds.), *Attachment: The fundamental questions* (pp. 39–45). Guilford.

Shaver, P. R., Schachner, D. A., & Mikulincer, M. (2005). Attachment style, excessive reassurance seeking, relationship processes, and depression. *Personality and Social Psychology Bulletin, 31*(3), 343–359.

Shear, K., & Shair, H. (2005). Attachment, loss, and complicated grief. *Developmental Psychobiology*, 47(3), 253–267. doi:10.1002/dev.20091.

Shear, M. K., & Gribbin Bloom, C. (2017). Complicated grief treatment: An evidence-based approach to grief therapy. *Journal of Rational-Emotive & Cognitive-Behavior Therapy*, 35(1), 6–25.

Shear, K., Boelen, P. A., & Neimeyer, R. A. (2011). Treating complicated grief converging approaches. In R. Neimeyer, D. L. Harris, H. R. Winokuer & G. F. Thompson (Eds), *Grief and bereavement in contemporary society: Bridging research and practice* (pp. 139–162). Routledge/Taylor & Francis Group.

Shear, K., Frank, E., Houck, P. R., & Reynolds, C. F. (2005). Treatment of Complicated Grief: A Randomized Controlled Trial. *JAMA: Journal of the American Medical Association*, 293(21), 2601–2608. doi:10.1001/jama.293.21.2601.

Shonkoff, J. P., Slopen, N., & Williams, D. R. (2021). Early Childhood Adversity, Toxic Stress, and the Impacts of Racism on the Foundations of Health. *Annual Review of Public Health*, 1(42), 115–134.

Shulman, L. (2018). *Before and After Loss*. Johns Hopkins Press.

Siegel, D. & Bryson, T. (2020). *The Power of Showing Up: How Parental Presence Shapes Who Our Kids Become and How Their Brains Get Wired*. Ballantine Books/Random House.

Siegel, D. J. (2010). *Mindsight: The new science of personal transformation*. Bantam.

Siegel, D. J. (2012a). *The developing mind: How relationships and the brain interact to shape who we are*. Guilford Press.

Siegel, D. J. (2012b). *Pocket Guide to Interpersonal Neurobiology: An Integrative Handbook of the Mind*. (Norton Series on Interpersonal Neurobiology) WW Norton & Company.

Siegel, D. (2020). *The Developing Mind. How Relationships and the Brain Interact to Shape Who We Are* (3rd ed.). Guilford Press.

Siegel, R. D. (2009). *The mindfulness solution: Everyday practices for everyday problems*. Guilford Press.

Simpson, J. A., & Belsky, J. (2008). Attachment theory within a modern evolutionary framework. In J. Cassidy & P. R. Shaver (Eds.), *Handbook of Attachment: Theory, Research, and Clinical Applications*. Guilford Press.

Simpson, J. A., & Rholes, W. S. (2017). Adult attachment, stress, and romantic relationships. *Current Opinion in Psychology*, 13, 19–24

Skritskaya, N. A., Mauro, C., Garcia de la Garza, A., Meichsner, F., Lebowitz, B., Reynolds, C. F., Simon, N. M., Zisook, S., & Shear, M. K. (2020). Changes in typical beliefs in response to complicated grief treatment. *Depression and Anxiety*, 37(1), 81 –89.

Slade, A. (2007). Reflective parenting programs: Theory and development. *Psychoanalytic Inquiry*, 26(4), 640–657.

Slade, A. (2008). The implications of attachment theory and research for adult psychotherapy: Research and clinical perspectives. In J. Cassidy & P. Shaver (Ed.), *Handbook of attachment: Theory, research, and clinical applications* (2nd ed.). Guilford Press.

Smigelsky, M., Bottomley, J., Relyea, G. & Neimeyer, R. (2019). Investigating risk for grief severity: Attachment to the deceased and relationship quality. *Death Studies*. 10.1080/07481187.2018.1548539.

Solomon, E. P., & Heide, K. M. (2005). The Biology of Trauma: Implications for Treatment. *Journal of Interpersonal Violence*, 20, 51–60.

Solomon, J., & George, C. (1996). Defining the caregiving system: Toward a theory of caregiving. *Infant Mental Health Journal*, 17(3), 183–197.

Solomon, R. M., & Rando, T. A. (2007). Utilization of EMDR in the treatment of grief and mourning. *Journal of EMDR Practice and research*, 1(2), 109–117.

Solomon, R. M. & Hensley, Barbara J. (2020). EMDR Therapy Treatment of Grief and Mourning in Times of COVID-19. *Journal of EMDR Practice and Research*, 14(3), 162–174.

Sonnby-Borgström, M. (2002), Automatic mimicry reactions as related to differences in emotional empathy. *Scandinavian Journal of Psychology, 43*: 433–443.

Sroufe, L. A. (2016). The place of attachment in development In Cassidy J. & Shaver P. R. (Eds.), *Handbook of attachment: Theory, research, and clinical applications* (3rd ed., pp. 997–1011). Guilford Press.

Sroufe, A. L., & Waters, E. (1977). Attachment as an organizational construct. *Child Development*, 1184–1199.

Stanton, R., & Reaburn, P. (2014). Exercise and the treatment of depression: a review of the exercise program variables. *Journal of Science and Medicine in Sport, 17*(2), 177–182.

Steele, H. & Steele, M. (2008). Ten Clinical Applications of the Adult Attachment Interview. In: H. Steele, & M. Steele (Eds.), *Applications of the Adult Attachment Interview* (pp. 3–30). Guilford Press.

Steele, H., & Steele, M. (2008). *Clinical applications of the adult attachment interview*. Guilford Press.

Steindl, S., & Matos, M. (2022). Compassion-Focused Imagery and Embodiment. In D. Harris, A. Ho, M. Stroebe, & H. Schut (1999). The Dual Process Model of Coping with BereavementL Rationale and Description. *Death Studies, 23*(3), 197–224.

Stevenson, J. Emerson, L. McKinnon, K., & Millings, A. (2022) Facets of Mindfulness Mediate the Relationship Between Attachment Orientation and Emotion Regulation in University Students. *Psychological Reports*, Epub ahead of print. PMID: 35947822.

Stroebe, M. S. (1992). Coping with bereavement: A review of the grief work hypothesis. *OMEGA Journal of Death and Dying, 26*(1), 19–42.

Stroebe, M. S., & Schut, H. (1999a). The dual process model of coping with bereavement: Rationale and description. *Death Studies, 23*(3), 197–224. doi:10.1080/074811899201046.

Stroebe, M. S., & Schut, H. (2010). The dual process model of coping with bereavement: A decade on. *OMEGA Journal of Death and Dying, 61*(4), 273–289.

Stroebe, M. S., Schut, H., & Stroebe, W. (2005). Attachment in Coping With Bereavement: A Theoretical Integration. *Review of General Psychology, 9*(1), 48–66. doi:10.1037/1089-2680.9.1.48.

Stroebe, M. S., Schut, H., & Stroebe, W. (2006). Who benefits from disclosure? Exploration of attachment style differences in the effects of expressing emotions. *Clinical Psychology Review, 26*(1), 66–85. doi:10.1016/j.cpr.2005.06.009.

Stroebe, M. S., Abakoumkin, G., Stroebe, W., & Schut, H. (2011). Continuing bonds in adjustment to bereavement: Impact of abrupt versus gradual separation. *Personal Relationships, 19*(2), 255–266.

Stroebe, M. S., Schut, H., & Finkenauer, C. (2013). Parents coping with the death of their child: From individual to interpersonal to interactive perspectives. *Family Science, 4*(1), 28–36.

Stroebe, M. S., Schut, H., & Van den Bout, J. (2013). *Complicated grief: scientific foundations for health care professionals* (1st ed.). Routledge.

Stroebe, M., Schut, H., & Boerner, K. (2017). Models of coping with bereavement: An updated overview. *Studies in Psychology, 38*(3), 582–607,

Stroebe, S., & Schut, H. (2016). Grief Overload: A missing link in the dual process model? *Omega, 74*(1), 96–109.

Stroebe, W., Zech, E., Stroebe, M. S., & Abakoumkin, G. (2005). Does social support help in bereavement? *Journal of Social & Clinical Psychology, 24*(7), 1030–1050. doi:10.1521/jscp.2005.24.7.1030.

Suzuki, S. (1973). *Zen Mind, Beginner's Mind*. Weatherhill.

Sveen, J., Eilegård, A., Steineck, G., & Kreicbergs, U. (2014). They still grieve – A nationwide follow-up of young adults 2–9 years after losing a sibling to cancer. *Psycho-Oncology, 23*(6), 658–664

Swain, J. E., Lorberbaum, J. P., Kose, S., & Strathearn, L. (2007). Brain basis of early parent–infant interactions: psychology, physiology, and in vivo functional neuroimaging studies. *Journal of Child Psychology and Psychiatry*, 48(3–4), 262–287. doi:10.1111/j.1469-7610.2007.01731.x.

Swain, J. E., Dayton, C., Kim, P., Tolman, R. M., & Volling, B. L. (2014). Progress on the paternal brain: Theory, animal models, human brain research, and mental health implications. *Infant Mental Health Journal*, 35(5), 394–408.

Szanto, K., Shear, K., Houck, P. R., Reynolds, C. F., Frank, E., Caroff, K., & Silowash, R. (2006). Indirect Self-Destructive Behavior and Overt Suicidality in Patients With Complicated Grief. *Journal of Clinical Psychiatry*, 67(2), 233–239.

Talia A. & Holmes, J. (2021). Therapeutic Mechanisms in Attachment- Informed Psychotherapy with Adults. In L. Berlin, J. Simpson, & R. Thompson, R. (Eds.). *Attachment: The Fundamental Questions*. The Guilford Press.

Talia, A., Miller-Bottom, M., Wyner, R., Lilliengren, P. & Bate, J. (2019). Patients' Adult Attachment Interview classification and their experience of the therapeutic relationship: are they associated? *Psychotherapy Research*, 22(2), 361.

Talia, A., Taubner, S., Miller-Bottome, M., Muurholm SD, Winther, A., Frandsen FW, Harpøth Talia, A. et. al. (2022). *Frontiers in Psychology*, 13, 985685.

Tang, Y.-Y., & Posner, M. I. (2013). Tools of the trade: theory and method in mindfulness neuroscience. *Social Cognitive and Affective Neuroscience*, 8(1), 118–120.

Taylor, N. & Robinson,W.D. (2016). The Lived Experience of Young Widows and Widowers. *The American Journal of Family Therapy*, 44(2), 67–79.

Taylor, S. E., Pham, L. B., Rivkin, I. D., & Armor, D. A. (1998). Harnessing the imagination: Mental simulation, self-regulation, and coping. *American Psychologist*, 53(4), 429.

Tedeschi, R. G., & Calhoun, L. G. (2003). *Helping Bereaved Parents: A Clinician's Guide*. Brunner-Routledge.

Teicher, M. H., Gordon, J. B., & Nemeroff, C. B. (2022). Recognizing the importance of childhood maltreatment as a critical factor in psychiatric diagnoses, treatment, research, prevention and education. Mol Psychiatry, 27(3), 1331–1338.

Teicher, M. H., & Samson, J. A. (2016). Annual Research Review: Enduring neurobiological effects of childhood abuse and neglect. *Journal of Child Psychology and Psychiatry, and Allied Disciplines*, 57(3), 241–266.

Teicher, M., Samson, J., Anderson, C. et al. (2016). The effects of childhood maltreatment on brain structure, function and connectivity. *Nature Reviews Neuroscience*, 17, 652–666.

Teicher, M. H., Ohashi, K., & Khan, A. (2020). Additional Insights into the Relationship Between Brain Network Architecture and Susceptibility and Resilience to the Psychiatric Sequelae of Childhood Maltreatment. *Adversity and Resilience Science*, 1(1), 4 –64.

Theisen, J. C., Fraley, R. C., Hankin, B. L., Young, J. F., & Chopik, W. J. (2018). How do attachment styles change from childhood through adolescence? Findings from an accelerated longitudinal Cohort study. *Journal of Research in Personality*, 74, 141–146.

Thoits, P. A. (2010). Stress and health major findings and policy implications. *Journal of health and social behavior*, 51(1 suppl), S41–S53.

Thompson, B. E. (2012). Mindfulness Training. In R. A. Neimeyer (Ed.), *Techniques of Grief Therapy: Creative Practices for Counseling the Bereaved* (pp. 39–41). Routledge.

Thompson, B. E., & Neimeyer, R. A. (Eds.) (2014). *Grief and the expressive arts: Practices for creating meaning*. Routledge.

Thompson, R. A. (2016). Early attachment and later development: Reframing the questions. In J. Cassidy & P. R. Shaver (Eds.), *Handbook of attachment* (3rd ed., pp. 330–348). Guilford.

Thompson, R.A. (2021). Internal Working Models as Developing Representations. In R. A. Thompson, J. Simpson, & L. Berlin, *Attachment: The fundamental questions* (pp.128–135). Guilford.

Thompson, R. A., Simpson, J. & Berlin, L. (2021). *Attachment: The fundamental questions*. New Guilford.

Thomson, P. (2010). Loss and disorganization from an attachment perspective. *Death Studies*, 34(10), 893–914. doi:10.1080/07481181003765410.

Tich Nhat Hanh (2010). Interview with Oprah Winfrey, www.oprah.com.

Trevarthen, C. (1993). The self born in intersubjectivity: The psychology of an infant communicating. In U. Neisser (Ed.), *The perceived self: Ecological and interpersonal sources of self-knowledge* (pp. 121–173). Cambridge University Press.

Trevarthen, C. (2009). The functions of emotion in infancy. In D. Fosha, D. Siegel & M. Solomon (Eds.), *The Healing Power of Emotion: Affective Neuroscience, Development & Clinical Practice* (pp. 55–85). W. W. Norton.

Vachon, M., & Harris, D. (2016). The Liberating Capacity of Compassion. In D. Harris, & T. Bordere (Eds.) *Handbook of Social Justice in Loss and Grief* (pp. 265–281). Routledge.

Vaillant, G. E. (1995). *The wisdom of the ego*. Harvard University Press.

Van der Hart, O., Nijenhuis, E. R. S., & Steele, K. (2006). *The haunted self: Structural dissociation and the treatment of chronic traumatization*. WW Norton & Company.

Van der Horst, F. C. P. (2011). *John Bowlby – from psychoanalysis to ethology: Unraveling the roots of attachment theory*. Wiley-Blackwell.

Van der Kolk, B.. (2014). *The Body Keeps the Score: Brain, Mind, and Body in the Healing of Trauma*. Viking Penguin.

Vanderwerker, L. C., & Prigerson, H. G. (2004). Social Support and Technological Connectedness as Protective Factors in Bereavement. *Journal of Loss & Trauma*, 9(1), 45–57.

Verhage, M., Schungel, C., Madigan, S., et. al. (2016). Narrowing the transmission gap: A synthesis of three decades of research on intergenerational transmission of attachment. *Psychological Bulletin*, 14, 337–366.

Vogel, D. L., Wade, N. G., & Hackler, A. H. (2008). Emotional expression and the decision to seek therapy: The mediating roles of the anticipated benefits and risks. *Journal of Social and Clinical Psychology*, 27(3), 254–278.

Vrtička, P., & Vuilleumier, P. (2012). Neuroscience of human social interactions and adult attachment style. *Frontiers in Human Neuroscience*, 6.

Vrtička, P., Bondolfi, G., Sander, D., & Vuilleumier, P. (2012). The neural substrates of social emotion perception and regulation are modulated by adult attachment style. *Society for Neuroscience*, 7(5), 473–493.

Walker, P. (2018). *PTSD: From surviving to thriving*. Azure Coyote Publishing.

Wallin, D. J. (2007). *Attachment in Psychotherapy*. Guilford Press.

Wallin, D. J. (2010). From the inside out: The therapist's attachment patterns as sources of insight and impasse. *Clinical pearls of wisdom: Twenty one leading therapists offer their key insights*. (pp. 245–256). W. W. Norton & Co.

Wallin, D. J. (2014). We Are the Tools of our Trade: The Therapist's Attachment History as a Source of Impasse, Inspiration, and Change. In A. N. Danqueth & K. Berry (Eds.), *Attachment Theory in Adult Mental Health*. Routledge.

Walsh, F., & McGoldrick, M. (2004). Loss and the Family: A Systemic Perspective Living beyond loss. *Death in the family* (2nd ed., pp. 3–26). W W Norton & Co.

Walter, T. (1996). A new model of grief: Bereavement and biography. *Mortality*, 1(1), 7–25. Doi:1 0.1080/713685822.

Waters, T. E., Ruiz, S. K., & Roisman, G. I. (2017). Origins of Secure Base Script Knowledge and the Developmental Construction of Attachment Representations. *Child Development*, 88(1), 198–209

Watson, J. C., & Greenberg, L. S. (2009). Empathic resonance: A neuroscience perspective. In J. Decety & W. Ickes (Eds.), *The Social Neuroscience of Empathy* (pp. 125–138). MIT Press.

Wayment, H. A., & Vierthaler, J. (2002). Attachment style and bereavement reactions. *Journal of Loss and Trauma*, 7(2), 129–149. Doi:10.1080/153250202753472291.

Weber Falk, M., Eklund, R., Kreicbergs, U., Alvariza, A., & Lövgren, M. (2022). Breaking the silence about illness and death: Potential effects of a pilot study of the family talk intervention when a parent with dependent children receives specialized palliative home care. *Palliative and Supportive Care, 20,* 512–518.

Wei, M., Russell, D. W., Mallinckrodt, B., & Vogel, D. L. (2007). The Experiences in Close Relationship Scale (ECR)-short form: Reliability, validity, and factor structure. *Journal of Personality Assessment, 88*(2), 187–204.

Wigren, J. (2014). *My voice will go with you: The teaching tales of Milton H. Erikson.* Norton.

Wijngaards-de Meij, L., Stroebe, M. S., Schut, H., Stroebe, W., van den Bout, J., van der Heijden, P., & Dijkstra, I. (2005). Couples at Risk Following the Death of Their Child: Predictors of Grief Versus Depression. *Journal of Consulting and Clinical Psychology, 73*(4), 617–623.

Wijngaards-de Meij, L., Stroebe, M. S., Schut, H., Stroebe, W., van den Bout, J., van der Heijden, P. G., & Dijkstra, I. (2007a). Patterns of attachment and parents' adjustment to the death of their child. *Personality and Social Psychology Bulletin, 33*(4), 537–548.

Wijngaards-de Meij, L., Stroebe, M. S., Schut, H., Stroebe, W., van den Bout, J., van der Heijden, P. G. M., & Dijkstra, I. (2007b). Patterns of Attachment and Parents' Adjustment to the Death of Their Child. *Personality and Social Psychology Bulletin, 33*(4), 537–548. doi:10. 1177/0146167206297400.

Winokuer, H. R., & Harris, D. L. (2012). *Principles and practices of grief counseling.* Springer Publishing Co.

Wiseman, H., & Egozi, S. (2021). Attachment theory as a framework for responsiveness in psycho-therapy. In J. C. Watson & H. Wiseman (Eds.), *The responsive psychotherapist: Attuning to clients in the moment* (pp. 59–82). American Psychological Association.

Wood, L., Byram, V., Gosling, A. S., & Stokes, J. (2012). Continuing Bonds After Suicide Bereavement in Childhood. *Death Studies, 36*(10), 873–898. doi:10.1080/07481187.2011.584025.

Worden, J. W. (1982). *Grief counseling and grief therapy: A handbook for the mental health practitioner.* Springer Publishing Company.

Worden, J. W. (2009). *Grief counseling and grief therapy: A handbook for the mental health practitioner* (4th ed). Springer Publishing Co.

Worden, W. (2018). *Grief Counseling and Grief Therapy* (5th ed.). Springer Publishing

Worden, W., Kosminsky, P., & Carverhill, P. (2021). Foundational Grief Theories. In H. Servaty-Saib, & H. S. Chapple, *Handbook of Thanatology* (3rd ed.). Association for Death Education and Counseling.

Wortman, C. B., & Silver, R. C. (1989). The myths of coping with loss. *Journal of Consulting and Clinical Psychology, 57*(3), 349–357.

Wright, P. M. (2016). Adult Sibling Bereavement: Influences, Consequences, and Interventions. *Illness, Crisis & Loss, 24*(1), 34–45.

Yogman, M., & Garfield, C. F. (2016). Committee on Psychosocial Aspects of Child and Family Health. Fathers' role in the care and development of their children: the role of pediatricians. *Pediatrics, 138*(1), e20161128

Yu, He, Xu, Wang & Prigerson (2016) How do attachment dimensions affect bereavement adjustment? A mediation model of continuing bonds. *Psychiatric Research, 238,* 93–99.

Zampitella, C. (2011). Adult Surviving Siblings: The Disenfranchised Grievers. *Siblings and Groups, 35*(4), 333–347.

Zech, E. (2016). The dual process model in grief therapy. In R. Neimeyer (Ed.), *Techniques of grief therapy* (Vol. 2, pp. 19–24). Routledge.

Zech, E., & Arnold, C. (2011). Attachment and coping with bereavement: Implications for therapeutic interventions with the insecurely attached. In R. Neimeyer, D. L. Harris, H. R. Winokuer & G. F. Thompson (Eds), *Grief and bereavement in contemporary society: Bridging research and practice.* (pp. 23–35). Routledge/Taylor & Francis Group.

Zech, E., Rimé, B., & Pennebaker, J. W. (2007). The effects of emotional disclosure during bereavement. In M. Hewstone & H. Schut (Eds.), *The scope of social psychology: Theory and applications* (pp. 277–292). Routledge.

Zech, E., Ryckebosch-Dayez, A.-S., & Delespaux, E. (2010). Improving the efficacy of intervention for bereaved individuals: Toward a process-focused psychotherapeutic perspective. *Psychologica Belgica*, 50(1–2), 103–124.

Zeegers, M. A. J., Colonnesi, C., Stams, G.-J. J. M., & Meins, E. (2017). Mind matters: A meta-analysis on parental mentalization and sensitivity as predictors of infant–parent attachment. Psychological Bullet

Zetumer S., Young I., Shear M. K., Skritskaya N., Lebowitz B., Simon N., Reynolds C., Mauro, C., Zisook, S. (2015). The impact of losing a child on the clinical presentation of complicated grief. *Journal of Affective Disorders*, 170(1), 15–21.

Zhao, X., Hu, H., Zhou, Y., & Bai, Y. (2020). What are the long-term effects of child loss on parental health? Social integration as mediator. *Comprehensive Psychiatry*, 100, 152182.

INDEX

Page numbers in bold refer to tables. Page numbers followed by 'n' refer to notes.

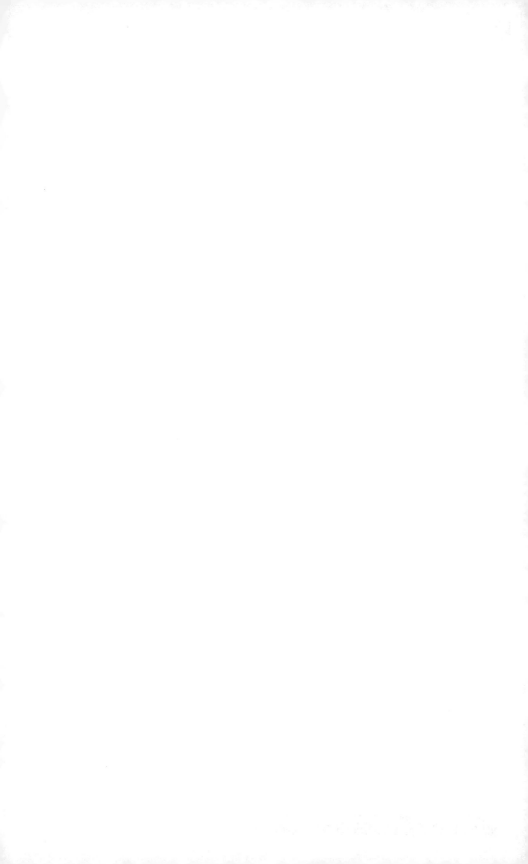

For Product Safety Concerns and Information please contact our EU
representative GPSR@taylorandfrancis.com Taylor & Francis Verlag GmbH,
Kaufingerstraße 24, 80331 München, Germany

Printed and bound by CPI Group (UK) Ltd, Croydon, CR0 4YY

08/06/2025

01897006-0006